Protein Abnormalities, Volume 2

PATHOLOGY OF IMMUNOGLOBULINS

DIAGNOSTIC AND CLINICAL ASPECTS

Protein Abnormalities

Volume 1
Physiology of Immunoglobulins: Diagnostic and Clinical Aspects
Stephan E. Ritzmann, *Editor*

Volume 2
Pathology of Immunoglobulins: Diagnostic and Clinical Aspects
Stephan E. Ritzmann, *Editor*

Protein Abnormalities, Volume 2

PATHOLOGY OF IMMUNOGLOBULINS
DIAGNOSTIC AND CLINICAL ASPECTS

Editor

Stephan E. Ritzmann, MD

Department of Pathology
Baylor University Medical Center
Dallas, Texas

ALAN R. LISS, INC., NEW YORK

About the Editor

Director, Clinical Chemistry and Proteinology
Department of Pathology
Baylor University Medical Center
Dallas, Texas

Clinical Professor of Pathology
The University of Texas Southwestern Medical School
Dallas, Texas

Adjunct Professor of Biology
Baylor University
Waco, Texas

Formerly, Professor of Internal Medicine and Pathology
The University of Texas Medical Branch
Galveston, Texas

Address all Inquiries to the Publisher
Alan R. Liss, Inc., 150 Fifth Avenue, New York, NY 10011
Copyright © 1982 Alan R. Liss, Inc.

Printed in the United States of America

Library of Congress Cataloging in Publication Data

Main entry under title:

Pathology of immunoglobulins.

(Protein abnormalities; v. 2)
Bibliography: p.
Includes indexes.
Contents: Measurement of viscosity/Jeffrey
Crawford & Harvey Jay Cohen—Imbalances of
kappa/lambda ratios of immunoglobulins/Frantisek
Skvaril, Andreas Morell, Silvio Barandum—Electrolyte
abnormalities and the anion gap in immunoglobulin
disorders/James J. Aguanno—[etc.]
    1. Gammopathies, Monoclonal. I. Ritzmann, Stephan E.
II. Series. [DNLM: 1. Immunoglobulins. W1 PR787
v.2/QW 601 P297]
RC647.H9P37 1982   616.07'93   82-18021
ISBN 0-8451-2801-9

Contents

Contributors

James J. Aguanno, PhD, Clinical Chemistry and Proteinology, Department of Pathology, Baylor University Medical Center, 3500 Gaston Avenue, Dallas, TX 75246 [37]

Samih Y. Alami, PhD, MD, Department of Laboratory Medicine, American University Hospital, P. O. Box 113-6044, Beirut, Lebanon [97]

Silvio Barandun, MD, Professor of Immunology, Institute for Clinical and Experimental Cancer Research, University of Bern. Tiefenau Hospital, 3004 Bern, Switzerland [21]

Harvey Jay Cohen, MD, Professor of Medicine, Duke University School of Medicine. Medical Service, Veterans Administration Medical Center, 508 Fulton Street, Durham, NC 27705 [13,237,293]

Jeffrey Crawford, MD, Associate in Medicine, Duke University School of Medicine. Geriatric Fellow, Veterans Administration Medical Center, 508 Fulton Street, Durham, NC 27705 [13,237,293]

Jerry C. Daniels, MD, PhD, Associate Professor in Internal Medicine and Microbiology, Division of Clinical Immunology, Department of Internal Medicine, The University of Texas Medical Branch, Galveston, TX 77550 [99]

Walter H. Hitzig, MD, Professor of Pediatrics, Kinderspital, Zurich, Steinweisstrasse 75, 8032 Zurich, Switzerland [111]

Robert A. Kyle, MD, William A. Donner Professor of Medicine and Laboratory Medicine, Mayo Medical School. Division of Hematology and Internal Medicine, Mayo Clinic and Mayo Foundation, Rochester, MN 55901 [261]

Andreas Morell, MD, Professor of Immunology, Laboratory of Cellular Immunology, Institute for Clinical and Experimental Cancer Research, University of Bern. Tiefenau Hospital, 3004 Bern, Switzerland [21]

Waldemar Pruzanski, MD, FRCP (C), FACP, Professor of Medicine, Immunology Diagnostic and Research Center, Department of Medicine, University of Toronto. The Wellesley Hospital, 160 Wellesley St. E., Toronto, Ontario, Canada M4Y 1J3 [325]

Jiri Radl, MD, PhD, Institute for Experimental Gerontology of the Organization for Health Research TNO, 151 Lange Kleiweg, 2280 HV Rijswijk, The Netherlands [55]

The number in brackets following each contributor's affiliation is the first page number of that contributor's chapter.

Stephan E. Ritzmann, MD, Clinical Professor of Pathology, The University of Texas Southwestern Medical School at Dallas. Adjunct Professor of Biology, Baylor University, Waco, TX. Clinical Chemistry and Proteinology, Department of Pathology, Baylor University Medical Center, 3500 Gaston Avenue, Dallas, TX 75246 **[ix,1]**

Gerald Shulman, MD, FF, Path (SA), MRC Path, Assistant Professor of Clinical Pathology, M.S. Hershey Medical College of the Pennsylvania State University, Hershey, PA 17033 **[71]**

Frantisek Skvaril, PhD, Immunochemical Laboratory, Institute for Clinical and Experimental Cancer Research, University of Bern. Tiefenau Hospital, 3004 Bern, Switzerland **[21]**

Marvin J. Stone, MD, Clinical Professor of Internal Medicine, The University of Texas Southwestern Medical School at Dallas. Charles A. Sammons Cancer Center, Baylor University Medical Center, 3500 Gaston Avenue, Dallas, TX 75246 **[161]**

Preface

The history of many classic biological disciplines has shown periods of extraordinary ferment accompanied by logarithmic increases in verifiable knowledge. A decade ago it became evident that biochemistry, cell physiology, genetics, endocrinology, and immunology were in such a garguantuan growth phase. Clinical and laboratory proteinology is emerging now as a functional discipline in its own right. It has provided insight into the biological roles of numerous proteins, such as the immunoglobulins, complement, oncofetal proteins, carrier proteins, and protease inhibitors. Together with immunological approaches, it has produced the modern diagnostic tools that aid in the detection and characterization of numerous proteins and their clinical effects. Many of the major advances of the past 10 years are presently in clinical use for the benefit of the patient, and many more are potentially applicable. This progress reflects the state of flux of a growing field.

In a series of books on protein abnormalities the multifaceted spectrum of proteinology will be presented by experts in basic, laboratory, and clinical fields. Volumes 1 and 2 deal with the physiologic, pathologic, diagnostic, and clinical aspects of the immunoglobulins. The monoclonal gammopathies—in particular, their usual and unusual manifestations, amyloidosis, hyperviscosity, and Bence Jones proteins—are extensively considered in this volume. These major immunoglobulin abnormalities are experiments of nature that have profound implications for both the healthy and the sick.

The increasing awareness of nutritional deficiencies and the affliction by parasitic infections of hundreds of millions of individuals worldwide have necessitated the inclusion of these subjects in later volumes. Likewise, the growing need for solid, basic information supportive of the diagnosis and treatment of pediatric and geriatric diseases warrants their special consideration. Further, the ever-increasing need for clinically relevant information concerning the amino acids and peptides and, in particular, their abnormalities in newborns has necessitated the addition of these relatively new topics.

This series reflects a concerted effort to present updated material in emerging areas of importance, without necessarily superseding the information presented in the earlier book *Serum Protein Abnormalities: Diagnostic and Clinical Aspects* [1]. These volumes are intended to provide the personnel involved in health care delivery with a distillation of current information on serum proteins and their counterparts in other biological fluids, as well as their relation to clinical and immunological aspects, in a practical and selective, rather than encyclopedic, fashion. The textual material is supplemented generously with illustrations and tables.

Foremost among the potential audience of this series are the clinician, clinical pathologist, clinical chemist, medical technologist, and other laboratory personnel, but a broader audience—medical students, house officers, practicing physicians, and educators—may find in it a spectrum of useful information. Emphasis has been placed on the complex relationship between human disease and protein pathophysiology, as it relates to diagnosis, therapy, and prevention. It is hoped that this attempt at bridging the widening gap between "bench" and "bed" will provide for the busy professional charged with the responsibility for patient care a valuable addition to his armamentarium and a reliable companion in times of need.

1. Ritzmann SE, Daniels JC: "Serum Protein Abnormalities: Diagnostic and Clinical Aspects," 2nd printing. New York: Alan R. Liss, Inc., 1982.

Stephan E. Ritzmann, MD

Acknowledgments

Acknowledgments are due the contributing authors for their cooperation and for sharing their expertise with their colleagues in the medical community. The publisher's extraordinary commitment to this project and the expeditious processing of its complex material are commendable. Special gratitude is expressed to Sandra K. Ritzmann, the editorial secretary, for her dedicated, resourceful, and diligent supervision of the laborious task of manuscript preparation, collation, communications with contributors and publisher, proofreading, and revisions. Without her dedication, this publishing endeavor would not have come to fruition.

Pathology of Immunoglobulins: Diagnostic and
Clinical Aspects, pages 1–10
© 1982 Alan R. Liss, Inc., 150 Fifth Avenue, New York, NY 10011

Introduction

Stephan E. Ritzmann, MD

The recognition of hypo-γ-globulinemia and its association with increased susceptibility to infections in a patient with chronic lymphocytic leukemia by Löffler in 1951 [1] and the demonstration of salutory effects of γ-globulin substitution therapy in a child with congenital A-γ-globulinemia by Bruton in 1952 [2,33] clearly presented the clinical need for practical quantitative and qualitative diagnostic assays for immunoglobulins (Igs) and their abnormalities. The introduction of radial immunodiffusion (RID) in 1965 by Mancini et al. [3] and Fahey and McKelvey [4] provided such a basic quantitative laboratory tool [6,9a,9b], which revolutionized the entire area of diagnostic protein quantitation in the clinical laboratory. Subsequently, other quantitative techniques, such as quantitative immunoelectrophoresis, nephelometry, and turbidimetry [10,16,21,28–31,34,36,43,46–49,53,64,65], have been introduced which were supplemented by powerful qualitative routine assays, mainly immunoelectrophoresis (IEP) [7,8,10,16–19,23,36,38–40, 43,48–50,52,61,62,68].

The term γ-globulin was initially equated with those proteins possessing antibody characteristics. The application of IEP has resulted in the demonstration of the electrophoretic distribution of antibody proteins within the entire γ-, β- and α$_2$-globulin ranges. Consequently, the functional and all-encompassing term immunoglobulin has been introduced by Hitzig [69] and Heremans [23] for those proteins possessing either antibody characteristics or the characteristic structure of antibodies. Quantum leaps of knowledge acquisition regarding Ig synthesis, regulation, structure, functions, and metabolism have subsequently occurred [5,8,10,16,20,27,32,35,40,53–58].

Immunoglobulin abnormalities are conventionally classified into three categories: hypo-γ-globulinemias, polyclonal gammopathies, and monoclonal gammopathies. These abnormalities are reflected by characteristic changes of serum protein electrophoresis (SPE) patterns [8].

HYPO-γ-GLOBULINEMIAS

Hypo-γ-globulinemias may be associated with a wide range of disorders of varied etiology (Table I). Decreases in the electrophoretic γ-globulin fraction and the IgG, A, M contained therein can result from either *decreased Ig synthesis, increased loss, hypercatabolism* or a *combination* of these factors [5a,5b,8,10,63].

Decreased Ig Synthesis

Primary Ig immunodeficiencies resulting from decreased Ig synthesis are most frequently detected during childhood. These include combined B/T-cell immunodeficiencies, sex-linked A-γ-globulinemia, selective IgA, IgM, κ- or λ-light (L) chain deficiencies, IgG subclass deficiencies, and others [8,10–13,32,33,35,63,66,67]. The mechanisms leading to these Ig deficiencies are diverse and incompletely understood. Defective B-cell differentiation appears to be the culprit in many of these patients.

Secondary Ig deficiencies due to decreased synthesis are principally encountered in adult patients. The majority of these Ig deficiencies cannot be unequivocally classified, and such disorders are therefore grouped under the heading "common, variable, unclassifiable hypo-γ-globulinemias" [5a,5b, 10,63]. Well-known causes of secondary hypo-γ-globulinemia include chronic lymphocytic leukemia and treatment with immunosuppressive agents, as well as severe protein malnutrition.

TABLE I. Partial List of Diseases Associated With Decreased Serum Immunoglobulin Levels

Diseases	IgG	IgA	IgM
Decreased synthesis			
Severe combined immunodeficiency	↓↓↔↓↓↓	↓↓↔↓↓↓	↓↓↔↓↓↓
Sex-linked A-γ-globulinemia	↓↓↔↓↓↓	↓↓↔↓↓↓	↓↓↔↓↓↓
Common variable hypo-γ-globulinemias	↓↔↓↓↓	↓↔↓↓↓	↓↔↓↓↓
Selective IgA deficiency	N	↓↓↓	N
Selective IgM deficiency	N	N	↓↓↓
Immunosuppressive therapy	N↔↓↓	N↔↓↓	N↔↓↓
Severe malnutrition	N↔↓↓	N↔↓	N↔↓
Increased loss			
Nephrotic syndrome	N↔↓↓↓	N↔↓↓	N
Protein-losing gastroenteropathies	N↔↓↓↓	N↔↓↓↓	N↔↓↓↓
Acute thermal burns	↓↔↓↓↓	↓↔↓↓↓	↓↔↓↓↓
Hypercatabolism			
Hyperthyroidism	↓↔↓↓	↓↔↓↓	↓↔↓↓
Myotonic dystrophy	↓↔↓↓↓	N	N
Antibodies to immunoglobulins	↓↔↓↓	↓↔↓↓	↓↔↓↓

N = Normal, ↓ = slight decrease, ↓↓ = moderate decrease, ↓↓↓ = marked decrease, ↔ = range.

Increased Ig Loss

Excessive Ig losses occur most commonly through the kidneys (nephrotic syndrome), the gastrointestinal tract (protein-losing gastroenteropathies), and the skin (acute thermal burns) [8]. Renal protein loss is characterized by a disproportionate decrease of low molecular weight serum proteins (e.g., albumin) but retention of large molecular weight proteins (e.g., IgM) and varying degrees of IgG decreases. In contrast, wastage of serum proteins into the gastrointestinal tract or through the skin results in "bulk" loss of all proteins irrespective of their molecular weight, with resultant deficiency of IgG, A, and M (and lymphocytes) [8,42].

Hypercatabolism of Ig

Hypermetabolic states occur in association with several disorders that result in decreased serum levels of one or more of the Ig classes. These conditions include hyperthyroidism, which can affect the levels of all Igs; myotonic dystrophy, which may be complicated by decreased levels of IgG due to its shortened half-life; and anti-Ig antibodies, which can affect any Ig class.

Serum concentrations of the five classes of immunoglobulins, G, A, M, D, and E, are age-dependent [5a,5b,8,10,32,33,35], and, therefore, their values in pediatric patients require reporting in age-adjusted terms. The *characterization of Ig deficiencies* is essential for etiologic, diagnostic, and therapeutic reasons.[1] For instance, the demonstration of a serum IgG concentration of 500 mg/dL in an adult patient mandates a search for the underlying etiology. On the other hand, an IgG level of < 100 mg/dL in such a patient may additionally necessitate γ-globulin substitution therapy to combat increased susceptibility to infections [5a,5b,8,20,22,63]. In general, adult serum IgG levels of < 200 mg/dL—i.e., less than one-fifth of the normal mean adult concentration—are often associated with an infectious diathesis.

HYPER-γ-GLOBULINEMIAS

Hyper-γ-globulinemias consist of essentially two varieties: the polyclonal and monoclonal gammopathies. These two categories can usually be distinguished by SPE analysis [8,21,39,40,43]. Unusual patterns of hyper-γ-globulinemia on SPE are often associated with circulating immune complexes [27,41].

Polyclonal Gammopathies (PG)

Hyper-γ-globulinemia of the polyclonal variety is generally characterized by a broad, diffuse, and heterogeneous increase mainly of the electrophoretic

[1]Ed. note: See also Chapter 7.

TABLE II. Partial List of Diseases Associated With Increased Serum Immunoglobulin Levels

Diseases	IgG	IgA	IgM
POLYCLONAL GAMMOPATHIES (PG)			
Infections	↑ ↔ ↑ ↑	N ↔ ↑	↑ ↔ ↑ ↑
Infectious mononucleosis			
Subacute bacterial endocarditis	↑ ↔ ↑ ↑	↓ ↔N	↑ ↔ ↑ ↑
Tuberculosis	↑ ↔ ↑ ↑	N ↔ ↑ ↑ ↑	↓ ↔N
Actinomycosis	↑ ↑ ↑	↑ ↑	↑ ↑ ↑
Deep fungus diseases	N	N ↔ ↑	N
Bartonellosis	↑	↓ ↔N	↑ ↑ ↔ ↑ ↑ ↑
Trypanosomiasis	N ↔ ↑	N ↔ ↑	↑ ↑ ↔ ↑ ↑ ↑
Liver diseases			
Infectious hepatitis (late stage)	↑ ↔ ↑ ↑	N ↔ ↑	N ↔ ↑ ↑
Laennec's cirrhosis	↑ ↔ ↑ ↑ ↑	↑ ↔ ↑ ↑ ↑	N ↔ ↑ ↑
Biliary cirrhosis	N	N	↑ ↔ ↑ ↑
Autoimmune disorders			
Lupus erythematosus	↑ ↔ ↑ ↑	N ↔ ↑	N ↔ ↑ ↑
Rheumatoid arthritis	N ↔ ↑ ↑ ↑	↑ ↔ ↑ ↑ ↑	N ↔ ↑ ↑
Sjögren's syndrome	N ↔ ↑	N ↔ ↑	N ↔ ↑ ↑
Scleroderma	N ↔ ↑	N	N ↔ ↑
Miscellaneous			
Sarcoidosis	N ↔ ↑ ↑	N ↔ ↑ ↑	N ↔ ↑
Hodgkin's disease	↓ ↔ ↑ ↑	↓ ↔ ↑	↓ ↔ ↑ ↑
Monocytic leukemia	N ↔ ↑	N ↔ ↑	N ↔ ↑ ↑
Cystic fibrosis	↑ ↔ ↑ ↑	↑ ↔ ↑ ↑	N ↔ ↑ ↑
Gluten-sensitive enteropathies	N	N ↔ ↑ ↑ ↑	N
Berger's disease (IgA nephropathy)	N ↔ ↑	↑ ↔ ↑ ↑ ↑	N ↔ ↑
Henoch-Schoenlein syndrome	N ↔ ↑	↑ ↔ ↑ ↑ ↑	N ↔ ↑
MONOCLONAL GAMMOPATHIES (MG)			
IgG-MG (myeloma or asymptomatic form)	N ↔ ↑ ↑ ↑	N ↔ ↓ ↓ ↓	N ↔ ↓ ↓ ↓
IgA-MG (myeloma or asymptomatic form)	N ↔ ↓ ↓ ↓	N ↔ ↑ ↑ ↑	N ↔ ↓ ↓ ↓
IgM-MG (macroglobulinemia or asymptomatic form)	N ↔ ↓ ↓ ↓	N ↔ ↓ ↓ ↓	N ↔ ↑ ↑ ↑
L chain disease (Bence-Jones myeloma)	N ↔ ↓ ↓ ↓	N ↔ ↓ ↓ ↓	N ↔ ↓ ↓ ↓
IgD-MG (IgD ↑ ↔ ↑ ↑ ↑)	N ↔ ↓ ↓ ↓	N ↔ ↓ ↓ ↓	N ↔ ↓ ↓ ↓
IgE-MG (IgE ↑ ↔ ↑ ↑ ↑)	N ↔ ↓ ↓ ↓	N ↔ ↓ ↓ ↓	N ↔ ↓ ↓ ↓
Heavy chain diseases (HCD)			
γ-HCD	N ↔ ↑ ↑ ↑	N ↔ ↓ ↓ ↓	N ↔ ↓ ↓ ↓
α-HCD	N ↔ ↓ ↓ ↓	N ↔ ↑ ↑ ↑	N ↔ ↓ ↓ ↓
μ-HCD	N ↔ ↓ ↓ ↓	N ↔ ↓ ↓ ↓	N ↔ ↑ ↑ ↑
(Chronic lymphocytic leukemia	N ↔ ↓ ↓ ↓	N ↔ ↓ ↓ ↓	N ↔ ↓ ↓ ↓)

N = normal, ↑ = slight increase, ↑ ↑ = moderate increase, ↑ ↑ ↑ = marked increase, ↔ = range.

γ-globulin fraction, as a result of increased proliferation of numerous plasma cell clones. Usually all major Ig classes are increased with their normal κ/ λ ratios preserved. Occasionally the Ig concentrations may reach extreme levels (e.g., IgG = 6.0–10.0 g/dL). *PG is, after hypoalbuminemia, the most frequently encountered serum protein abnormality, as detected by SPE.* No pathognomonic, diagnostic pattern can be obtained from the SPE pattern or the quantitation of these elevated Igs in individual patients, although on a statistical basis, such changes may be of diagnostic and clinical value. Nevertheless, monitoring of these Igs often provides useful and sometimes essential parameters in the therapeutic and prognostic follow-up of certain patients with PG. The spectrum of diseases associated with a PG is extremely varied; it includes numerous subacute and chronic infections, chronic liver diseases, autoimmune disorders, and others (Table II). It should be noted, however, that these Ig profiles in the various disorders may be secondary rather than primary in nature. For instance, sarcoidosis associated with PG may be a reflection of hepatic involvement by this disease, whereas sarcoidosis without liver affection may not be characterized by PG.

In certain diseases, the PG may be restricted to one class [24,36,67] (Table III). For instance, IgG is selectively increased in chronic active (lupoid) hepatitis and lymphogranuloma venereum with IgA and IgM being relatively normal [8,24]. IgA is selectively increased in a polyclonal fashion in certain patients with gluten-sensitive enteropathy, Aldrich syndrome, ataxia telangiectasia, familial thrombocytopenia or neutropenia, hereditary sensory neuropathy, and alcoholism. Furthermore, selective increases of polyclonal serum dimeric IgG_2-subclass, as well as glomerular deposits of IgA_2 immune complexes, have been demonstrated in Berger's disease (primary IgA nephropathy), alcoholic cirrhosis, and Henoch-Schoenlein purpura [26]. Selective polyclonal hyper-IgM is associated with early infectious hepatitis, recent viral infections, African trypanosomiasis, and neonatal or intrauterine infections.

Selective polyclonal increases of IgD may be encountered with staphylococcal skin infections, while selective polyclonal IgE increases occur with parasitic infections and the hyperimmunoglobulinemia E syndrome with undue susceptibility to infections (Buckley Syndrome) [37].

Polyclonal gammopathies are encountered much less frequently in children than in adult patients with comparable underlying diseases. For instance, during late stages of thermal burn injuries, the degree of secondary PG eventually evolving after the initial hypo-γ-globulinemia due to Ig loss (Table I) is less pronounced than in adult patients [8,24,42]. Likewise, PG developing in response to certain infections is usually less marked in children than in adults. Notable exceptions, however, do occur. For instance, toxocariasis (visceral larva migrans syndrome) may cause marked PG with increases of IgG, IgM, and IgE [24,25].

Elevated polyclonal IgM levels in cord serum may reflect nonspecifically the presence of overt or lanthanic intrauterine infections [14,15]. The fetus and the newborn can elaborate IgM earlier and at higher rates than IgG and IgA. Consequently, cord IgM concentrations are increased in almost all symptomatic neonates with congenital infections. The "TORCH" diseases— *T*oxoplasmosis, *R*ubella, *C*ytomegalovirus disease, *H*erpes simplex, and *O*thers (syphilis, listeriosis, aseptic meningitis, enteroviral infections, etc.)—are frequently accompanied by increased cord IgM. The finding of increased cord IgM in such a wide range of diseases necessitates the use of more specific diagnostic measures for these TORCH agents, including appropriate serologic tests, immunofluorescence with IgM specific antibodies, and other assays.

TABLE III. Partial List of Diseases Associated With Selective Polyclonal Increases of Serum IgG, A, M, D, or E

IgG
  Chronic active (lupoid) hepatitis
IgA
  Aldrich syndrome
  Ataxia-telangiectasia
  Gluten-sensitive enteropathy
  Early hepatic cirrhosis
  Alcoholic cirrhosis
  Familial thrombocytopenia
  Hereditary sensory neuropathy
  Carcinoma of nasopharynx
  Lactating women (11S-IgA)
IgM
  Early hepatitis
  Primary biliary cirrhosis
  Recent viral infection
  Neonatal or intrauterine infection (cord serum)
  African trypanosomiasis
  Immunodeficiency with hyper-IgM
  Leprosy
  Lupus erythematosus
  Rheumatoid arthritis
IgD
  Staphylococcal dermatitis
IgE
  Aldrich syndrome
  Parasitic infestation
  Asthma
  Idiopathic hyper-IgE (Buckley Syndrome)

Monoclonal Gammopathies (MG)

Hyper-γ-globulinemia of the monoclonal variety is usually characterized by a rather narrow, restricted Ig increase primarily in the γ-globulin region, resulting in a monoclonal "spike," due to the M-protein, structurally consisting of one Ig class and one L chain type. The MG represents the expression of disordered synthesis reflected by the triad of excessive proliferation of single B-cell clones, the elaboration of electrophoretically, structurally, and antigenically homogeneous Igs or L chain moieties (i.e., M-proteins), and often a deficiency of the normal background Ig [38]. Currently, a definitive laboratory diagnosis of MG can be made by the application of SPE, IEP, and Ouchterlony analysis, immunofixation [45,59,60], with IEP being the method of choice [8,17,21,23,38,43,44].

In this context it must be realized that the demonstration of an M-protein by these techniques only allows the *laboratory diagnosis of a monoclonal gammopathy* (e.g., IgG-λ monoclonal gamgammopathy or IgA-κ + Bence Jones protein [BJP]-κ monoclonal gammopathy), whereas the clinical diagnosis of monoclonal gammopathy allows the separation into a "malignant" form (e.g., myeloma, macroglobulinemia [Waldenström] or an asymptomatic state (i.e., without any clinical manifestations of myeloma, etc.). Only M-proteins obtained from patients with the clinical manifestations of myeloma qualify for the designation "myeloma proteins".

The quantitative *monitoring of M-proteins* is an important aspect of the staging of the disease and assessment of the efficacy of therapy [9a,9b,16,54]. Furthermore, the quantitation of the normal (polyclonal) background IgG may become essential in such patients with increased susceptibility to infections.

PROJECTIONS

The subject of Igs, as part of diagnostic and clinical immunology and proteinology, has matured into its own discipline, permeating all aspects of medicine. Quantitative and qualitative characterization of Igs is desirable, if not essential, in numerous clinical situations in order to assess the general immunological homeostasis and to uncover specific defects in the immunological orchestration of vital protective functions. Thus, in patients with hypo-γ-globulinemia, the characterization of Igs in serum and other body fluids aids in the assessment of possible risk of infections, as well as in the elucidation of underlying etiopathogenic factors; and in patients with hyper-γ-globulinemia, it allows the monitoring of progression of disease and therapeutic efficacy. Clearly, during this time of transition, the proven basis of Ig assays [21] provides the rationale for the emergence of a new, advanced diagnostic methodology. The need for diagnostic and prognostic Ig profiles, with the aid of computerized and automated facilities, is clearly on the horizon.

REFERENCES

1. Löffler H: Skoda im Wendepunkt der Medizin. Wien Med Wochenschr 63:771, 1951.
2. Bruton OC: Agammaglobulinemia. Pediatrics 9:722, 1952.
3. Mancini G, Carbonara AO, Heremans JF: Immunochemical quantitation of antigens by single radial immunodiffusion. Immunochemistry 2:235, 1965.
4. Fahey JL, McKelvey E: Quantitative determination of serum immunoglobulins in antibody-agar plates. J Immunol 94:84, 1965.
5a. Committee Report—Bulletin WHO 45:125, 1971.
5b. Immunodeficiency. Report of a WHO Scientific Group. Clin Immunol Immunopathol 13:296–359, 1978.
6. Becker W, Rapp W, Schwick G, Störiko K: Methoden zur quantitativen Bestimmung von Plasmaproteinen durch Immunopräzipitation. Z Klin Chem 6:113, 1968.
7. Penn GM, Davis T: "Identification of Myeloma Proteins." Chicago: American Society of Clinical Pathologists, 1975.
8. Ritzmann SE, Daniels JC (eds): "Serum Protein Abnormalities, Diagnostic and Clinical Aspects." Boston: Little, Brown Co., 1975.
9a. Ritzmann SE: Radial Immunodiffusion Revisited. Part 1. ASCP Laboratory Medicine 7:23–33, 1978.
9b. Ritzmann SE: Application and Interpretation of RID Assays, Part 2. ASCP Lab Med 8:27–40, 1978.
10. Fudenberg HH, Stites DP, Caldwell JL, Wells JV (eds): "Basic and Clinical Immunology." 2nd ed. Palo Alto, CA: Lange Med Publ, 1978.
11. Hobbs JR, Milner RD, Watt PJ: Gamma M deficiency predisposing to meningococcal septicaemia. Br Med J 4:583, 1967.
12. Bernier GM, Gundermann JR, Ruyman FB: Kappa-chain deficiency. Blood 40:795, 1972.
13. Barandun S, Morell A, Skvaril F, Oberdorfer A: Deficiency of κ- or λ-type immunoglobulins. Blood 47:79–89, 1976.
14. Alford CA, Stagno S, Reynolds DW: Diagnosis of chronic perinatal infections. Am J Dis Child 129:455–463, 1975.
15. Nahmias AJ: The TORCH Complex. Hosp Practice 9:65–72, 1974.
16. Ritzmann SE (ed): "Physiology of Immunoglobulins", New York: Alan R. Liss, Inc., 1982.
17. Grabar P, Williams CA: Méthode permettant l'étude conjugée des propriétés électrophorétiques immunochimiques d'un mélange de protéines. Application du sérum sanguin. Biochim Biophys Acta 10:193, 1953.
18. Poulik MD: Filter paper electrophoresis of purified diphtheria toxoid. Can J Med Sci 30:417, 1952.
19. Schultze HE, Heremans JF: "Molecular Biology of Human Proteins with Specific Reference to Plasma Proteins, Vol I, Nature and Metabolism of Extracellular Proteins." Amsterdam, London, New York: Elsevier Publ Co., 1966.
20. Hanson LÅ, Björklander J, Wadsworth C, Bake B: Intravenous Immunoglobulin in Antibody Deficiency Syndromes. Lancet I:396, 1982.
21. Seligmann M (Chairman), Bentwich Z, Bianco N, et al: Use and Abuse of Laboratory Tests in Clinical Immunology: Critical Considerations of eight widely used diagnostic procedures. Report of an IUIS/WHO Working Group. Clin Exp Immunol 46:662, 1981.
22. Ochs HD, et al: Safety and patient acceptibility of intravenous immune globulin in 10% maltose. Lancet II:1158, 1980.

23. Heremans JF: Immunochemical Studies on Protein Pathology. The Immunoglobulin Concept. Clin Chim Acta 4:639, 1959.
24. Ritzmann SE: Personal observations.
25. Fanning M, Hill A, Lauger HM, Keystone JS: Visceral Larva Migrans (toxocariasis) in Toronto. Can Med Assoc J 124:21–26, 1981.
26. André C, Berthoux FC, André F, et al: Prevalence of IgA$_2$ Deposits in IgA Nephropathies. A Clue to their Pathogenesis. New Engl J Med 303:1343–1346, 1980.
27. Ritzmann SE, Daniels JC: Immune Complexes: Characteristics, Clinical Correlations, and Interpretive Approaches in the Clinical Laboratory. Clin Chem 28:1259–1271, 1982.
28. Ritchie RF (ed): "Automated Immunoassays." Parts 1 and 2. New York and Basel: M. Dekker, Inc., 1978.
29. Ritchie RF: Automated immunoprecipitation analysis of serum proteins. In Putnam FW (e d): "The Plasma Proteins, Structure, Function and Genetic Control." 2nd ed, Vol II. New York: Academic Press, 1975, pp 375–425.
30. Nakamura RM, Dito WR, Tucker ES III (eds): "Immunoassays in the Clinical Laboratory." New York: Alan R. Liss, Inc., 1979.
31. Keitges PW, Nakamura RM (eds): "Diagnostic Immunology. Current and Future Trends." Skokie, IL: College of American Pathologists, 1980.
32. Bellanti JA (ed): "Immunology II." Philadelphia: W.B. Saunders, 1978.
33. Bergsma D, Good RA, Finstad J, Miescher PA, Smith RT (eds): Immunologic Deficiency Diseases in Man. Birth Defects IV(1), The National Foundation, March of Dimes, 1968.
34. Nakamura RM, Dito WR, Tucker ES III (eds): Immunoassays. Clinical Laboratory Techniques for the 1980's. New York: Alan R. Liss, Inc., 1980.
35. Good RA, Fisher DW (eds): "Immunobiology: Current Knowledge of Basic Concepts in Immunology and their Clinical Applications." Stamford, CT: Sinauer Assoc., Inc., 1975.
36. Hong R: Evaluation of the immunoglobulins. In Bach FH, Good RA (eds): "Clinical Immunobiology." Vol 3. New York: Acad Press, 1976, pp 1–19.
37. Buckley RH, Sampson HA: The hyperimmunoglobulinemia E syndrome. In Franklin EC (ed): "Clinical Immunology Update: Reviews for Physicians." New York: Elsevier Publ, 1981, pp 147–167.
38. Osserman EF, Takatsuki K: Considerations regarding the pathogenesis of the plasmacytic dyscrasias. Ser Hematol 4:28, 1965.
39. Cawley LP: "Electrophoresis and Immunoelectrophoresis." Boston: Little, Brown and Co., 1969.
40. Waldenström JG: "Monoclonal and Polyclonal Hypergammaglobulinemia, Clinical and Biological Significance." Nashville, TN: Vanderbilt University Press, 1968.
41. Kelly RH, Scholl MA, Harvey VS, Devenyi AG: Qualitative testing for circulating immune complexes by use of zone electrophoresis on agarose. Clin Chem 26:396–402, 1980.
42. Ritzmann SE, Daniels JC: Serum protein abnormalities in thermal burns. In Lynch JB, Lewis SR (eds): "Symposium on the Treatment of Burns." Vol 5. St. Louis, MO: C.V. Mosby Co., 1973, pp 31–41.
43. Franklin EC: Electrophoresis and immunoelectrophoresis in the evaluation of homogeneous immunoglobulin components. In Bach FH, Good RA (eds): "Clinical Immunobiology." Vol 3. New York: Academic Press, 1976, pp 21–36.
44. McLaughlin H, Hobbs JR: Clinical Significance of Bence Jones Proteinuria. In Peeters H (ed): "Proteins and Related Subjects: Protides of the Biological Fluids." Vol 20. Amsterdam: Elsevier Publ, 1972, pp 251–254.
45. Ritchie RF, Smith R: Immunofixation I, Clin Chem 22:497, 1976; Immunofixation II, Clin Chem 22:1735, 1976; Immunofixation III, Clin Chem 22:1982, 1976.
46. Axelsen NH (ed): Quantitative immunoelectrophoresis, new developments and applications. Scand J Immunol [Suppl] 2, 1975.

47. Axelsen NH, Krøll, J, Weeke B (eds): "A Manual of Quantitative Immunoelectrophoresis. Methods and Applications." Scand J Immunol 2 [Suppl 1], 1973.
48. Rose NR, Friedman H (eds): "Manual of Clinical Immunology." 2nd ed. Washington, DC: American Soc Microbiol. 1980.
49. Englhardt A, Lommel H (eds): "Serumproteine." Weinheim, Germany: Verlag Chemie, 1974.
50. Heremans J: "Les Globulines Sériques dy Système Gamma Leur Nature et Leur Pathologie." Arscia SA (ed). Paris: Bruxelles and Masson et cie, 1960.
51. Ouchterlony Ö: "Handbook of Immunodiffusion and Immunoelectrophoresis." Appendices by Hirschfield J, Clausen J, Sewell MMH. Ann Arbor, MI: Ann Arbor Science Publ, Inc., 1968.
52. Schneider W, Berndt H: "Praktikum und Atlas der Immunoelektrophorese." Munich: J.F. Lehmanns, Verlag, 1960.
53. Roitt I: "Essential Immunology." 4th ed. Oxford: Blackwell Scientific, 1980.
54. Salmon SE (ed): "Myeloma and Related Disorders." Philadelphia: W.B. Saunders, Clinics in Haematol II:1–238, 1982.
55. Kochwa S, Kunkel HG (eds): Immunoglobulins. Annals NY Acad Sci 190:1–584, 1971.
56. Good RA, Day SB (series eds): Comprehensive Immunology. Vol 5. In Litman GW, Good RA (eds): "Immunoglobulins." New York: Plenum Publ Corp, 1978.
57. Merler E (ed): "Immunoglobulins. Biologic Aspects and Clinical Uses." Washington, DC: National Academy of Sciences, 1970.
58. Putnam FW: "The Plasma Proteins, Structure, Function and Genetic Control." 2nd ed, Vol III. Chapter 1: Immunoglobulins I. Structure, pp 1–153; Chapter 2: Immunoglobulins II. Antibody Specificity and Genetic Control, pp 155–221; Chapter 3: Immunoglobulins III: Comparative Biochemistry and Evolution, pp 223–284; Chapter 4: Antibodies with Molecular Uniformity, pp 285–332. New York: Academic Press, 1977.
59. Cawley LP, Minard BJ, Tourtellote, et al: Immunofixation electrophoretic techniques applied to identification of proteins in serum and cerebrospinal fluid. Clin Chem 22:1262, 1976.
60. Sun T: Immunofixation electrophoresis. In Ritzmann SE (ed): "Physiology of Immunoglobulins." New York: Alan R. Liss, Inc., 1982, pp 97–115.
61. Engle RL Jr, Wallis LA: "Immunoglobulinopathies—Immunoglobulins, Immune Deficiency Syndromes, Multiple Myeloma and Related Disorders." Springfield, IL: C.C. Thomas, 1969.
62. Kawai T: "Clinical Aspects of the Plasma Proteins." Philadelphia: J.B. Lippincott, 1973.
63. Hitzig WH: Immunoglobulin deficiencies, Chapter 7, this volume.
64. Dito WR: Quantitation of serum proteins by centrifugal fast analyzer. In Ritzmann SE (ed): "Physiology of Immunoglobulins." New York: Alan R. Liss, Inc., 1982, pp 119–137.
65. Ritzmann SE, Aguanno JJ, Finney MA, Hughes RC III: Quantitation of normal and abnormal serum immunoglobulins G, A, and M by radial immunodiffusion, nephelometry and turbidimetry. In Ritzmann SE (ed): "Physiology of Immunoglobulins." New York: Alan R. Liss, Inc., 1982, pp 139–156
66. Frantisek S, Morell A, Barandun S: Imbalances of κ/λ ratios of immunoglobulins, Chapter 2, this volume.
67. Hobbs JR: Secondary antibody deficiency. Proc R Soc Med 61:883, 1968.
68. Scheidegger JI: Une microméthode de l'immunoélectrophorèse. Int Arch Allergy Appl Immunol 7:103, 1955.
69. Hitzig WH: Die Physiologische Entwicklung der "Immunoglobuline" (Gamma and Beta$_2$-Globuline). Helv Paediatr Acta 12:596, 1959.

DIAGNOSTIC METHODOLOGY AND INTERPRETATION

Pathology of Immunoglobulins: Diagnostic and
Clinical Aspects, pages 13–19
© 1982 Alan R. Liss, Inc., 150 Fifth Avenue, New York, NY 10011

1

The Measurement of Viscosity

Jeffrey Crawford, MD, and Harvey Jay Cohen, MD

In this chapter we will discuss the methods used for the measurement of serum viscosity.[1] In order to understand these measurements and their interpretation, certain definitions and concepts are important. These will be presented here, while the relationships of viscosity to blood flow will be discussed in Chapter 9. Viscosity is a measurement of a fluid's resistance to flow. It can be determined by the ratio:

$$\text{viscosity (centipoise)} \cong \frac{\text{shear stress (dynes/cm}^2) \times 100}{\text{shear rate (s}^{-1})}$$

Shear stress is the force per unit area applied in the direction of flow required to make one plane of fluid slide over another. Shear rate is the difference in the velocities of two fluid planes measured in centimeters per second divided by the distance between them (Fig. 1).

These relationships form the basis of the measurement of viscosity by a rotational viscometer. Different geometric designs have been used, but one of the most popular is the cone-and-plate model such as the Wells-Brookfield micro-viscometer [1] (Fig. 2). The fluid to be studied is placed between the cone and plate and the cone is driven at different speeds of rotation, or different shear rates. The resistance a sample fluid exerts on the rotation of the cone is the shear stress created in that fluid. It can be measured with a torque-measuring device and the viscosity can then be calculated. A major utilization of the rotational viscometer has been in the study of fluid viscosity over a wide range of shear rates. Such studies have increased our knowledge of the relationship of viscosity to rheology, the study of the flow of fluids.

The relationship of viscosity to flow was first studied by Poiseuille in 1843 using a capillary tube system [2]. A similar capillary tube remains the

[1]Ed. note: See also [14].

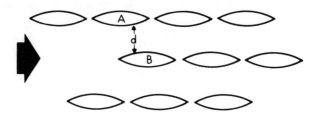

Fig. 1. A shear stress (arrow) is applied resulting in the movement of fluid plane B relative to A. The difference in the rate of movement of these two fluid planes divided by the distance (d) between them is the shear rate of the fluid.

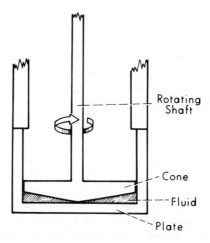

Fig. 2. Diagrammatic view of a cone-and-plate viscometer. By varying the speed of rotation (arrow), a range of shear rates can be created and compared to the resultant shear stresses of the fluid studied.

standard clinical method for the measurement of viscosity today. The Poiseuille equation states

$$\eta = \frac{\Delta P}{Q} \times \frac{\pi r^4}{1}$$

where η = viscosity, ΔP = pressure gradient, Q = flow rate, r = radius, and l = length of tube.

Simple fluids such as water maintain a constant viscosity despite wide variations in capillary radius, length, flow, or pressure. The homogeneity

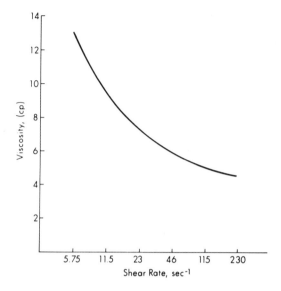

Fig. 3. The relationship of viscosity to shear rate for whole blood; cp = centipoise.

and small size of the fluid elements result in uniform frictional forces between fluid planes. Thus the shear stress of a simple fluid remains constant despite variations in the shear rate. This rheological property is termed Newtonian behavior. Blood does not conform to the laws of simple fluids and is, therefore, non-Newtonian. This suspension of cellular elements, plasma proteins, and lipids in an electrolyte solution results in varying internal frictional forces between fluid planes. Therefore, as the shear rate decreases, blood viscosity increases (Fig. 3). Shear rates decrease with decreasing vessel size. Blood flow through the aorta has been estimated to have a shear rate between 100 and 300 s^{-1} while flow through the arterioles has a shear rate between 11 and 25 s^{-1} [3]. Studies of conjunctival blood flow suggest that in some pathologic circumstances, flow can occasionally approach zero and, therefore, so would shear rate [4].

A major factor in the non-Newtonian increase in blood viscosity with decreasing shear rate appears to be the increased red cell aggregation, or rouleaux formation, that occurs as a result of the increased interaction between plasma proteins and red cells at lower flow rates. Physiologic dilution of red cells with plasma in the microcirculation attenuates this effect somewhat. However, pathologic changes in plasma proteins or red cells can dramatically increase rouleaux formation and viscosity at low rates of shear.

Rotational viscometers have the ability to measure fluids at low shear rates. The cone-and-plate viscometer can measure shear rates of plasma from

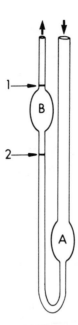

Fig. 4. Ostwald viscometer. The flow time (in seconds) of serum at 37°C is determined between marks 1 and 2. The viscometer is placed in a water bath (37°C) and 5 mL of serum is delivered into reservoir A. After equilibration at 37°C, suction is applied until the upper meniscus of serum fills reservoir B at mark 1. The serum is then allowed to flow freely back into reservoir A. The time required for the upper meniscus of the serum to pass between markers 1 and 2 is measured with a stopwatch.

450 s^{-1} to 45 s^{-1}. Another instrument, the Couette cylindrical viscometer, can measure shear rates from 100 s^{-1} to less than 0.1 s^{-1} [5]. The capillary tube has the disadvantage of a high fixed shear rate in the range of 450 s^{-1}. Even within the capillary tube shear rates vary between the wall and the center. In addition to its inability to reflect the shear rates existing in the microcirculation, another disadvantage is that most clinical studies with the capillary tube have used serum or plasma rather than whole blood and have thereby negated the important effects of red cell-protein interaction. Despite all these apparent inadequacies and inaccuracies, the measurement of serum viscosity by the capillary tube remains the most useful and common clinical tool for the evaluation and diagnosis of hyperviscosity.

The most popular capillary tube used is the Ostwald viscometer (Fig. 4). This is a simple, inexpensive apparatus which can be easily standardized and is reproducible in determining relative viscosities. This measurement is derived by measuring the flow time of the patient's serum relative to the flow

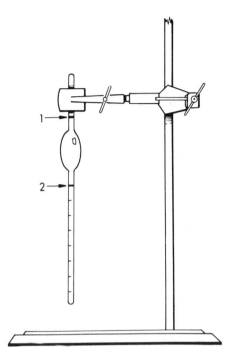

Fig. 5. A red cell pipette made stationary with a ring stand. See text for description of use.

time of distilled water at 37° C. The answer is expressed as η rel^{37}. Values for normal serum are in the range of 1.6 to 2.0, but each viscometer must be standardized because of variations in bulb volume, capillary diameter, water bath temperature, etc. To estimate the contribution of a cryoprotein to viscosity, determinations can be repeated at varied temperatures including 25° and 4° C (i.e., thermoviscosimetry).

As a bedside procedure, a red cell pipette (Fig. 5) can be substituted for the Ostwald viscometer [6]. Plasma is generally substituted for serum, eliminating the time delay for clot reaction, and the test is performed at room temperature, eliminating the need for a water bath. A 1 mL sample volume is sufficient rather than the usual 5 mL sample needed for the Ostwald viscometer. Samples are pipetted into a stationary red cell pipette and the flow time is measured between the lines immediately above and below the bulb reservoir. An elevated value must be verified at 37°C in order to eliminate the influence of a cryoprotein, but otherwise correlation between the two techniques is good. In order to obtain reliable longitudinal studies with either procedure, however, conditions such as the pipette and temperature must be kept constant. Other variations of the measurement of relative viscosity have been suggested; using a disposable needle-syringe system for ward use [11] or a Cannon-Manning semi-microviscometer when sample volume is limited [12].

Despite being a rather simple and straightforward procedure, measurement of serum or plasma viscosity has generally been reserved for the specialized evaluation of hyperviscosity syndromes. The development of an automated standardized capillary viscometer by Harkness has led to studies of other possible clinical uses of plasma viscosity measurements [7]. Plasma viscosity has been correlated with the erythrocyte sedimentation rate in detecting subtle changes in protein patterns in disease (8,9,10,13). Both tests reflect increases in fibrinogen and globulins. Decreases in albumin will increase the sedimentation rate, but not the viscosity, which may be low with isolated hypoalbuminemia. The plasma viscosity is unaffected by anemia or polycythemia. Also unlike the sedimentation rate, which frequently reaches a maximum value, the viscosity remains proportional to the degree of protein elevation. These advantages merit further clinical studies to clarify the usefulness of routine viscosity measurements as compared to the sedimentation rate.

In the management of patients with dysproteinemias, a capillary viscosity measurement provides the most useful screening tool for hyperviscosity. Once the presence of hyperviscosity has been established, a rotational viscometer, if available, provides a useful tool to study the changes in viscosity at various temperatures with varying shear rates for both serum or plasma and whole blood. Such measurements may be helpful in dissecting the pathophysiologic basis for the increased viscosity. This will be discussed further in Chapter 9.

ACKNOWLEDGMENTS

This work was partially supported by the Mallinckrodt and VA Geriatrics Fellowship Programs.

REFERENCES

1. Fareed J, Messmore HL, Gawlick GM, Bermes EW: Physical methods for the measurement of serum viscosity and protein concentration. In Sunderman FW (ed): "Proteins and Proteinopathies." Philadelphia: Institute for Clinical Science, 1977.
2. Poiseuille JCM: Ann Chim Phys 16:60, 1843.
3. Van der Elst CW, Malan AF, De V Heese H: Blood viscosity in modern medicine. South Afr Med J 52:526, 1977.
4. Wells R, Edgerton H: Blood flow in the microcirculation of the conjunctival vessels of man. Angiology 18:699, 1967.
5. Graf C, Barras J-P: Rheological properties of human blood plasma—a comparison of measurements with three different viscometers. Experientia 35:224, 1979.

6. Wright DJ, Jenkins DE: Simplified method for estimation of serum and plasma viscosity in multiple myeloma and related disorders. Blood 36:516, 1970.
7. Harkness J: A new instrument for the measurement of plasma viscosity. Lancet 2:280, 1963.
8. Harkness J: The viscosity of human blood plasma: Its measurement in health and disease. Biorheology 8:171, 1971.
9. Hutchinson RM, Eastham RD: A comparison of the erythrocyte sedimentation rate and plasma viscosity in detecting changes in plasma proteins. J Clin Pathol 30:345, 1977.
10. Bradlow BA, Haggan JM: A comparison of the plasma viscosity and erythrocyte sedimentation rate as screening tests. South Afr Med J 55:415, 1979.
11. Leonard RCF: Simple technique for measuring serum or plasma viscosity with disposable apparatus. Br Med J 283:1154, 1981.
12. Kley HV, Lathrop PE: Easy measurement of viscosity of semi-micro serum samples. Clin Chem 27:1142, 1981.
13. Pickup ME, Dixon JS, Hallet C, Bird HA, Wright V: Plasma viscosity—a new appraisal of its use as an index of disease activity in rheumatoid arthritis. Ann Rheum Dis 40:272, 1981.
14. Wolf RE, Levin WC, Ritzmann SE: Thermoproteins. In Ritzmann SE, Daniels JC (eds): "Serum Protein Abnormalities: Diagnostic and Clinical Aspects," 2nd printing. New York: Alan R. Liss, Inc., 1982, pp 487–512.

Pathology of Immunoglobulins: Diagnostic and
Clinical Aspects, pages 21–35
© 1982 Alan R. Liss, Inc., 150 Fifth Avenue, New York, NY 10011

2

Imbalances of κ/λ Ratios of Immunoglobulins

Frantisek Skvaril, PhD, Andreas Morell, MD, and Silvio Barandun, MD

INTRODUCTION

Human immunoglobulin (Ig) molecules are composed of two heavy (H) and light (L) polypeptide chains. Heavy chains are class-specific, and presently, five classes are recognized: IgG, IgA, IgM, IgD, and IgE. In addition, H chain subclasses have been characterized. Two types of L chains, κ and λ, are bound to each of the five H chains. All H chains and both L chains have a characteristic antigenic structure, and therefore, specific antisera can be prepared in various animal species. Antisera specific for κ- or λ-L chains are usually employed for the L chain typing of monoclonal Ig of the various classes, and for the detection of Bence Jones proteins (BJP). Monoclonal proteins are visualized by a characteristic curvature of the precipitin line with the corresponding antiserum on immunoelectrophoresis (IEP).

The quantitative relation of normal IgG Igs of κ- and λ-type is about 1.8 ± 0.3 as determined in single radial immunodiffusion (RID) by means of L chain specific antisera [3,4]. The distribution of κ and λ molecules within monoclonal Igs has shown that there may be some differences: The κ/λ ratio of IgG paraproteins was found to be about 1.6, of IgA paraproteins 1.3, of IgM proteins 4.0, and of IgD myeloma proteins 0.05. Very little is known about the κ/λ Ig distribution in biological fluids other than serum.

Four methods can be used for the detection of Ig light (L) chain imbalances:

1) κ/λ imbalances are detectable by *double immunodiffusion* with anti-κ and anti-λ sera mixed in appropriate ratios (the so-called double-line (DL) κ/λ method [19]). The distance between the two parallel lines precipitated in the unknown sample is compared macroscopically with the distance in a normal or reference serum. Deviations from κ/λ ratio in the normal or

reference serum are expressed as "κ/λ imbalances in favor of κ (or λ) Igs."

2) κ and λ Igs can be measured directly by *RID* and the κ/λ ratio can be calculated and compared with the κ/λ ratio in a normal or reference serum.

3) IgG-κ and IgG-λ have been recently determined in *turbidimetric analysis* by means of monoclonal antibodies against κ-chain (and λ-chain, respectively) in mixture with a monoclonal antibody against Fc-γ [23].

4) κ and λ Igs can also be detected with *hemagglutination techniques* [10]. The method is applicable to a variety of clinical situations and antisera which fail to give satisfactory precipitin reactions, can also be used.

The double immunodiffusion (DL κ/λ method) is less expensive and less time-consuming than the RID and it is the preferred method for screening of a large number of samples. In addition to one of the methods for κ/λ assays, serum protein electrophoresis and IEP [16,17] should be performed to obtain the necessary basic information regarding the serum protein distribution in the sample.

METHODOLOGY

Preparation of Antisera

For the detection of κ/λ imbalances in Igs, potent antisera against both L chain types are necessary. They can be raised in rabbits by immunization with BJP of both types [6]. The absorption of the crude antisera is carried out with suitable serum or urine fractions. The specificity of the final preparations is tested by IEP with several sera containing monoclonal IgG, IgA, and IgM proteins and urines with BJP. Specific antibodies in the antisera are then determined quantitatively [7].

The immunoreagent used for screening sera for L chain imbalances represents a mixture of such anti-κ and anti-λ sera containing approximately 1 mg/mL of anti-κ and 1.7 mg/mL of anti-λ antibodies (DL κ/λ antiserum).[1]

Immunoprecipitation Methods

Double immunodiffusion in agar [12] is performed in two types of hexagonal or rosette patterns. For the so-called *macro-method,* a Shandon Agar Cutter is used: the central well is 9 mm and the peripheral well 6 mm in diameter, with 10 mm in between. For the *micro-method,* patterns are cut out with the central well 3.5 mm and peripheral well 2.0 mm in diameter;

---

[1]This antiserum is not yet commercially available. A limited amount can be obtained upon request from the Institute of Cancer Research, Tiefenau-Hospital, 3004 Bern, Switzerland.

the distance in between is 5.5 mm. Immunodiffusion plates with macro-rosettes are incubated for 48 hours at 37°C; with micro-rosettes for 24 hours at room temperature. Both types of rosettes are found to be convenient and practical. After precipitation the plates are washed, dried, and stained as usual for immunodiffusion methods.

IEP [5] is performed on 5 × 12 cm slides. The antigen wells are 1 mm in diameter and they are placed at a distance of 1.7 mm from the antiserum trough (1.5 mm in width). Similar results, however, can be obtained by IEP on microscopic slides [18] in a suitable laboratory apparatus. For double immunodiffusion as well as for IEP, 1.5% agar with a low electroendosmosis in barbital buffer pH 8.6 (e.g., 0.05) is used.

Quantitative determination of κ/λ ratios may be achieved by using RID plates [9] containing either κ- or λ-specific antisera separately, or in plates with a DL κ/λ antiserum. In the latter, two precipitin rings are formed.

INTERPRETATION OF RESULTS

A mixture of anti-κ and anti-λ sera, using double immunodiffusion with dilutions of normal human serum, forms two parallel precipitin lines. At an anti-κ and anti-λ antibody ratio of 1.0/1.7, λ Ig precipitate in a line closer to the peripheral antigen well and κ Ig form a line closer to the antiserum well. The precipitin lines can be identified by comparing the reactions with BJP of both types with those obtained by normal serum (Fig. 1). A reverse position of the precipitin lines can be achieved by mixing the antisera in inverse proportions. The described dilution arrangement, however, appears preferable since it reflects the normal concentration trends in serum: The

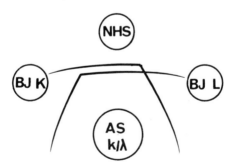

Fig. 1. Schematic representation of double immunodiffusion of pooled normal human serum (NHS) (in 1:6 dilution) and of Bence Jones proteins of κ and λ types (in 2 mg/mL concentration) against a mixture of specific anti-κ and anti-λ sera. This antiserum mixture contains 0.97 mg of anti-κ and 1.68 mg of anti-λ antibody per mL. (Reproduced with permission from Skvaril and Barandun [19].)

higher concentration of κ Ig causes a higher diffusion rate, and consequently, the κ line occurs more distant from the antigen well than the λ precipitin line.

Both precipitin lines are detectable in normal human serum over a wide dilution range. The clearest results, however, are obtained within the range of 1:3 to 1:8 (Fig. 2). The optimal dilution of a normal serum should be determined whenever a new DL κ/λ serum lot is used. An appropriately diluted normal human serum specimen is analyzed in each rosette, together with the sera to be tested. The distance between the two lines precipitated with the normal serum represents the "reference value" to which the distances, obtained with the test sera, are compared. In the majority of normal sera, the distance between two precipitin lines is identical. In sera with distorted κ/λ ratios, shifting of one or of the other line occurs in accordance with the principles of immunodiffusion [12]. At a κ Ig predominance, the κ line will be closer to the antiserum well and the distance between both lines will increase. On the other hand, in the case of an L chain imbalance in favour of λ Ig, a "convergence" of both lines should occur. In extreme cases, the λ line will superimpose or cross the κ line.

The limits of the method for detecting imbalances of the κ/λ-Ig ratios can be established by adding a mixture of purified IgG, IgA, and IgM myeloma proteins of κ and λ L chain types in various proportions to normal serum. These mixtures are then diluted and tested in double immunodiffusion. Both

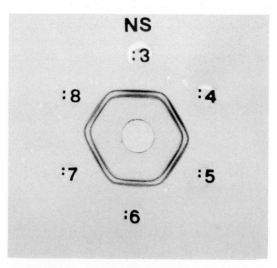

Fig. 2.   Double immunodiffusion of normal human serum (NS) at various dilutions (peripheral wells) with the κ/λ DL antiserum (central well). NS 1:3, :4, :5, :6, etc., diluted 1:3, :4, :5, etc. (Reproduced with permission from Skvaril and Barandun [19].)

divergence and convergence of precipitin lines can be observed when κ or λ monoclonal proteins of these various Ig classes are added to normal serum. However, the sensitivity of the test system is not equal for all Ig classes: A clear shift of precipitin lines is detectable when 1 mg of IgG is added to 1 mL of normal serum; but for a comparable effect, the addition of 3 mg of either IgA or IgM per mL of serum is necessary.

The decreased reaction of IgA with anti-L chain antibodies has been explained to be due to steric hindrance of L chains bound to α-H chains [11,13]. For IgM, the reason for the lower sensitivity in the DL κ/λ system is different: The IgG diffuses, due to its lower molecular weight and higher absolute concentration, much more rapidly than the IgM and precipitates all anti-L chain antibody in front of the diffusion field. When the IgG is eliminated from the reaction by testing the macromolecular fraction isolated from the serum, instead of the whole serum, a substantially higher sensitivity in the detection of IgM L chain imbalances can be achieved. Another, less time-consuming alternative method consists of pretreatment of the whole serum with a reducing agent, such as mercaptoethanol or dithiothreitol; the treated IgM behaves in the diffusion reaction similarly to the IgG and influences the position of κ or λ precipitin lines more markedly than the monoclonal 19S IgM in the untreated serum.

Two clearly separated, parallel precipitin lines appear also on IEP of a normal human serum precipitated with a "double-line κ/λ" antiserum, and imbalances in the κ/λ Ig ratios also result in changes of the distances between the two lines. IEP, however, is more suitable for the detection and typing of a monoclonal protein than for the detection of κ/λ imbalances in a serum with heterogeneous (polyclonal) Igs.

Imbalances in κ/λ Ig ratios can be measured quantitatively in the RID [9] by using a mixture of isolated monoclonal IgG proteins of κ and λ L chain types as calibrators, and antisera to both L chain types incorporated in the gel. Although the participation of Igs other than IgG has not been fully evaluated in this type of analysis, it may be assumed that with regard to the concentration ratios, molecular weight differences, or hindrance of the L chain reactivity, the IgG will also in this method be the predominantly participating Ig class.

κ/λ Ig RATIOS IN NORMAL AND PATHOLOGICAL SERA

Analyses of Normal Sera

In a preliminary screening of sera from children and adults with the DL κ/λ method for κ/λ imbalances it has been shown that this ratio is subject to slight variations during life [14,15,20,22]. In children a κ/λ imbalance in favor of λ-Igs was found (Fig. 3). Therefore, a quantitative study was performed with the RID of sera from individuals at various age groups.

The distribution of κ/λ ratios in groups of sera from children, young adults, blood donors, and aged individuals (over 95 years) is shown in Figure 4. A marked difference can be observed between values obtained in children and in young adults. Also a significant difference can be seen between the κ/λ ratio in young adults and a more heterogeneous group of blood donors (male and female, 20–60 years). A broad distribution range was found in the group of aged persons. It should be noted that none of these sera contained M-proteins; no clinical symptoms of immunodeficiency were demonstrable in any of the individuals tested. With the exception of the aged people, the Ig levels were within a normal range. Arithmetical mean values, standard deviations, and ranges of κ/λ-Ig ratios in groups of these sera are given in Table I.

For further analyses all children (1–24 months) were divided into groups of 4-month intervals. The distribution of κ/λ ratios in these groups is shown in Figure 5. In all four groups, the κ/λ ratio is significantly lower than 1.6, a value found in the young male adults. Thus, the relative concentration of λ-Igs in the sera from children is higher than in the sera from adults. In the youngest group (1–3 months), the κ/λ ratio is somewhat higher than in other age groups (1.45 ± 0.2). This is probably due to the passively transferred

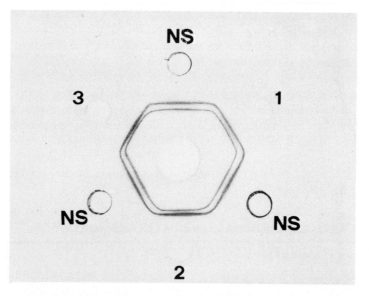

Fig. 3.   Analysis of three sera from children (Nos. 1,2,3) by the DL κ/λ method with normal serum (NS) as reference. All sera were analyzed in 1:6 dilutions.

maternal IgG. In the last group (13–14 months), a slight trend for increasing κ/λ ratios is observed.

Paraproteinemic Sera

Sera with monoclonal Igs are characterized by a markedly distorted κ/λ-Ig ratio. When such sera are reacted by immunodiffusion with the κ/λ DL

TABLE I. κ/λ **Ratios in Sera of Individual Groups**

		κ/λ ratios		
Sera from	No. of subjects	Mean values ± 1 SD	Range	Significance of differences from young adult values
Children	111	1.25 ± 0.20	0.8–1.8	P < 0.001
Young adults	139	1.68 ± 0.26	1.2–2.7	—
Blood donors	197	1.91 ± 0.32	1.2–2.8	P < 0.001
Aged individuals	45	1.62 ± 0.33	1.2–2.9	N.S.[a]

[a]Not significant.
Reproduced by permission from Skvaril et al. [22].

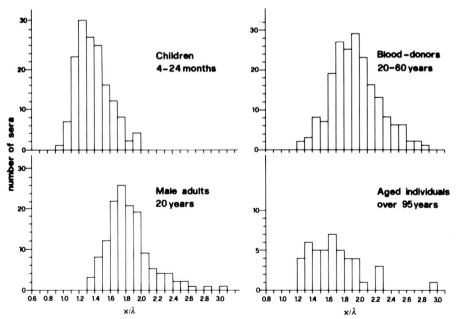

Fig. 4. Distribution of κ/λ immunoglobulin ratios in sera from children, young male adults, blood donors, and aged people. (Reproduced with permission from Skvaril et al. [20].)

antiserum, the monoclonal protein will influence the position of the precipitin line of the corresponding L chain type by shifting it into the antigen excess zone. The second line reflects Igs of the opposite L chain type, i.e., non-myeloma or "normal" background Igs.

Precipitin patterns of sera with myeloma proteins of any class (except IgM) developed with the κ/λ DL antiserum are shown in Figure 6. Similar clear-cut patterns were obtained when sera containing free L chains were tested.

For reasons mentioned above, monoclonal IgM proteins do not cause an appropriate shifting of the corresponding precipitin line as do the other monoclonal Igs. The applicability of the DL κ/λ method for the detection of the L chain type of a monoclonal IgM (or for the detection of the κ/λ imbalance in the IgM class) can, however, be improved by prior treatment of the serum with reducing agents (Fig. 7). Both untreated and treated sera are tested in the same arrangement: κ/λ imbalances of the IgG class are detected in the analysis of the untreated and of the IgM class in the treated sample [21].

In some patients with lymphoproliferative disorders, two or even more monoclonal Igs can be found. Such sera require analysis by IEP, using the same κ/λ DL antiserum. The reaction of a serum with a double M-component

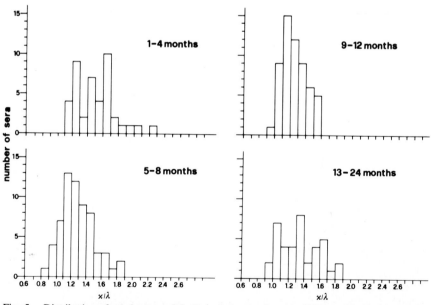

Fig. 5. Distribution of κ/λ immunoglobulin ratio in sera from children up to 2 years of age. (Reproduced with permission from Skvaril et al. [20].)

is demonstrated in Figure 8. In sera with γ-, α-, or μ-H chain disease proteins, the precipitation patterns developed with the κ/λ DL antiserum represent the background Igs, since these particular proteins lack the L chains.

The results of the analysis of more than 2000 sera with a monoclonal Ig, employing both the conventional techniques and the DL κ/λ method, agreed without exception. An added advantage of the κ/λ DL method is the fact that an M-protein is recognized and typed and the background IgG is visualized simultaneously.

Sera From Hypogammaglobulinemic Patients

On routine analysis of sera from patients with primary immune deficiency with the κ/λ method, it was observed that L chain imbalances occurred more

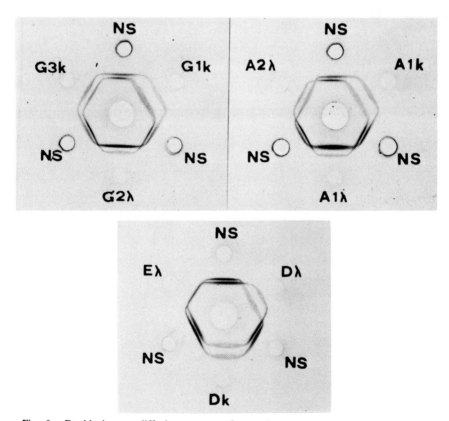

Fig. 6. Double immunodiffusion patterns of normal serum (NS) and myeloma sera with monoclonal proteins of IgG, IgA, IgD, and IgE classes and κ or λ L chain types developed with the κ/λ DL antiserum. All sera were diluted 1:6. (Reproduced with permission from Skvaril and Barandun [19].)

frequently than in other groups of nonmonoclonal gammopathy patients. A broad distribution of the κ/λ ratio can be seen in these patients (Fig. 9).

In addition to these cases, a marked κ/λ imbalance was observed in two male adults—in one in favor of κ- and the other in favor of λ-Igs—with primary hypogammaglobulinemia [1]. These patients (not included in Figure 9) are reported in detail.

CASE REPORT 1 (κ-CHAIN DEFICIENCY)

A 38-year-old male (BP) suffered from chronic diarrhea and pernicious anemia (Hb 4.7 g/100 mL) since the age of 14 years. Hypogammaglobulinemia was detected with a selective deficiency of κ-chain Ig at the age of 28. The patient was successfully treated with Vitamin B_{12} and antibiotics, which rapidly improved his condition. The immunologic abnormalities (hypogammaglobulinemia, κ-chain deficiency) still persist today (1982). Serum Ig concentrations, κ/λ ratio, and other characteristics are summarized in Tables II and III, respectively.

CASE REPORT 2 (λ-CHAIN DEFICIENCY)

A 39-year-old man (RW) was hypogammaglobulinemic with typical antibody deficiency syndrome. Since infancy he suffered from chronic pansinusitis, bronchitis, and pneumonia, requiring repeated treatment with antibiotics. A deficiency of λ-chain Ig and a moderate hypochromic anemia (Hb 11.0 g/100 mL) were found at age 31. Although his general condition improved with the appropriate therapy, his immunologic status remains unchanged (1982) (Tables II and III).

Three other cases with similar disorders of Ig synthesis have been reported in the literature. A young girl with recurrent infections and diarrhea was

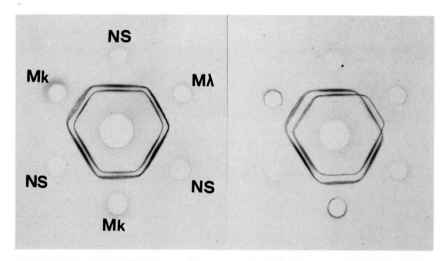

Fig. 7. Double immunodiffusion reaction of normal serum (NS) and three sera containing monoclonal IgM with the κ/λ DL antiserum. Left: untreated samples. Right: samples treated with dithiothreitol. All sera were diluted 1:6 (For details see text.)

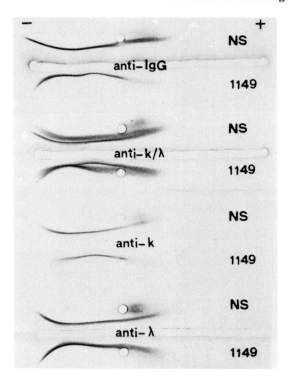

Fig. 8. Immunoelectrophoretic analysis of a serum with a double M-component (No. 1149, diluted 1:2) precipitated with an anti-IgG (γ-chain specific), anti-κ/λ DL serum and with L chain-specific antisera (anti-κ, anti-λ). For comparison, a normal human serum (NS) (undiluted) was assayed. The slow moving component represents a monoclonal IgG of λ-type and the faster component, a monoclonal IgG of κ-L chain type (Reproduced with permission from Skvaril and Barandun [19].)

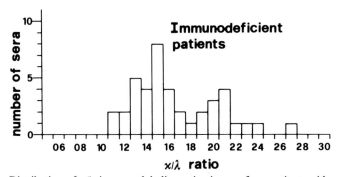

Fig. 9. Distribution of κ/λ immunoglobulins ratios in sera from patients with primary hypogammaglobulinemia. (Reproduced with permission from Skvaril et al. [22].)

TABLE II. Serum Immunoglobulins of Patients BP and RW

	Total serum protein (g/100mL)	IgG (mg/100mL)	IgA (mg/100mL)	IgM (mg/100mL)	IgD (mg/100mL)	IgE (U/mL)	IgG subclasses			
							G1 (mg/mL)	G2 (mg/mL)	G3 (mg/mL)	G4 (mg/mL)
Patient BP										
1970–1974	6.4[a] (5.2–7.1)[b]	555 (375–760)	39 (28–54)	21 (<20–32)	6 (5–8)	120 (80–180)	5.2 (5.0–5.5)	0.3 (0.1–0.4)	1.0 (0.9–1.0)	0.04 (0.007–0.08)
Patient RW										
1972–1974	6.2 (6.0–6.4)	440 (390–530)	< 10	48 (40–60)	< 5	41 (35–45)	2.6[c]	1.5	0.25	0.005
Normal controls	7.2 (6.5–8.4)	1200 (900–1500)	210 (120–400)	190 (90–260)	(5–30)	(100–250)	6.6 (3.5–11.5)	3.2 (1.3–6.8)	0.6 (0.1–2.1)	0.5 (0.03–2.9)

[a]Mean.
[b]Range
[c]Determinations in one serum sample.
Reproduced with permission from Barandun et al. [1].

TABLE III. κ/λ Ratio of Serum Immunoglobulins of Patients BP and RW

Method	Specific antiserums to	Total serum	Isolated serum IgG	Isolated serum IgM
Patient BP				
Immunoelectrophoresis	κ	(+)[a]	(+)	0
	λ	+	+	+
	α/κ	0		
Radial immunodiffusion[b]	κ	0.05 mg/mL (1.2%)		
	λ	4.0 mg/mL (98.8%)		
Quantitative precipitation[c]	κ	0.1 mg/mL (1.8%)		
	λ	5.6 mg/mL (98.2%)		
Patient RW				
Immunoelectrophoresis	κ	+	+	+
	λ	(+)	(+)	(+)
	α/κ	(+)		
Radial immunodiffusion	κ	3.55 mg/mL (87.2%)		
	λ	0.55 mg/mL (12.8%)		
Quantitative precipitation	κ	3.65 mg/mL (84.5%)		
	λ	0.67 mg/mL (15.5%)		

[a]+ = distinct precipitin line; (+) = weak precipitin line; 0 = no reaction.
[b]Normal values: κ/λ ratio in serum of 300 adult individuals 1.8 ± 0.3.
[c]Normal values: serum pool κ = 7.0 mg/mL (65.5%), λ = 4.05 mg/mL (34.5%).
Reproduced with permission from Barandun et al. [1].

deficient in κ-chain Igs, had decreased IgG, IgA, and IgE serum levels [2]. κ-Chain deficiencies were observed also in two children, one boy and one girl, suffering from mucoviscidosis. The IgG levels in both patients were normal [8].

CONCLUSIONS

This chapter has focused on the diagnostic methodology and clinical interpretation of L chain (κ/λ) imbalances of Igs.

Moderate L chain imbalances may be encountered physiologically and may be due to either asynchronous maturation of κ- and λ-Ig-producing cells during infancy, or to exogenous immunogenic influences, genetic factors etc., during adulthood. In aged persons above 95 years, there is a trend toward increasing levels of IgG and IgA: In these individuals the imbalanced synthesis of Igs may be the cause for the distorted κ/λ ratios.

The most *excessive L chain imbalances* are found in sera from patients with monoclonal gammopathies. In these cases, the analysis for κ/λ imbalances offers a sensitive method for the detection of monoclonal Igs present at relative low concentrations in sera with normal or even elevated concentration of the residual, background Ig. In hypogammaglobulinemias a broad distribution of κ/λ ratios is encountered: in five unusual cases reported thus far, polyclonal or heterogeneous Igs belonging almost exclusively to one L chain type were identified. A developmental defect of the B-cell system has been postulated as the most probable cause for this immunological disturbance.

REFERENCES

1. Barandun S, Morell A, Skvaril F, Oberdorfer A: Deficiency of κ- or λ-type immunoglobulins. Blood 47:79, 1976.
2. Bernier GM, Gunderman JR, Ruymann FB: Kappa-chain deficiency. Blood 40:795, 1972.
3. Eickhoff K, Heipertz R: The determination of serum immunoglobulin concentrations on the basis of their light chain antigenic properties. Clin Chim Acta 78:343, 1977.
4. Fahey JL: Two types of 6.6 S γ-globulins, β2A globulins and 18S γ₁-microglobulins in normal urine. J Immunol 91:438, 1963.
5. Grabar P, Burtin P: "Immunoelectrophoretic Analysis. Application to Human Biological Fluids." Amsterdam: Elsevier, 1964.
6. Hijmans W, Schuit HRE, Klein F: An immunofluorescence procedure for the detection of intracellular immunoglobulins. Clin Exp Immunol 4:457, 1969.
7. Kabat BA, Mayer MM: "Experimental Immunochemistry." Springfield: ChC Thomas, 1964.
8. Maertzdorf W, Stoop JW, Mul NAJ, Zegers BJM, Ballieux RE: A child with mucoviscidosis (cystic fibrosis of the pancreas), diabetes mellitus and a disorder of immunoglobulins. Eur J Clin Invest 2:294, 1972.
9. Mancini G, Carbonara AG, Heremans JF: Immunochemical quantitation of antigens by single radial immunodiffusion. Immunochemistry 2:235, 1965.
10. Mason DY: Measurement of kappa: lambda light chain ratios by haemagglutination techniques. J Immunol Methods 6:273, 1975.
11. Osterland CK, Chaplin H: Atypical antigenic properties of a IgA myeloma protein. J Immunol 96:842, 1966.
12. Ouchterlony O: Diffusion-in-gel methods for immunological analysis. Prog Allergy 5:1, 1958.
13. Prendergast RA, Grey HM, Kunkel HD: Recombination of heavy and light chains of human γA-myeloma proteins: Formation of hybrid molecules and configurational specificity. J Exp Med 124:185, 1966.
14. Rádl J, Sepers JM, Skvaril F, Morell A, Hijmans W: Immunoglobulin pattern in humans over 95 years of age. Clin Exp Immunol 22:84, 1975.
15. Riesen W, Keller H, Skvaril F, Morrell A: Restriction of immunoglobulin heterogeneity, autoimmunity, and serum protein levels in aged people. Clin Exp Immunol 26:280, 1976.
16. Ritzmann SE, Daniels JC: Serum electrophoresis and total serum proteins. In Ritzmann SE, Daniels JC (eds): "Serum Protein Abnormalities." Boston: Little Brown, 1975, pp. 3–25.
17. Ritzmann SE, Lawrence M: Qualitative immunoelectrophoresis. In Ritzmann SE, Daniels JC (eds): "Serum Protein Abnormalities." Boston: Little Brown, 1975, pp 27–53.
18. Scheidegger JJ: Une microméthode de l'immunoelectrophorèse. Int Arch Allergy Appl Immunol 7:103, 1955.

19. Skvaril F, Barandun S: A simple method for the simultaneous detection of human immunoglobulins of both light chain types. J Immunol Methods 3:127, 1973.
20. Skvaril F, Barandun S, Kuffer F, Probst M: Veränderung des κ/λ Verhältnisses der menschlichen Serumimmunglobuline im Verlaufe der Entwicklung. Blut 33:281, 1976.
21. Skvaril F: Unpublished results.
22. Skvaril F, Barandun S, Morell A, Kuffer F, Probst M: Imbalances of κ/λ immunoglobulin light chain ratios in normal individuals and in immunodeficient patients. In Peeters H (eds): "Protides of Biological Fluids, 23th Colloquium." Oxford: Pergamon Press, 1976, pp 415–420.
23. Jefferis R, Deverill I, Ling NR, Reeves WG: Quantitation of human total IgG, kappa IgG and lambda IgG in serum using monoclonal antibodies. J Immunol Methods 39:355, 1980.

Pathology of Immunoglobulins: Diagnostic and
Clinical Aspects, pages 37–51
© 1982 Alan R. Liss, Inc., 150 Fifth Avenue, New York, NY 10011

3

Electrolyte Abnormalities and the Anion Gap in Immunoglobulin Disorders

James J. Aguanno, PhD

INTRODUCTION

Proper interpretations of serum electrolyte values requires not only an understanding of the underlying pathophysiology but also knowledge and appreciation of possible analytic factors which can alter test results. Patients with multiple myeloma may develop fluid and electrolyte disorders secondary to the renal involvement, such as nephrotic and Fanconi syndromes. The nephrotic syndrome is commonly encountered in patients with multiple myeloma, and as a consequence they can develop a dilutional hyponatremia due to edema formation. Clinically, it appears imperative to distinguish true hyponatremia from pseudohyponatremia due to high concentrations of serum M-proteins.

Hypercalcemia is also a frequent complication of multiple myeloma which in most instances represents true hypercalcemia, i.e., an elevation in both total and ionic calcium concentrations. In some patients, however, the total calcium is elevated but the ionic calcium is normal. These patients are asymptomatic and, therefore, may require no treatment for hypercalcemia. These as well as other conditions must be recognized before the correct diagnosis and treatment can be instituted. Other electrolyte aberrations in patients with immunoglobulin (Ig) abnormalities include hypercupremia and deviations of the anion gap.

SODIUM AND POTASSIUM

Numerous disease states may result in a true lowering of plasma sodium (Na) and/or potassium (K) concentrations [1–3]. However, there are circumstances in which the measured plasma concentrations of these electrolytes are falsely low, resulting in pseudohyponatremia and pseudohypokalemia.

The major factors which contribute to spuriously low values (Table I) include both intrinsic properties of the sample (e.g., increased concentration of proteins and lipids and increased viscosity) and the method by which the sample is analyzed (e.g., flame photometry and indirect potentiometry). Both Na and K are affected to an unequal extent, since the plasma concentration of Na is approximately 35-fold greater than that of K, the absolute decrease in the number of mmol/L of Na is greater and, therefore, more obvious. For example, a sample having a total protein concentration of 10 g/dL may be expected to show a 10% decrease in the measured Na and K. If the true values are 140 mmol/L and 4.0 mmol/L for Na and K, respectively, the Na would be lowered by 14 mmol/L to new level of 126 mmol/L, while K would be lowered by only 0.4 mmol/L to a level of 3.6 mmol/L. In this example, the Na fell below the lower limit of normal (135–145 mmol/L) while K remained within the normal range (3.5–4.5 mmol/L). For this reason, more attention has been given to pseudohyponatremia than to low K concentrations.

The pseudohyponatremia associated with hyperproteinemic and hyperlipidemic conditions is best explained on a plasma-water basis. The plasma portion of blood contains both electrolytes and nonelectrolytes consisting primarily of dissolved and suspended lipids and proteins. Since Na and the other ionic constituents are confined to the aqueous phase of plasma, their concentrations are directly proportional to the plasma water content of the sample, which decreases as the concentration of protein and lipid increases. Therefore, due to the space-occupying properties of proteins and lipids, the serum of patients with hyperproteinemia or hyperlipidemia may exhibit a pseudohyponatremia, depending somewhat on the analytic technique used. Pseudohyponatremia has been reported in patients with uncontrolled diabetes mellitus with severe hyperlipidemia [4], and with hyperproteinemia due to the presence of an M-protein in the serum [5–7]. In patients with elevated levels of plasma lipids, the pseudohyponatremia appears to be primarily due to the volume-displacing properties of the lipids. It seems unlikely however that the pseudohyponatremia in patients with hyperproteinemia is solely due to plasma water effects (Table I). There is sufficient experimental evidence to support the contention that pseudohyponatremia can be the consequence of the volume-displacing properties of proteins [8,9]. Shyr and Young [9] showed the effects of increasing protein (bovine serum) on the measurement of Na and K by both flame photometry and direct potentiometry (Fig. 1). These results clearly indicate a decrease in the Na and K concentrations as measured by flame photometry with increasing total protein levels, although there was little or no difference in the measurement of Na or K in the same samples as determined by ion-selective electrode (ISE). The methodological bias between the two techniques is best explained on a plasma water basis. Measurement of protein-containing samples by direct potentiometry yields a

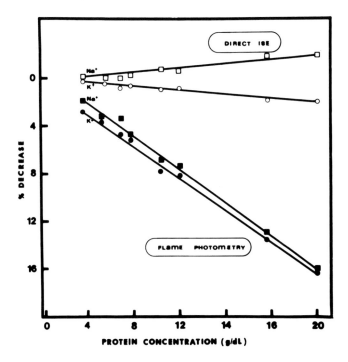

Fig. 1. Effect of protein concentration (bovine serum albumin) on the measurement of Na^+ and K^+ using direct ion-selective electrode (ISE) method (open symbols) and by flame photometry (closed symbols). (Reproduced with permission from Shyr and Young [9].)

TABLE I. Causes of Spuriously Low Sodium and Potassium Concentrations

Intrinsic properties of the sample

    Hyperproteinemia
        Displacement of plasma water
        Cationic nature of the M-protein
        Sodium binding to the M-protein
    Hyperlipidemia
    Hyperviscosity

Analytic factors

    Flame Photometry
    Indirect Potentiometry

concentration expressed on a plasma water basis while flame photometry presents data on a total plasma basis. Therefore, the bias between direct ISE and flame photometry may be a function of lipid and protein concentrations in the sample [10]. Since direct ISE measurement is only sensitive to the water phase of plasma, the concentration obtained by this technique is independent of the amount of nonelectrolyte components in the sample. This is not the case for flame photometry or indirect (diluted) ISE procedures, which use an aliquot of the sample that contains both electrolyte and nonelectrolyte phases, thus yielding a concentration based on the total volume of the plasma sample. Consequently, all results of electrolyte measurements involving a dilution step (including those which measure by ISE) will decrease as the lipid and protein concentrations increase.

The relationship between the decrease in Na and K concentrations as a function of total protein in normal subjects as in patients with hyperproteinemia is shown in Figure 2 [8]. The observed concentrations of Na and K clearly tend to decrease as the protein concentrations increase. However, there exists a rather broad range of values, making it difficult to predict accurately, solely on the basis of protein concentrations and water content of the serum, the extent of the decrease in the measured serum Na or K concentrations in individual patients. A numerical correction table may allow a better prediction of actual Na values suggested by indirect methods in samples containing elevated lipid and/or protein levels [11].

Other factors must also be considered. For example, it has been postulated that M-proteins can act as cations causing hyponatremia by displacing serum Na [6,7]. All other serum cations will also be lowered by this mechanism but a significant reduction is also manifest for Na because it is the major serum cation.

It has been suggested, but not conclusively proved, that Na and K appear to interact with or bind to a nonprotein, protein-bound plasma constituent. Although both Na and K show this interaction, the magnitude is greater for Na [8].

Finally, the influence of serum viscosity on the determination of Na and K must be considered. Although the hyperviscosity syndrome occurs most frequently in Waldenström's macroglobulinemia (see Chapter 5), it may also be associated with IgG and IgA multiple myeloma and various serum immune-complex disorders [12,13].

In addition to their perplexing clinical challenges and potentially fatal outcome, patients with hyperviscosity syndrome also present problems to the clinical chemistry laboratory that may lead to the inappropriate administration of intravenous fluids if these pitfalls are not recognized. It has been shown that roller-pump dilutors, which are widely used in combination with a flame photometer for the determination of Na and K, can yield spuriously low

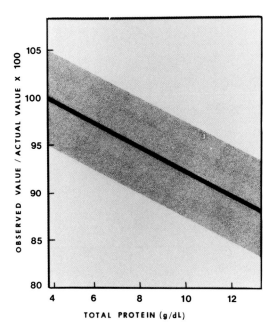

Fig. 2. Effect of increasing protein concentration in both normal patients and in patients with a polyclonal gammopathy on the measurement of Na^+ and K^+. (Modified and reproduced with permission. From Ladenson [8].)

results [14]. The magnitude of this error appears to be directly correlated with the relative serum viscosity (Fig. 3). Therefore, the recognition of this analytical error, rather than its misinterpretation as true hyponatremia, is essential for the appropriate treatment of such patients.

The clinical implications of pseudohyponatremia are obvious. On the one hand, if the low concentration of serum Na is thought to represent true hyponatremia, inappropriate fluid therapy may be instituted, and conversely, a normal value of serum Na in a patient with severe hyperproteinemia may mask a true hypernatremia, which would require prompt treatment.

CALCIUM

Hypercalcemia has long been recognized as a complication of malignant disease including multiple myeloma [15,20]. Although the specific mechanisms responsible for cancer-associated hypercalcemia remain uncertain, a

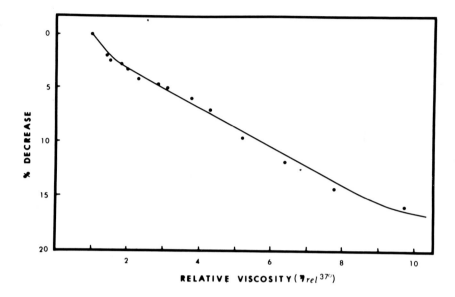

Fig. 3. Effect of relative viscosity on the measurement of Na^+ and K^+. (Modified and reproduced with permission from Vader and Vink [14].)

number of possible etiologic factors have been suggested [16–19]; they include the elaboration of osteoblastic activity factors, prostaglandins, parathyroid hormone, etc. In a review of 869 cases of multiple myeloma, Kyle [20] found the initial serum Ca concentrations to be elevated in 30% of the patients, while hypocalcemia was present in only 1%.

In most patients with multiple myeloma the increase in serum Ca represents true hypercalcemia, i.e. elevation of total and free (ionic) Ca, the latter being the metabolically active fraction and comprising approximately 47% of total serum Ca. It is this free Ca fraction which appears responsible for clinical manifestations of hypercalcemia [21]. Hypercalcemia per se is not necessarily pathogenic, and clinically asymptomatic hypercalcemia has been recognized in patients with multiple myeloma [22–26], as illustrated in the following case report.

CASE REPORT

This 59-year-old black male was admitted to the hospital for evaluation of hypercalcemia, hyperproteinemia, and anemia that were found on routine physical examination. Areas of diffuse osteopenia were seen on both chest and spinal x-rays, and a skull series showed multiple lytic lesions. The patient admitted to a 5-kg weight loss over the past

2 months and right upper arm pain for the past 8 months. He denied anorexia, nausea, constipation, lethargy, or change in mental status. Laboratory data included a Ca of 14.4 mg/dL (normal, 9.0–10.3 mg/dL), total serum protein of 12.4 g/dL (normal, 6.0–8.5 g/dL), albumin of 2.7 g/dL (normal, 3.5–5.0 g/dL), hemoglobin of 10.3 g/dL (normal, 14–18 g/dL) and an erythrocyte sedimentation rate (ESR) of 142 mm/h (normal, 0–9 mm/h). Serum protein electrophoresis revealed a large M-protein in the γ-region. Immunoelectrophoresis of the serum and urine showed the M-protein to be an IgG (λ) monoclonal gammopathy with a Bence Jones protein in the urine.

A diagnosis of multiple myeloma was made, and treatment was started with saline and furosemide for hypercalcemia, and melphalan and prednisone for the malignancy. Despite this therapy, the Ca values appeared to fluctuate between 9.3 and 14.5 mg/dL (Fig. 4). On the 12th hospital day, the patient was treated with mithramycin and discharged 16 days after admission.

This case exemplifies a fairly typical presentation of multiple myeloma with associated hypercalcemia. However, the hypercalcemia seen in this patient would appear to have been totally asymptomatic but was nevertheless treated rather aggressively with diuretics and mithramycin. Subsequently, it was determined that the ionized Ca was always within the normal range (i.e., 4.5–5.0 mg/dL) and that changes in total serum Ca paralleled the amount of total serum proteins (Table II).

These data can be explained on the basis of Ca binding the M-protein in this patient. Although the binding of Ca by an M-protein is not a common finding, there are at least five reports in the literature which support and

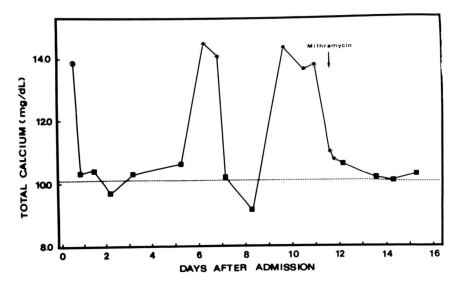

Fig. 4. Total calcium concentration as a function of time in a patient with an IgG (λ) M-protein which binds calcium. (Reproduced with permission from Ladenson et al. [22].)

confirm this observation [22–26]. All patients had an IgG monoclonal gammopathy; three had κ- and two λ-light chain IgG M-proteins. In 1973, Lindgarde and Zettervall [25] first demonstrated that an M-protein had significant Ca binding ability. The isolated γ-globulin fraction from a patient with multiple myeloma and asymptomatic hypercalcemia with normal ionic Ca concentrations was shown to bind Ca to a greater extent than the γ-globulin fraction from normal subjects or from other patients with multiple myeloma. The Ca binding activity was later conclusively proven to be associated with the Fab fragment of IgG [26].

The determination of total Ca using two separate samples from the patient described above are summarized in Table III. The three non-ACA methods (atomic absorption spectroscopy [AAS], SMA 12/60 and EGTA titration) gave similar results for total Ca but were distinctly lower for those samples analyzed with the ACA. Although the chemical basis for the measurement of Ca differs among the non-ACA methods, this was not considered to be a likely source of the discrepancy because in both the ACA and the SMA 12/60, cresolphthalein complexone is used to detect Ca. Thus, the most likely explanation for the method discrepancy is the manner in which protein-bound

TABLE II. Relationship between total and ionic calcium in a patient with a calcium-binding M-protein

Sample	Protein, g/dL (normal, 6.0–8.5 g/dL)	Total calcium, mg/dL (normal, 9.0–10.3 mg/dL)	Ionic calcium, mg/dL (normal, 4.5–5.0 mg/dL)
1	10.7	13.2	4.52
2	7.4	11.1	4.55
3	ND[a]	11.5	4.95
4	8.1	12.1	4.90
5	8.5	11.9	4.85

[a]Not done.
Reproduced with permission from Ladenson et al. [22].

TABLE III. Methodologic Differences in the Measurement of Total Calcium in a Patient with a Calcium-Binding M-Protein

Sample	Protein (g/dL)	Albumin (g/dL)	Total calcium, mg/dL			
			AAS	SMA 12/60	EGTA titration	Dupont ACA
1	10.7	2.9	13.2	14.0	13.7	10.8
2	7.4	2.8	11.1	10.9	ND[a]	9.5

[a]Not done.
Reproduced with permission from Landenson et al. [22].

Ca is released. The AAS and SMA 12/60 methods both release protein-bound Ca by the addition of acid to the serum sample. The DuPont ACA and the Corning titrator (EGTA titration) methods rely on a competition for Ca between protein (albumin and M-protein) and the cresolphthalein complexone or EGTA, respectively. This principle is based on the assumption that either the complexone or the EGTA has a higher affinity for Ca than does protein. The problem lies in the fact that the cresolphthalein complexone was not able to release all of the Ca from the M-protein, which has a higher affinity constant for Ca than does albumin [24]. EGTA, however, is a stronger Ca chelating agent than cresolphthalein complexone and presumably can remove all the Ca from the M-protein.

The binding of Ca to an M-protein can explain the apparent asymptomatic severe hypercalcemia seen in certain patients with multiple myeloma. Prompt recognition of this abnormal Ca binding is important to avoid potentially injurious therapeutic measures for hypercalcemia, and the measurement of either ultrafiltrable or ionized Ca in patients with hypercalcemia and multiple myeloma constitutes an important laboratory aspect in the management of such patients. These analytes should be measured at least once during the hospital course of such patients in order to rule out the presence of a Ca-binding M-protein.

COPPER

Copper (Cu) is an essential trace element and it functions as a co-factor for certain important enzymes such as cytochrome oxidase, tyrosinase, monamine oxidase, ascorbic acid oxidase, uricase, and others. In normal human serum at least 95% of Cu is associated with ceruloplasmin, which is an α_2-globulin capable of binding eight Cu molecules [27].

Elevated levels of serum Cu have been reported in two cases of multiple myeloma [28,29]. The first case, reported by Goodman et al. in 1967 [29], was a 69-year-old woman who presented with the typical features of multiple myeloma in addition to corneal pigmentation suggestive of the Kayser-Fleischer ring seen in Wilson's disease. She was found to have an IgG (κ) monoclonal gammopathy with an M-protein concentration of 3.2 g/dL. The serum Cu concentration was 3350 mg/dL (normal, 70–160 mg/dL) with a normal ceruloplasmin level. Penicillamine therapy did not produce a significant increase in urinary Cu excretion, which indicated that the Cu was being tightly bound. Subsequent investigation showed that the Cu migrated with the γ-globulin fraction on serum protein electrophoresis.

The second case of hypercupremia, reported by Levin et al. in 1976 [28], was found in a patient with an IgG (λ) monoclonal gammopathy and clinical features of multiple myeloma. Corneal discoloration was also noted in this patient. Serum IgG concentrations ranged between 2350–3200 mg/dL. Serum Cu was 1250 mg/dL and the ceruloplasmin averaged 41.2 mg/dL (normal, 25–35 mg/dL). Penicillamine therapy promptly increased the urinary Cu excretion by more than 20-fold of baseline with a concomitant fall in the serum Cu concentration. In an attempt to localize the protein fraction responsible for Cu-binding the patient was given ^{64}Cu intravenously. Approximately 20 hours after the administration, serum protein electrophoresis revealed that 80% of the radioactivity was associated with the γ-globulin fraction. More recently, the M-protein from this patient has been purified to homogeneity and it has been shown that Cu was bound only to the Fab fragment [30,31].

THE ANION GAP

The anion gap is most commonly defined as the difference between the serum concentration of Na and the sum of chloride and bicarbonate concentrations. In actuality, there is no anion gap, i.e., the total concentration of cations must be equal to the total concentration of anions in order to preserve electrical neutrality. Therefore, as defined, the anion gap actually represents the net difference between unmeasured cations and unmeasured anions. The constituents of unmeasured cations and unmeasured anion and their normal serum concentrations are shown in Table IV [32]. The normal anion gap is 12 mmol/L with a 2 SD range of 8–16 mmol/L [33]. The diagnostic importance of an increased anion gap in the evaluation of acid-base disorders is well known [32,33], and the significance of a decreased anion gap has also received much attention. Some of the causes of decreased anion gap are listed in Table V.

The frequency and pathogenesis of the decreased anion gap seen in patients with a monoclonal gammopathy was investigated by Murray et al. [34]. In this retrospective study, 50 patients with multiple myeloma were found to have a mean anion gap of 9.2 ± 0.4, which was significantly less than the 12.2 ± 0.4 mmol/L found in hospitalized controls. In addition, one third of the myeloma patients had anion gaps of ≤ 6.0 mmol/L, whereas only two of 102 control samples were below that value. Moreover, these authors found an inverse relationship between the anion gap and the concentration of the monoclonal protein with a tendency for the anion gap to be lowered as the concentration of the M-protein increased. There is, however, enough scattering of data points to prevent the accurate prediction of the anion gap from the M-protein level by itself. This situation is analogous for Na (see Fig. 2). Murray et al. [34] attributed the decrease in the anion gap to the net cationic charge of the monoclonal protein at physiological pH, resulting in increased unmeasured cations and thereby lowering the anion gap.

TABLE IV. Normal Concentration of "Unmeasured Cations" and "Unmeasured Anions"

Unmeasured cations (mmol/L)		Unmeasured anions (mmol/L)	
K$^+$	4.5	Protein	15
Ca^{++}	5.0	Phosphate	2
Mg^{++}	1.5	Sulfate	1
		Organic acids	5
Total	11	Total	23

Reproduced with permission from Oh and Carroll [32].

TABLE V. Causes of Decreased Anion Gap

Laboratory error
  Pseudohyponatremia
  Overestimation of chloride (bromism)
Decreased concentrations of unmeasured anions
  Hypoalbuminemia
  Analbuminemia
Increased concentration of unmeasured cations
  Hyperkalemia
  Hypercalcemia
  Hypermagnesemia
  Lithium toxicity
  Monoclonal and polyclonal gammopathies

Reproduced with permission from Emmett and Narins [33].

Consistent with the above hypothesis, DeTroyer et al. [35] found that the anion gap was significantly decreased in patients with IgG, but not IgA, multiple myeloma (Fig. 5). IgG M-proteins have isoelectric points higher than the physiologic pH and thus are positively charged. Therefore, in order to maintain electrical neutrality in the serum, the accumulation of positive charge as seen in patients with IgG monoclonal gammopathies, must be counterbalanced by a compensatory increase of anions (chiefly chloride). The net result is a decrease in the anion gap. On the other hand, IgA M-proteins have isoelectric points slightly below the physiologic pH and therefore behave as anions at a normal pH. Consequently, large amounts of circulating IgA can be expected to increase the anion gap. This was in fact demonstrated by Paladini and Sala [36], who showed that the anion gap was increased in patients with IgA multiple myeloma and decreased in patients with IgG myeloma (Fig. 6). Furthermore, it has been suggested that a confirmed low anion gap should alert the laboratory to perform serum protein electrophoresis on such samples [37].

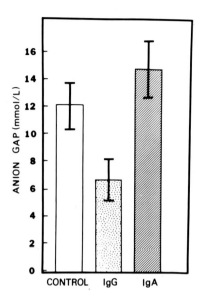

Fig. 5. Effect on the measured anion gap seen in patients with an IgG or an IgA M-protein. (Modified and reproduced with permission from Paladini and Sala [36].)

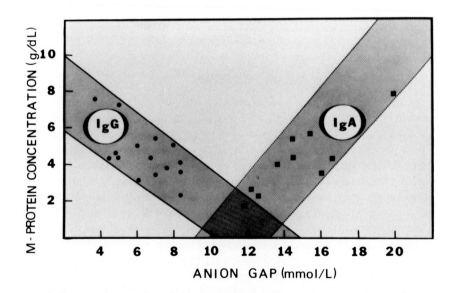

Fig. 6. Effect of IgG and IgA M-protein concentrations on the anion gap. (Modified and reproduced with permission from DeTroyer et al. [35].)

The decrease in anion gap is not restricted to patients with the overt clinical manifestations of multiple myeloma. Schnur et al. [38] demonstrated that patients with an asymptomatic monoclonal gammopathy can also exhibit a decrease in the anion gap; they failed, however, to document a correlation with either the class of Igs or the concentration of the monoclonal proteins. The correlations between total protein and the anion gap appear rather tenuous [39], whereas polyclonal increases of the γ-globulin fraction can decrease the anion gap [39,40] above γ-globulin concentrations of 3 g/dL [40]. This decrease in the anion gap could simply be the result of hyperproteinemia causing a pseudohyponatremia by a volume-displacing mechanism as discussed earlier. Superimposed on the polyclonally increased γ-globulin is a relative increase in IgG, which is positively charged and thereby lowers the anion gap through a mechanism analogous to that seen in patients with an IgG monoclonal gammopathy, i.e., a compensatory increase in the serum concentration of cations to counterbalance the increase in positive charges due to the presence of IgG.

The clinical significance of a low anion gap in the presence of a high Ig concentration, whether monoclonal or polyclonal, are similar. For example, the presence of a low anion gap may be the initial indication of an increased Ig concentration [37], while a normal anion gap, on the other hand, does not exclude the presence of high Ig levels. On the other hand, the finding of a normal anion gap in a patient with hyperimmunoglobulinemia may mask the presence of a high anion gap metabolic acidosis.

REFERENCES

1. Burke MD: Electrolyte studies. 1. Sodium and water. Postgrad Med 64:147–153, 1978.
2. Burke MD: Electrolyte studies. 2. Potassium, chloride, and acid-base. Postgrad Med 64:205–210, 1978.
3. Swezey CB, Jacobson W: Computer-based diagnostic reporting for serum electrolytes. Am J Clin Pathol 74:812–819, 1980.
4. Frier BM, Steer CR, Baird JD, Bloomfield S: Misleading plasma electrolytes in diabetic children with severe hyperlipidemia. Arch Dis Child 55:771–775, 1980.
5. Tarail Q, Buchwald KW, Holland JF, Selawry OS: Misleading reductions of serum sodium and chloride associated with hyperproteinemia in patients with multiple myeloma. Proc Soc Exp Biol Med 110:145–148, 1962.
6. Frich PG, Schmid JR, Kistler HJ, Hitzig WH: Hyponatremia associated with hyperproteinemia in multiple myeloma. Helv Med Acta 33:317–329, 1967.
7. Bloth B, Christensson T, Mellstedt H: Extreme hyponatremia in patients with myelomatosis. Acta Med Scand 203:273–275, 1978.
8. Ladenson JL: Direct potentiometric analysis of sodium and potassium: Evidence for electrolyte interaction with a nonprotein, protein-associated substance(s). J Lab Clin Med 90:654–665, 1977.
9. Shyr C, Young CC: Effect of sample protein concentration on results of analyses for sodium and potassium in serum. Clin Chem 26:1517, 1980.

10. Czaban JD, Cormier AD: More on direct potentiometry: the ion–selective electrode vs. flame photometry. Clin Chem 26:1921–1922, 1980.
11. Levy BG: Determination of sodium with ion-selective electrodes. Clin Chem 27:1435–1438, 1981.
12. Wolf RE, Levin WC, Ritzmann SE: Thermoproteins. In Ritzmann SE, Daniels JC (eds): "Serum Protein Abnormalities: Diagnostic and Clinical Aspects." Boston: Little, Brown and Co., 1975, pp 487–512.
13. Stites DP: Clinical laboratory methods for detection of antigens and antibodies. In Fudenberg HH, Stites DP, Caldwell JL, Wells JV (eds): "Basic and Clinical Immunology." 3rd ed. Los Altos, CA: Lange Med Publ, 1980, pp 343–381.
14. Vader HL, Vink CLJ: The influence of viscosity on dilution methods its problems in the determination of serum sodium. Clin Chim Acta 65:379–388, 1975.
15. Gutman AB, Tyson TL, Gutman EB: Serum calcium, inorganic phosphorus and phosphatase activity in hyperparathroidism, Paget's disease, multiple myeloma and neoplastic disease of the bones. Arch Intern Med 57:413, 1936.
16. Skrabanek P, McPartlin J, Powell D: Tumor Hypercalcemia and ectopic hyperparathyroidism. Medicine 59:262–282, 1980.
17. Clinicopathologic Conference of Barnes Hospital. Malignant hypercalccmia. Am J Med 67:486–494, 1979.
18. Sherwood LM: The multiple causes of hypercalcemia in malignant disease. N Engl J Med 303:1412–1413, 1980.
19. Besarab A, Caro JF: Mechanisms of hypercalcemia in malignancy. Cancer 41:2276–2285, 1978.
20. Kyle RA: Multiple myeloma: Review of 869 cases. Mayo Clin Proc 50:29–40, 1975.
21. McLean FC, Hastings AB: The state of calcium in the fluids of the body: 1. The conditions affecting the ionization of calcium. J Biol Chem 108:285–322, 1935.
22. Ladenson JL, McDonald JM, Aguanno JJ, Goren M: Multiple myeloma and hypercalcemia? Clin Chem 25:1821–1825, 1979.
23. Soria J, Soria C, Dao C, James JM, Bousser J, Bilski-Pasquier G: Immunoglobulin bound calcium and ultrafiltrable serum calcium in myeloma. Br J Haematol 34:343–344, 1976.
24. Jaffe JP, Mosher DF: Calcium binding by a myeloma protein. Am J Med 67:343–346, 1979.
25. Lindgarde F, Zettervall O: Hypercalcemia and normal ionized serum calcium in a case of myelomatosis. Ann Intern Med 78:396–399, 1973.
26. Spira G, Silvian J, Tatarsky I, Hazani A: Calcium binding IgG myeloma protein. Scand J Haematol 24:193–198, 1980.
27. Daniels JC: Carrier Protein Abnormalities. In Ritzmann SE, Daniels JC (eds): "Serum Protein Abnormalities: Diagnostic and Chemical Aspects." Boston: Little Brown and Co., 1975, pp 213–241.
28. Levin RA, Hultquist DE, Baker BL, Falls HF, Gershowitz H, Penner JA: Hypercupremia associated with a monoclonal immunoglobulin. J Lab Clin Med 88:375–388, 1976.
29. Goodman SI, Rodgerson DO, Kauffman J: Hypercupremia in a patient with multiple myeloma. J Lab Clin Med 70:57–62, 1967.
30. Baker BL, Hultquist DE: A Copper-binding immunoglobulin from a myeloma patient. J Biol Chem 253:1195–1200, 1978.
31. Baker BL, Hultquist DE, Gershowitz H: Studies of the copper-binding site of an immunoglobulin isolated from a myeloma patient with hypercupremia. Fed Proc 37:1278, 1978 (Abstract).
32. Oh MS, Carroll HJ: The anion gap. N Engl J Med 297:814–817, 1977.
33. Emmett M, Narins RG: Clinical use of the anion gap. Medicine 56:38–54, 1977.

34. Murray T, Long W, Narins RG: Multiple myeloma and the anion gap. N Engl J Med 292:574–575, 1975.
35. DeTroyer A, Stolarozyk A, DeBeyl DZ, Stryckmans P: Value of anion gap determination in multiple myeloma. N Engl J Med 296:858–860, 1977.
36. Paladini G, Sala PG: Anion gap in multiple myeloma. Acta Haematol 62:148–152, 1979.
37. Frohlich J, Adam W, Golhey MJ, Bernstein M: Decreased anion gap associated with monoclonal and pseudomonoclonal gammopathy. CMA Journal 114:231–232, 1976.
38. Schnur MJ, Appel GB, Karp G, Osserman EF: The Anion gap in asymptomatic plasma cell dyscrasias. Ann Intern Med 86:304–305, 1977.
39. Keshgegian AA: Anion gap and immunoglobulin concentration. Am J Clin Pathol 74:282–286, 1980.
40. Keshgegian AA: Decreased anion gap in diffuse polyclonal hypergammaglobulinemia. N Engl J Med 299:99–100, 1978.

PATHOPHYSIOLOGIC CONSIDERATIONS

Pathology of Immunoglobulins: Diagnostic and
Clinical Aspects, pages 55–69
© 1982 Alan R. Liss, Inc., 150 Fifth Avenue, New York, NY 10011

4

Effects of Aging on Immunoglobulins

Jiri Radl, MD, PhD

Aging is characterized by a declining capacity of the individual to maintain homeostasis of his biological systems. Changes which appear in the immune system with age reveal a pattern of a gradually developing immunodeficiency. Thymus-derived or -dependent (T)-cell-mediated functions have been demonstrated to be the first to decline, probably reflecting involution of the thymus and a selective decrease in certain T-cell populations. This decline precedes a decrease in bone marrow-derived (B)-cell functions and the appearance of most aging phenomena [1]. It is believed that this immunodeficiency may play a causative role in the pathogenesis of some age-related disorders [14] such as autoimmune diseases, increased susceptibility to infections, some forms of amyloidosis, and malignancy within the lymphoid system and perhaps of some other tissues as well.

When searching for these age-related abnormalities, immunoglobulins (Igs) in the serum are an obvious choice for analysis, since blood samples are readily and repeatedly available and only a small amount of serum is needed for the investigation. The Ig levels in serum directly reflect the activity of the B immune system and also indirectly that of the T immune system. Thousands of different B-cell clones are continuously active in response to the many diverse stimuli to which everyone is exposed at any one time; however, the vast majority of these responses can take place only in cooperation with T-helper cells and under the control of T-suppressor cells. Each individual B-cell clone produces only one homogeneous population of Igs (antibodies) at a given time. Under normal conditions, the sum of the products of the immense numbers of various clones pooled in the blood yields a heterogeneous (polyclonal) Ig spectrum, with a relatively constant proportion of Igs of various individual classes, subclasses, and light (L) chain types.

During aging, the serum Igs exhibit some deviations that mirror changes occurring in the immune system. These include quantitative changes, restriction of the heterogeneity of Ig, and the appearance of transient and persistent homogeneous Ig components.

IMMUNOGLOBULIN LEVELS

Cross-sectional studies in aging humans have demonstrated that the overall Ig levels do not decrease with age. No substantial changes in IgM and IgD and increases in IgG and IgA levels were common findings [8,10,13,16,22,30].

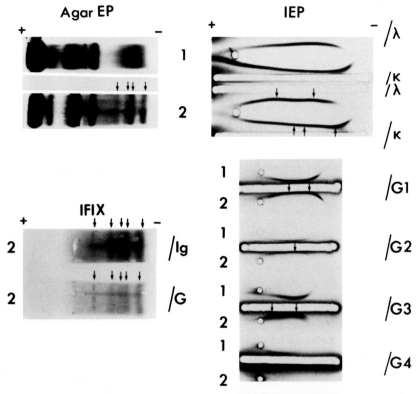

Fig. 1. Immunoglobulins of restricted heterogeneity of marked intensity in the serum of an aged patient (2) demonstrated by means of agar gel electrophoresis (AGAR-EP), immunofixation (IFIX) and immunoelectrophoresis (IEP). Antisera used: Rabbit anti-κ(/κ) and λ(/λ)-L chains, swine (IgG fraction) anti-IgG (/G), swine and sheep anti-IgG subclasses (/G1 - /G4); rabbit antihuman Ig(/Ig). Note the "washboard" pattern in the electrophoretic plates, the symmetric deviations of the precipitin lines (h-Ig) revealed by IEP and indicated by arrows, and the absence of a distinct line of the IgG₄ subclass. As a control, a pooled normal human serum (1) was used.

In a longitudinal study [5], about two thirds of the aging subjects investigated showed increasing values for IgG and IgA classes, and in only a small proportion of the group were the Ig levels decreased. The quantitation of IgG subclasses [22] in a group of over-95-year-old humans showed normal values of IgG_2 and IgG_4 but significantly increased levels of IgG_1 and IgG_3 when compared with a control group of young adults.

Progressively increasing variations among Ig levels of different individuals with age is a characteristic finding in both human and rodent species [22,11,20].

IMMUNOGLOBULINS OF RESTRICTED HETEROGENEITY AND TRANSIENT HOMOGENEOUS Ig COMPONENTS

Reports on investigations into qualitative changes in the serum Ig spectrum during aging are scarce. By the use of sensitive electrophoretic and immunodiffusion techniques, such as agar electrophoresis according to Wieme [34], immunoelectrophoresis (IEP), immunoselection, immunofixation, and double-line immunodiffusion [28], a number of deviations from the normal pattern was demonstrated in two groups of people over 80 and over 95 years of age, respectively [30,22]. An aberration of the normal κ/λ ratio of Ig was found in a high frequency in both groups investigated (49% and 40%, respectively). In 14% of the sera from the latter group, the Ig spectrum showed changes compatible with a pattern of restricted heterogeneity [28]. When analyzed in detail, such sera reveal (usually multiple) inconspicuous partial or selective Ig deficiencies, which are often accompanied, however, by the appearance of several small mono- or oligoclonal Ig components (Fig. 1). Because these homogeneous Ig components are transient, of low concentration, and superimposed on a relatively high background of normal heterogeneous Ig, they are only rarely detected in most routine laboratories using conventional electrophoretic techniques.

BENIGN MONOCLONAL GAMMOPATHY (IDIOPATHIC PARAPROTEINEMIA)[1]

While the age-related deviations in the serum Ig spectrum described in the previous paragraph are often very subtle and change with time, there is another abnormality which is pronounced, persistent, and clearly related to aging. It has been reported under several terms [31] but most frequently as benign or idiopathic monoclonal gammopathy (MG). Since its first description by Waldenström in 1944 [32], numerous case reports and clinical and

---

[1]Ed. note: See also [36].

laboratory studies on idiopathic MG (IMG) have been published and repeatedly reviewed [2,6,12,17,19,31,33,35]. On the basis of these data, the major features of this condition can be summarized as follows:

1) There exist in serum one or more homogeneous Ig components (monoclonal Ig = M-protein) which persist at a generally constant concentration over many years, usually until the individual's death. The M-protein level is usually lower than 2 g/dL, but well documented case reports with an M-protein concentration above this value have also been published.

2) The class-distribution of the M-proteins is approximately 60%, 20%, and 20% for IgG, IgA, and IgM, respectively. IMG of IgD or IgE class has not been conclusively proved up to now. Bence Jones proteinemia and/or proteinuria is very rare in IMG.

3) Igs of classes and subclasses other than that of the M-protein may show various changes but they are never so severely depleted as in myeloma or Waldenström's macroglobulinemia.

4) Accordingly, investigation of the bone marrow cells by immunofluorescence may reveal an increased monoclonal cell proliferation; however, these cells are not morphologically abnormal, and they do not reach such a dominance as is found in plasma cell malignancies. In general, appreciable numbers of lymphoid cells producing Ig of other classes and L chain types are usually present. The benign character of the cell proliferation is also reflected in the absence of skeletal abnormalities, as revealed by x-ray examination.

5) The occurrence of IMG is clearly age-related. Beginning in the fourth decade, the frequency increases up to 19% in the tenth decade of life (Fig. 2).

6) IMG is regarded as being essentially "benign." From case histories of large numbers of persons with IMG who were followed up for long periods, it became obvious that the development of a B-cell malignancy arising from IMG is an extremely rare event. The ratio of the incidence of IMG to that of M-proteinemias due to a B-cell malignancy (i.e., benign vs. malignant MG) can be estimated as about 100:1.

7) Findings of an increased incidence of IMG within the families of individuals with IMG indicate that genetic predisposition for IMG has to be considered a probability.

A large body of clinical and laboratory data on a number of aspects of IMG has been accumulated in the last two decades. However, the etiology, pathogenesis, and significance of IMG remain essentially unknown. Some questions are still of practical urgency. What is the relationship between IMG and plasma cell malignancy? Does IMG represent a premyeloma stage? What role does aging play in the development of IMG? Is there any relationship between IMG and other nonmalignant MG? All of these questions are relevant in daily clinical practice for making the correct differential diagnosis and for the initiation and follow-up of specific treatment. New clues for the improvement of our understanding of IMG and other age-related Ig abnormalities have recently been offered by results obtained in experimental studies in an animal model.

Studies in Animals

In investigating sera from mice of different strains [23], M-proteins were detected in increasing frequency with age in all mouse strains tested (Fig. 3). However, mice of different strains showed a different onset, frequency, and class distribution of the M-proteins. The lowest frequency of M-protein was seen in CBA/BrARij and BALB/c mice, the highest in the C57BL/KaLwRij mouse. Follow-up studies and postmortem examinations demonstrated that only a small percentage of the M-proteins were transient MG or MGs due to a B-cell malignancy. Additional comparative study showed that, except for some quantitative differences, most of the features of human and C57BL mouse IMG were essentially identical. Therefore, the aging C57BL mouse was used for further studies on the etiology and pathogenesis of IMG.

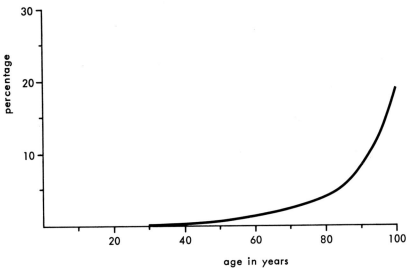

Fig. 2. Frequency of idiopathic monoclonal gammopathies in man in relation to age (combined data from the literature). (Reprinted from van Camp and Radl [6a].)

Successful transplantation of M-protein-producing clones from old mice to young healthy recipient mice by bone marrow or spleen cell transfers (while maintaining their nonprogressive character) indicated that IMG represents an intrinsic B-cell abnormality expressed as an autonomic monoclonal proliferation [24]. However, in subsequent transplantations, the "take" frequency of IMG gradually decreased and propagation of the condition for more than four generations was never achieved. This was in contrast with transplantation experiments using myeloma or B lymphoma cells, where both neoplasms could be propagated continuously with a high "take" frequency and shortened survival times of the recipient mice. Thus, IMG in the C57BL

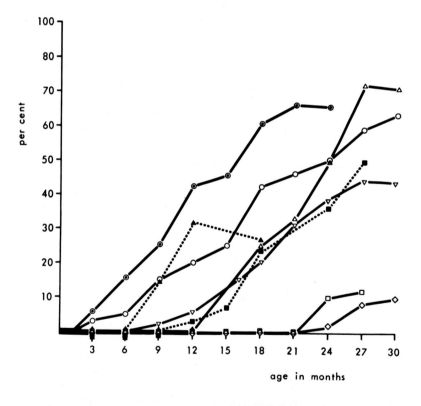

Fig. 3. Frequency of homogeneous immunoglobulins in the sera of mice of different strains in relation to age. (Reprinted with permission from Radl et al. [23].)

mouse shows a pattern of a "benign" monoclonal proliferative disorder, a clearly distinct counterpart of a B-cell malignancy.

Further investigations on factors which may contribute to the development of IMG demonstrated that a deficiency in the T immune system plays a crucial role in this respect [27]. Thymectomy performed in young adult C57BL mice substantially increased the frequency of age-related Ig abnormalities, including the pattern of Ig of restricted heterogeneity and the appearance of transient and persistent homogeneous Ig. Even more pronounced changes during aging were observed in mice which were neonatally thymectomized. A similar effect of thymectomy on the development of these Ig abnormalities was also seen in CBA mice that show only a few and a late onset of homogeneous Ig in their sera with age under normal conditions. While thymectomy caused a clear-cut increase in the frequency of IMG, the incidence of B-cell malignancies was not influenced in these experimental groups. The studies on Ig abnormalities in the aging nude mouse [29] were in accordance with the results of previous observations. These congenitally athymic mice developed a broad spectrum of selective Ig deficiencies, Ig of restricted heterogeneity, and high numbers of transient and persistent (probably IMG) homogeneous Ig on aging. Animals with a higher antigenic load had significantly more homogeneous Ig than specific-antigen-free and barrier maintained nude mice.

The findings from these experimental studies can be interpreted as indicating that the extent of the antibody repertoire, as reflected in the heterogeneity of the serum antibody pool, becomes altered during aging. Actually, a progressive decrease in the heterogeneity of the plaque-forming cell response has been demonstrated in aging mice [7,9]. It seems likely that most of the Ig abnormalities are only secondary consequences of an impairment in the T immune system. Several lines of evidence obtained from reconstitution experiments and from clinical observations in patients with selective T-cell deficiency [25] support the suggestion that the T immune system plays an important role in the regulation of the Ig heterogeneity and that the appearance of Ig with restricted heterogeneity and of transient homogeneous Ig may be very sensitive indicators of an impairment in the T immune system and the consequent imbalance in the T-B immune system network. Impaired helper and control T-cell functions can be expected to reduce the numbers of responding B-cell clones and to allow overshoot reactions of some of the clones, leading to these deviations in the serum Ig spectrum. However, the appearance of persistent IMG cannot be explained in such simplistic fashion. From animal studies it is known that this abnormality is actually the result of an intrinsic defect within one B-cell clone, which is irreversible. Nevertheless, it is possible that this condition also evolves as a consequence of aging in the immune system, as is suggested by the following hypothesis [26].

Three-Stage Hypothesis on the Development of Idiopathic Monoclonal Gammopathy

IMG, a benign proliferative disorder of a B-cell clone, develops as a consequence of an age-related immunodeficiency in three successive stages:

Stage 1. During aging, involution of the thymus and genetically determined selective decreases in certain T-cell subpopulations lead to an impairment in the T-cell mediated immune functions. The onset, extent, and progress of this malfunction can be influenced by some extrinsic factors, such as environment, chronic antigenic stimulation, virus infections, and others.

Stage 2. As a consequence of improper helper and control T-cell functions, an impairment in the B-cell activities will occur. The resulting imbalance in the T-B immune system network will be manifested as restriction of heterogeneity of the immune response and excessive clonal proliferations with an overshoot production of homogeneous Ig. The changes in this stage are still reversible.

Stage 3. The repeated mono- or oligoclonal expansions result in a higher probability for either a spontaneous or a virus-inducted mutation of the regulatory genes within an affected B-cell clone. Such a clone will then become autonomous and independent of normal control mechanisms and will continue to proliferate and secrete its antibody product even without further antigenic stimulation.

Similar mono- or oligoclonal proliferative disorders may also affect individual T-cell clones by similar mechanisms. Depending on their specific functions, such T-cell clones would further magnify the imbalance in the immune system network and could lead to suppression of some or to expansion of other related B- or T-cell clones via any of the regulatory circuits (e.g., the idiotype/anti-idiotype network system).

It is possible that IMG and B-cell neoplasias involve similar steps in their development (e.g., previous clonal expansions or genetic predisposition). However, in its final stage, IMG shows clear-cut differences, indicating that the defect in the intrinsic cell regulation occurs at a different subcellular level in the two proliferative disorders.

DIAGNOSTIC ASPECTS

Normal Ig Values in the Aged

The determination of Ig levels is undoubtedly a valuable contribution to the making of the diagnosis in certain diseases. For example, increased levels of serum Ig are found in various infections and in autoimmune and liver diseases. A selective or an overall decrease in serum Ig is an important symptom of a number of immunodeficiency diseases. The interpretation of the results of Ig determinations in an elderly patient, however, may present some problems. Because of the increasing variability in the normal values of several laboratory parameters among aging individuals, it is often difficult to properly evaluate results of the investigation. Sometimes certain individual values which would be considered to be abnormal in young persons or adults may still be normal for an older person. Application of a broader range of normal values obtained from determinations in a large group of healthy aged individuals is pertinent, but it leads to minimizing the value of such an investigation. This is because many actually abnormal values would still fall within this broad "normal" range in individual cases. A proper way of evaluation in this respect seems to be to assess results of the tests performed in case of a disease in each old patient against that person's own reference values obtained during periodic check-ups. *While Ig levels vary widely among individuals, they are relatively stable within the normal individual, even for a prolonged period of time.* This seems to also be true for the aging population. At first sight, such a procedure would seem to add extra costs to the health care and therefore not be justified; however, it may pay off by increasing the value of the laboratory tests and by avoiding the repetition of the investigations because of the uncertainty in their interpretation.

Evaluation of the Ig Heterogeneity

As described above, a restriction of the Ig heterogeneity and the appearance of homogeneous Ig in the serum seems to be a sensitive indicator for various clinical and even subclinical immunodeficiencies. Screening for such abnormalities could be done on a routine basis by simple laboratory techniques [28]. A sensitive agar electrophoresis [34], immunofixation with a polyvalent anti-Ig serum, and IEP using an antiserum specific for all Ig classes and L chains proved to yield satisfactory results in this respect. More detailed investigations using sophisticated and more costly techniques to specify the type of the abnormality should be done only in individual and specific situations where the results are indispensable for making the correct diagnosis.

DIFFERENTIAL DIAGNOSIS OF MONOCLONAL GAMMOPATHIES

The finding of homogeneous Ig, M-proteins, in the serum of elderly patients is definitely not a rare event and it is not restricted to a malignancy of the B immune system. On the contrary, "benign" disorders of the immune system accompanied by an MG are far more frequent, and their prevalence can be estimated to be about 100 times that of myeloma. Most of the conditions in which homogeneous Ig have frequently been reported to appear are listed in Table I. Our attempt at classification of these conditions is only

TABLE I. Occurrence of Homogeneous Immunoglobulins in Sera of Man and Some Animal Species

Condition	Human	Animal model	Monoclonal Ig component in serum					
			Frequency	Concentration (g/dL)	Duration	Ig class	Bence Jones Protein in urine (serum)	Remark
1. B-cell malignancies	Multiple myeloma, Waldenström's macroglobulinemia, lymphoma	Myeloma: dog, cat, cow, mouse. Induced plasmacytoma: mouse, rat	Obligatory	> 2 progressive	Persistent	G > A > D > E M	Frequent	Low frequency of "nonsecretory" and Bence Jones types
	Lymphosarcoma, chronic lymphocytic leukemia (amyloidosis, heavy chain disease—some forms)	Lymphoma, lymphosarcoma: mouse	Facultative	< 2	Persistent	M > G	Rare	(L chains, incomplete H chains, respectively)
2. B-cell benign proliferative disorders	Benign monoclonal gammopathy (idiopathic paraproteinemia, benign immunocytoma)	Mouse (C57BL)	Increase with aging	< 2 constant	Persistent	G > A = M (D, E?)	Rare exceptions	Probably as a consequence of age-related immunodeficiency
3. Immunodeficiencies								
Primary	Wiskott-Aldrich, DiGeorge, Nezelof syndromes; SCID	Nude athymic mice, thymectomized mice	Frequent	< 1	Transient	Mainly G, M	0	T-B immune system imbalance
Secondary	Due to aging	Aging mice	Increase with aging	< 1	Transient	Mainly G, M	0	T-B immune system imbalance

Category	Human associations	Animal models	Notes	Amount (g/L)	Duration	Immunoglobulin class	Frequency of ≥ 2	Proposed mechanism
4. Early ontogenesis with excessive antigenic stimulation	Intrauterine infections		Rare	Usually < 1	Transient	Mainly G, M	0	T-B immune system imbalance
5. Reconstitution of the immune system after bone marrow transplantation	SCID, aplastic anemia, leukemia, pretreatment with immunosuppressive agents	Irradiated mice, irradiated monkeys	Often between 2nd and 12th mo after transplant	< 1	Transient	Mainly G, M	0	T-B immune system imbalance
6. Autoimmune diseases	Chronic cold agglutinin diseases, chronic autoimmune liver diseases, occasionally other autoimmune diseases	Mouse (NZB)		< 2	Usually persistent	Mainly M, G	0	Autoantibody activity or unknown
7. Subacute and chronic infections, tumors	Lichen myxedematosus, mycosis fungoides, SSPE, MS	Aleutian mink disease, EAE?	CSF > serum	< 2	Persistent or transient	Mainly G, M	0	Reactive paraproteinemia? Some cases may belong to categories 1, 2, 3, or 8
8. Homogeneous response to polysaccharides	e.g., dextran, levan, bacterial polysaccharides	Rabbits, mice		< 1	Transient	Mainly G, M	0	Genetically determined

Abbreviations: SCID = severe combined immunodeficiency; MS = multiple sclerosis; CSF = cerebrospinal fluid; SSPE = subacute sclerosing panencephalitis; EAE = experimental allergic encephalomyelitis.

tentative, because the information on the etiology and pathogenesis is insufficient in a number of the disorders. When similar disorders have been observed or could be induced in animals, they are mentioned as experimental models. The major characteristics of the MG in each of the groups which are helpful in differential diagnosis are briefly mentioned.

On the basis of this classification, several questions arise concerning the differential diagnosis of M-protein in an elderly patient: 1) Is it a product of an autonomous B cell proliferative disorder? If so, is it benign or malignant (categories 1 or 2)? 2) If not, does the M-protein reflect an immune system disorder (categories 3, 5, 6, or possibly 7)? 3) If not, is it only an excess homogeneous response to some special (mainly bacterial polysaccharide) antigens (category 8 or possibly 7)?

It is obvious that a correct answer to the first question is the most important one for the patient's sake. Incorrect evaluation of the clinical and laboratory findings may lead to not only unnecessary but often harmful treatment modes, such as cytostatic agents in patients with a benign condition or an immunodeficiency. Conversely, the proper time for initiation of specific treatment for B-cell malignancy can be missed if inappropriate investigation or evaluation lead to release of the patient from the regular controls. Detailed discussion of the clinical and laboratory features of the individual conditions listed in Table I is beyond the scope of this chapter. Diagnostic approaches employing presently available modern clinical, hematological, and immunological techniques usually will allow the establishment of the correct diagnosis in the vast majority of patients. Only occasional situations may present special problems, such as the so-called "slow" or "smoldering" myeloma [18]. It is extremely difficult to distinguish it from benign monoclonal gammopathy. However, this form of myeloma is mostly of the IgG class and may, therefore, be amenable to an analysis of the J chain positive M-protein-producing cells [3,3a,15]. If confirmed, this approach may offer a promising discriminator between the two conditions.

PROGNOSTIC AND THERAPEUTIC ASPECTS

Age-related abnormalities in serum Ig, as described in the previous paragraphs, reflect a gradually developing immunodeficiency, which may in turn, play a causative role in the origin of some age-related diseases. The findings of such abnormalities in the serum of an elderly patient should therefore receive careful medical attention. If present in combination with other symptoms and other abnormal laboratory results, they usually are valuable indicators of an immune system disorder, as well as of its progression or regression. If present without any other symptomatology, appropriate follow-up studies of such patients appear indicated. There is still too little information available on the significance of this mostly selective, age-related immunodeficiency in man to justify more detailed investigations by the clinician or any attempts at preventive treatment in such patients.

In addition to these practical considerations, emanating from the findings of M-proteins or other Ig abnormalities, there are numerous aspects of age-related Ig abnormalities that warrant further investigative efforts. While there is a clear indication for a correlation between longevity and the absence of serum Ig abnormalities and immune system disorders among different strains of mice, very little is known on this subject in man. Well-documented follow-up studies in man are desirable to confirm the presumption of the role of the age-related immunodeficiency with respect to the development of autoimmune diseases, amyloidosis, and proliferative disorders. As far as the latter are concerned, the differences between the benign and malignant forms, as found in animal studies, require confirmation and extensions in man. The general assumption that the "benign" MG has no influence on the health condition or survival time of its host may need confirmation by appropriate studies or, at least, a reevaluation. To increase our understanding of the etiology and pathogenesis of IMG, it is useful not only for more accurate and timelier differential diagnosis between this condition and B-cell malignancies, but also for the following reason: It is likely that the mechanisms leading to monoclonal proliferative disorders during the aging process are similar and operative at multiple sites within different tissues. When involving tissues of vital importance, such as the arterial walls, some of these "benign" tumors may endanger the life of the host. In this respect, the theory of the monoclonal origin of atherosclerotic plaques [4,21] is of possible significance. The advantage of using IMG as a model for studies on age-related mechanisms governing the development of benign proliferative disorders lies in the fact that there is a great amount of information available on the physiology and pathology of the immune system and that functional parameters of its component cells are readily assessable.

REFERENCES

1. Adler WH, Jones KH, Nariuchi H: Ageing and immune function. In Thompson R (ed): "Recent Advances in Clinical Immunology." Edinburgh, London, New York: Churchill Livingstone, 1977, p 77.
2. Axelsson U: An eleven-year follow-up on 64 subjects with M-components. Acta Med Scand 201:173, 1977.
3. Bast EJEG, Wiringa G, van Camp B, Ballieux RE: Malignancy associated lymphoid cell markers in monoclonal gammopathy. In Peeters H (ed): "Protides of Biological Fluids." Oxford, New York: Pergammon Press, 1979, p 351.
3a. Bast EJEG, van Camp B, Boom S, Jaspers SCA, Ballieux RE: Differentiation between benign and malignant monoclonal gammopathies by the presence of the J-chain. Clin Exp Immunol 44:375, 1981.

4. Benditt EP, Benditt JM: Evidence for a monoclonal origin of human atherosclerotic plaques. Proc Natl Acad Sci 70:1753, 1973.
5. Buckley CE, Buckley EG, Dorsey FC: Longitudinal changes in serum immunoglobulin levels in older humans. Fed Proc 33:2036, 1974.
6. Camp van B: Clinical and Experimental Studies on the Nature of Monoclonal Gammopathies. Dissertation, Free University in Brussels, Belgium, 1980.
6a. van Camp B, Radl J: Studies on the humoral immune response during aging. Ned T Gerontol 9:237, 1978.
7. Doria G, D'Agostaro G, Pontti A: Age-dependent variations of antibody avidity. Immunology 35:601, 1978.
8. Finger H, Emmerling P, and Hof H: Serumimmunglobulin-Spiegel in Senium. Dtsch Med Wochenschr 98:2455, 1973.
9. Goidl EA, Innes JB, Weksler ME: Loss of IgG and high-avidity plaque-forming cells and increased suppressor cell activity in aging mice. J Exp Med 144:1037, 1976.
10. Grundbacher FJ, Schreffler DC: Changes in human serum immunoglobulin levels with age and sex. Z Immun-Forsch 141:20, 1970.
11. Haaijman JJ, van den Berg P, Brinkhof J: Immunoglobulin class and subclass levels in the serum of CBA mice throughout life. Immunology 32:923, 1977.
12. Hällen J: Discrete gammaglobulin (M-)components in serum. Acta Med Scand (Suppl) 462:1, 1966.
13. Haferkamp O, Schlettwein-Gsell D, Schwick HG, Störiko K: Serumproteine im hohen Lebensalter unter besonderer Berücksichtigung der Immunglobuline und Antikörper. Klin Wochenschr 44:725, 1966.
14. Hijmans W, Hollander CF: The pathogenic role of age-related immune dysfunctions. In Makinodan T, Yunis E (eds): "Immunology and Aging. Vol. 1. Series-Comprehensive Immunology." New York, London: Plenum Medical Book Company, 1977, p 23.
15. Isaacson P: Immunochemical demonstration of J chain: A marker of B-cell malignancy. J Clin Pathol 32:802, 1979.
16. Kalff MW: A population study on serum immunoglobulin levels. Clin Chim Acta 28:277, 1970.
17. Kyle RA, Bayrd ED: "The Monoclonal Gammopathies, Multiple Myeloma And Related Plasma-cell Disorders." Kugelmass IN (ed). Springfield, IL: C. C. Thomas, 1976, p 284.
18. Kyle RA, Greipp PR: Smoldering multiple myeloma. N Engl J Med 302:1347, 1980.
19. Kyle RA: Monoclonal gammopathy of undetermined significance. Am J Med 64:814, 1978.
20. Mink JG: Serum Immunoglobulin Levels And Immunoglobulin Heterogeneity In The Mouse. Dissertation, Erasmus University in Rotterdam, The Netherlands, 1980.
21. Pearson TA, Wang A, Solez K, Heptinstall RH: Clonal characteristics of fibrous plaques and fatty streaks from human aortas. Am J Pathol 81:379, 1975.
22. Radl J, Sepers JM, Skvaril F, Morell A, Hijmans W: Immunoglobulin patterns in humans over 95 years of age. Clin Exp Immunol 22:84, 1975.
23. Radl J, Hollander CF, Van den Berg P, De Glopper E: Idiopathic paraproteinemia. I. Studies in an animal model—the ageing C57BL/KaLwRij mouse. Clin Exp Immunol 33:395, 1978.
24. Radl J, De Glopper E, Schuit HRE, and Zürcher C: Idiopathic paraproteinemia. II. Transplantation of the paraprotein-producing clone from old to young C57BL/KaLwRij mice. J Immunol 122:609, 1979.
25. Radl J: The influence of the T immune system on the appearance of homogeneous immunoglobulins in man and experimental animals. In Karcher D, Lowenthal A, and Strosberg AP (eds): "Humoral Immunity in Neurological Disorders." New York, London: Plenum Press, 1979, p 517.

26. Radl J: Idiopathic paraproteinemia—A consequence of age-related deficiency in the T immune system. Three-stage development - A hypothesis. Clin Immunol Immunopathol 14:251, 1979.

27. Radl J, De Glopper E, Van den Berg P, Van Zwieten MJ: Idiopathic paraproteinemia. III. Increased frequency of paraproteinemia in thymectomized aging C57BL/KaLwRij and CBA/BrARij mice. J Immunol 125:31, 1980.

28. Radl J: Immunoglobulin levels and abnormalities in aging humans and mice. In Adler WH, Nordin AA (eds): "Immunological Techniques Applied to Aging Research." Boca Raton, FL: CRC Press, 1981, p 121.

29. Radl J, Mink JG, Van den Berg P, Van Zwieten MJ, Benner R: Increased frequency of homogeneous immunoglobulins in the sera of nude athymic mice with age. Clin Immunol Immunopathol 17:469, 1980.

30. Riesen W, Keller H, Skvaril F, Morell A, Barandun S: Restriction of immunoglobulin heterogeneity, autoimmunity and serum protein levels in aged people. Clin Exp Immunol 26:280, 1976.

31. Ritzmann SE, Loukas D, Sakai H, Daniels JC, Levin WC: Idiopathic (Asymptomatic) Monoclonal Gammopathies. Arch Intern Med 135:95, 1975.

32. Waldenström JG: Incipient myelomatosis or essential hyperglobulinemia with fibrinogen-openia—a new syndrome? Acta Med Scand 117:216, 1944.

33. Waldenström JG: Benign Monoclonal Gammapathies. In Azar A, Potter M (eds): "Multiple Myeloma and Related Disorders." Vol. 1. Hagerstown, MD: Harper and Row, 1973, p 247.

34. Wieme, RJ: "Studies On Agar Gel Electrophoresis. Techniques-Applications." Brussels: Arscia, 1959.

35. Zawadski ZA, Edwards GA: Nonmyelomatous Monoclonal Immunoglobulinemia. In Schwartz RS (ed): "Progress In Clinical Immunology." Vol. 1. New York: Grune & Stratton, Inc., 1972, p 105.

36. Ritzmann SE: Immunoglobulin Abnormalities. In Ritzmann SE, Daniels JC: "Serum Protein Abnormalities: Diagnostic and Clinical Aspects," 2nd printing. New York: Alan R. Liss, Inc., 1982, pp 351–486.

Pathology of Immunoglobulins: Diagnostic and
Clinical Aspects, pages 71–96
© 1982 Alan R. Liss, Inc., 150 Fifth Avenue, New York, NY 10011

5

Ethnic Differences in Immunoglobulins and Their Abnormalities

Gerald Shulman, MD

HISTORICAL BACKGROUND

The essential features of the disease now known as multiple myeloma were described in a series of papers published between 1846 and 1850 [7,15,46].[1] These publications covered the clinical aspects of the disease, the properties of Bence Jones protein, and postmortem, and histopathological features. The authors considered this hitherto undescribed disease "essentially malignant in nature" affecting the "osseous system." Dr. William MacIntyre noted and later described all the important characteristics of a urinary protein known subsequently, and with little justice, as Bence Jones protein. Perplexed by finding these changes in the urine of one of his patients, MacIntyre referred the specimen to a specialist with an established reputation as a chemical pathologist, Dr. Henry Bence Jones, who proceeded to examine the urine in some detail. Bence Jones documented the properties and significance of this protein [7]; MacIntyre described the clinical features of the disease, which included severe bone pains [46]. The patient died and at autopsy the ribs, sternum, and cervical, thoracic, and lumbar vertebrae were found softened, fragile, and easily cut, with the interior replaced with a soft "gelatiniform, blood-red substance." Some of this material was referred for histological examination to Dr. John Dalrymple, whose publication on the subject was illustrated with woodcuts which were credible drawings of the cells described [15]. The next basic contribution appeared in 1944, one hundred years later, when Dr. Jan Waldenström described macroglobulinemia [97]. The most

---

[1]Ed. note: See also [109] for an account of this first case of myeloma.

striking feature was high serum viscosity at room temperature, with gelling of the serum upon refrigeration and liquefaction upon warming to 37°C. Electrophoretic and chemical analysis demonstrated hyperglobulinemia. The proteins were compared with very high molecular weight proteins with sedimentation properties resembling, on ultracentrifugation, some of the antibodies.

As methods applicable to the study of molecular structure and substructure of immunoglobulins (Igs) have become available to medical scientists, investigation has proceeded at a rapid rate. The resulting body of information on both normal Igs and molecules, or subunits thereof, that characterize immunoglobulin abnormalities has become of great interest to immunologists, protein biochemists, geneticists, and epidemiologists and to clinicians responsible for the care of patients afflicted with various neoplastic disorders of B cells. The importance of ethnic differences in Igs and their abnormalities thus became apparent.

PHYSIOLOGICAL CONSIDERATIONS

Despite the belief that many illnesses are a consequence of some imbalance of immunity, it is often difficult to interpret observed serum Ig levels in relation to the disease in which they occur. A part of the problem may be related to uncertainty about the effect of physiologic variation in humoral immunity on estimates of confidence intervals in apparently healthy controls. Significant age-, sex-, and race-related differences in Ig levels occur throughout the lifespan of apparently healthy individuals [71,79,80,89].[2] Another part of the problem may be related to the heterogeneous mixture of proteins that constitutes the Igs; dominant elevation of one subtype may be masked by borderline low-normal levels of another Ig subtype.

TECHNICAL CONSIDERATIONS

Standards for Ig measurements have also fallen short of requirements for quantitative science. In spite of efforts to encourage adoption of acceptable standards, imprecisely standardized work has frequently been published. Nevertheless, the work has been valid and useful, since each report contained its own reference ranges and quality control. A research standard for human Igs was studied by the World Health Organization (WHO) International Reference Center for Immunoglobulins in an international collaborative survey [70]. On the basis of these tests the material was considered to be suitable for use as a standard for estimation of serum Igs G, A, and M for clinical

[2]Ed. note: See also Ritchie RF [68a].

purposes. Greater uniformity of results than previously obtained was made possible by general introduction of the research standard, with more meaningful interlaboratory comparison of results. *Best results are obtained with antisera produced with as heterogeneous an antigen preparation as possible and when the standard is heterogeneous and closely similar to the Ig in the material being studied.* Thus, use of a whole serum standard is preferable to use of purified material as both secondary and primary calibrating standards. When the international reference preparation was used as primary calibration in a collaborative study, variation in results obtained in different laboratories was substantially reduced [22] and better uniformity of reporting became possible. Manufacturers of commercially available standards adopted the WHO's recommendation that working standards should be calibrated in terms of the international reference preparation. However, comparison of major sources of commercial quality control materials has shown that there still is lack of agreement in expressing concentrations of specific proteins [30,77,81]. Results reported in various studies should therefore be interpreted with these standardization problems borne in mind.

ETHNIC DIFFERENCES IN EXPRESSION OF IMMUNOGLOBULINS IN HEALTH

Serum Immunoglobulins in Adults in Different Countries

Significant variations in serum Ig concentrations in apparently healthy subjects in different ethnic groups have often been reported [69,71,79,80,89,106]. The majority of reports have been in African populations of developing countries in the tropics. Little work has appeared on ethnic differences in people in the tropics outside the African region [101,106]. It has generally been pointed out [69,71,79,80,89,101,106], although adequate proof is lacking [29,53,54], that environmental factors, including high incidence of protozoal and helminth infections, are responsible for raised serum Igs in the tropics. While environmental factors could explain some results [53], it seems more probable that raised Igs in African and New Guinean peoples may be due to inherited capacity to produce higher quantities of Igs during infections. Observation that serum Ig levels of Americans of African origin are higher than those of Caucasian or Oriental origin lends some support to this view [29,43].

Malaysia

In Malaysia, which has a typical tropical climate, data have been reported showing that while levels of plasma Igs in the three constituent races (Malays, Indians, Chinese) did not differ significantly, levels were comparable to those observed in Caucasians and other peoples in temperate climates [106]. Plasma samples from 121 healthy adult blood donors resident in Kuala Lumpur were assayed for Igs G, A, and M by radial immunodiffusion (RID) [48] using standards from the World Health Organization [70]. Mean values reported ($\pm$ 1 SD) in IU/mL of IgG, IgA, and IgM were for males 133 $\pm$ 55, 123 $\pm$ 58, and 154 $\pm$ 96, respectively; and for females, 143 $\pm$ 44, 134 $\pm$ 76, and 278 $\pm$ 112, respectively. These values fall within ranges reported for Caucasians [69,101] but are significantly lower than those reported for Nigerians [60,94], New Guineans [101], Zaireans [60], and Gambians [71] (Table I). As reported previously [29], IgM levels found in Malaysian females of all three races were greater than in the males, and there was no sex difference in IgA and IgG levels [106].

Eleven Different Countries

The same WHO standard [70], related to the international reference preparation for human serum Ig, was employed in a method of single RID to assay IgG, IgA, and IgM in an international collaborative study in eleven different countries [69]. Results, expressed in IU/mL, provided a basis for establishment of ranges of normal values for these proteins, and for comparison of levels between different populations. Values estimated in this way were comparable when assayed by different laboratories [22]. Samples were obtained on young male blood donors aged 20–29 years, who were believed to be healthy. Blood, obtained without use of a tourniquet, was defibrinated by stirring with wooden sticks. Concentrations of serum Igs were estimated, after appropriate dilution, by direct comparison with the international reference preparation 69/97 [70]. All measurements were made in laboratories in the locality where serum was collected.

Improved definition of population reference ranges. Results were expressed as geometric means and 95% confidence intervals owing to lognormal distributions [34,69], which renders reference ranges meaningful as compared with 2 SD spread around arithmetic mean. Ig concentrations in general populations do not conform to normal gaussian distribution [69]. To normalize distribution and achieve equality of group variance, concentrations require conversion to logarithms for statistical analyses. Means and SDs are then calculated for logarithmic values. For presentation, logarithms are converted back to original arithmetic form; means thus expressed are geometric means and the SDs (variances), as a result, are proportional (exponential) values about the mean. The 95% confidence interval, referred to as "reference range" may be obtained by taking the antilogarithms of the log means $\pm$ twice the SD of these logs. These limits are not symmetrical about the geometric means; Student's t-test may be used on log transformations for evaluation of significance.

As expected, all groups showed a rather broad range of levels for each Ig (Table I). The geometric mean in IU/mL (95% confidence intervals) for IgG and IgM (287 [146–567] and 211 [34–1413], respectively) were highest in Nigeria; but surprisingly, IgA levels (80 [31–207]) were lowest [69]. This agreed in part with previous reports of elevated levels of these proteins in serum of West African adults [71,94]. At the same time, the lowest values were reported from Mexico, with geometric means (95% confidence intervals) for IgA and IgM of 97 (29–327) and 63 (12–333), respectively [69]. Among the highest concentration of IgM were those reported from Australia (191 [86–425]) and from Algeria (190 [84–429]), the latter also showing high IgA (164 [84–317]). Comparatively moderate increases of all three Igs were reported from Chile: IgG, 156 (83–292); IgA, 163 (73–365); and IgM, 158 (109–228) [69]. Results from West Germany, Japan, Netherlands, Sweden, and Switzerland were essentially similar to those reported from the United Kingdom, where levels were IgG, 123 (73–207); IgA, 115 (46–289); and IgM, 133 (47–372) [69].

Black and White Subjects in South Africa

Blood donor populations. In South Africa [80], the same WHO standard (international reference preparation 69/97) was used in a method of RID to assay serum IgG, IgA, and IgM in blood donors. Samples were obtained in approximately equal numbers of both sexes in 784 volunteers living in the Johannesburg metropolitan area. White donors attended the donor drawing center of the South African Blood Transfusion Service, whereas black donors were drawn by the mobile unit of the Blood Transfusion Service of the South African Institute for Medical Research in Johannesburg. Also, the mobile unit drew blood samples from 150 male volunteer donors aged between 20–29 years, employed in the gold mining industry in the Johannesburg area. These men were migrant black workers from Malawi. Significantly greater levels of the three Igs were found in urbanized black male and female donors as compared with corresponding groups of whites [80] (Table I). Geometric means (95% confidence intervals) for serum IgG, IgA, and IgM in black males were 183 (129–260), 217 (112–421), and 184 (100–339), respectively. Similarly, values for white males were 128 (85–194), 115 (53–249), and 147 (68–318), respectively, which agreed well with published results in Caucasians from European countries [69]. Geometric means (95% confidence intervals) for serum IgG, IgA, and IgM in black females was 189 (125–287), 162 (77–341), and 197 (106–365), respectively. Similarly, values for white females were 117 (65–211), 104 (48–226), and 170 (74–387), respectively. It was interesting to note a significant difference in serum Igs of black males from Malawi; while they had slightly greater levels of IgG and IgM (199

TABLE I. Concentrations of serum immunoglobulins in different ethnic groups

Author / Town and country	Sex	Number of observations (n)	Age (yr)	IgG (IU/mL)[a]	IgA (IU/mL)[a]	IgM (IU/mL)[a]
Yadav and Shah [106]						
Malaysia	Males	121		133 ± 55	123 ± 58	154 ± 96
	Females			143 ± 44	134 ± 76	278 ± 112
Rowe [69]						
Algiers, Algeria	Males	100	20–29	97–143–213	84–164–317	84–190–429
Perth, Australia	Males	94[b]	20–29	94–143–219	56–127–286[b]	86–191–425
Santiago, Chile	Males	100	20–29	83–156–292	73–163–365	109–158–228
Birmingham, England	Males	51	20–29	73–123–207	46–115–289	47–133–372
Offenbach, Germany	Males	45	20–29	86–124–178	48–108–244	59–133–298
Osaka, Japan	Males	98	20–29	102–146–210	70–129–237	68–144–308
Mexico City, Mexico	Males	100	20–29	82–127–196	29–97–327	12–63–333
Utrecht, Netherlands	Males	100	20–29	65–116–206	40–94–223	48–127–334
Ibadan, Nigeria	Males	100	20–29	146–287–567	31–80–207	34–211–1413
Uppsala, Sweden	Males	94	20–29	90–126–177	57–126–282	52–135–345
Lausanne, Switzerland	Males	100	20–29	87–135–208	56–136–334	81–176–380

Shulman [80] Johannesburg, South Africa						
Males						
	Black BD[c]	172	28	129–183–260	112–217–421	100–184–339
	H[d]	77	42	105–183–317	69–194–544	83–172–356
	White BD	232	38	85–128–194	53–115–249	68–147–318
	H	160	53	77–133–230	58–137–322	64–140–302
Females						
	Black BD	191	28	125–189–287	125–162–287	106–197–365
	H	59	38	117–184–290	117–177–290	94–189–379
	White BD	189	37	65–117–211	48–104–226	74–170–387
	H	155	49	71–125–218	50–121–290	78–162–334
Economidou [19]						
Thessaly, Greece						
	Males	225	30–50	88–143–232	56–133–316	49–136–378
	Females	165	30–50	90–146–237	62–133–282	67–221–721
Athens, Greece						
	Males	102	30–50	95–140–205	43–124–358	49–156–490
	Females	102	30–50	100–146–215	45–121–325	70–253–907
Buckley [11] Durham, NC, USA						
Males						
	Black					
	White			White 37% less P < 0.001	White 18% less P = 0.010	P.N.S.
Females						
	Black	819				
	White			White 23% less P < 0.001	White 14% less P = 0.029	White 38% more P < 0.001

Results are expressed in international units per milliliter (IU/mL) as lower 95% confidence interval—geometric mean (median)—upper 95% confidence interval with the exception of those from Malaysia, which appear as mean ± 1 SD.

[a] Results converted from mg/dL to IU/mL using Calbiochem-Behring conversion factors of 0.115 for IgG, 0.595 for IgA, and 1.15 for IgM.

[b] n = 95 for IgA.

[c] BD = blood donors.

[d] H = hospital in-patients.

and 174 IU/mL, respectively), IgA levels were less (176 IU/mL) than in the Johannesburg black males. Dominant IgA elevation occurs with micronodular Laennec type of cirrhosis, which typically results from uniform toxic damage from alcohol, iron (hemochromatosis, hemosiderosis), or from Wilson's disease [34]. Since the liver is of gut origin, it is not surprising that its most common reaction is IgA in type [34]. Greater concentration of serum IgA in the Johannesburg black male population may, therefore, reflect the high incidence of liver disease associated with chronic alcoholism, malnutrition, hemosiderosis, and associated cirrhosis [10,36].

Hospital in-patients. A similar study of serum Igs G, A, and M in 451 randomized hospital in-patients in Johannesburg was compared with results in sex- and race-matched blood donors (Table I) [80]. Average age of each patient group was at least a decade greater than the corresponding blood donor group. In general, no differences were noted in concentrations of serum IgG and IgM. However, serum IgA was found to be significantly greater in the hospital patient population in all groups of subjects studied, segregated on basis of race and sex. Greater concentration of IgA was also shown to occur with increasing age in multiple group comparison [80]. Significantly greater IgM was found in females, while significantly greater IgA was found in males.

Rural and Urban Greece

Serum Igs G, A, and M, measured by RID [48], using commercially obtained immunoplates and standard serum (Meloy laboratories) were compared in 390 inhabitants aged between 30–50 years, of a rural community, and in 204 age- and sex-matched residents of an urban area in Greece [19]. Persons tested were selected at random and given a complete physical examination. Any previous history of infections was recorded, with specific reference to brucellosis, typhoid, and diarrhea. Only assumedly healthy individuals were included in the study. The rural population was chosen first becaue of its poor hygienic conditions—the water supply is pumped from open wells and there is no sewage system. Second, originating from these village communities were two cases of α-chain disease, which may be related to environmental factors providing sustained antigenic stimulation of the gut. No sex effect or difference based on rural or urban residence was noted on IgG levels; the rural sample showed elevated IgA ($P < 0.05$); and IgM was greater in females. Geometric mean values (log normal ranges) of serum IgG in urban males and females (expressed in IU/mL related to the WHO International reference standard 67/95) were 140 (95–205) and 146 (100–215), respectively; corresponding IgA levels were 124 (43–358) and 121 (45–325) and those of IgM were 156 (49–490) and 253 (70–907), respectively. Results in rural males and females likewise for IgG were 143 (88–232) and 146

(90–237), respectively; IgA levels were 133 (56–316) and 133 (62–282) and IgM levels were 136 (49–378) and 221 (67–721), respectively. Comparisons of these results with other ethnic groups are shown in Table I.

Concentrations in North America Adjusted for Physiological Variation

A new method for characterizing mean and confidence intervals for IgG, IgA, and IgM has made it possible to evaluate observations in a single patient independent of confounding physiologic variation [11]. Derived confidence intervals and categories of altered IgG, IgA, and IgM observed in healthy subjects in Chapel Hill, North Carolina, were shown to be comparable between all age, race, and sex groups. Further, bounded by 2 SDs about the mean, only 5% of apparently healthy controls were excluded. The data presented provided a basis for evaluation and interpretation of serum Ig levels in patients throughout life. Generation of normative data was achieved using a biomathematical model based on the curvilinear cumulative frequency distribution observed in the data. This was plotted against logarithmically transformed serum Ig concentrations, rendering the distribution approximately linear. The SD of each serum Ig was computed on the basis of $\log_e$ of the ratio of observed concentration to its respective age-, race-, and sex-adjusted peer means. All data were expressed in potency units of the WHO serum Ig international reference standard. Any laboratory having access to a comparable reference standard may use the same methods in interlaboratory comparison of results. In the course of the study [11] serum IgG levels were found to be the same in white males and females. Average (geometric mean) serum IgA concentration in white males was 24% greater than white females and IgM concentration was 11.8% lower. Average concentration of IgG in black males was 26% greater, IgA 29.7% was greater, and IgM averaged 40.8% greater than in black females. All tests of statistical difference were highly significant ($P < 0.006$). Contrasts of race-related differences showed white males to have 37.9% less IgG and 18.7% less IgA than black males ($P < 0.01$), but IgM did not differ significantly. White females had 23.5% less IgG, 14.9% less IgA, and 38.8% more IgM than black females. All differences were highly significant ($P < 0.02$).

Immigrant Populations

The environmental challenge mainly maintains normal levels. Natives of developing countries were found typically to have greater concentrations of IgG and IgM than British controls, but after having lived in Britain for some years, levels more closely approximated British levels [14]. Residual elevation was called *racial* and presumably reflects genetic survival values in the country of origin. Serum IgA levels were suggested to be the same presumably because there is little difference in the leak-back from the gut, where antigenic challenges are always at a high level [34]. IgE levels are usually much greater in areas with high rates of helminth infection [34].

Serum Immunoglobulins From Birth Through Adolescence

Premature infants. As first described by Hitzig [31], the premature infant can develop severe A-γ-globulinemia. This is because transplacental transfer of IgG occurs largely during the last trimester of pregnancy [32] (Fig. 1). A prophylactic dose of γ-globulin given to premature infants can reduce subsequent infection and death rate [5,88]. In any given subject, individual variation in Ig concentration usually remains within ± 20% over time periods of years [32]. Studies in healthy twins have indicated that the actual normal levels of IgG and IgA have only a small genetic contribution [32].

Children and adolescents. There are a number of contradictory reports dealing with Ig concentrations in normal children [25,61,87,102]. However, when presented as geometric mean values with 95% confidence intervals and also as percentages of mean normal adult levels, close uniformity of results has been demonstrated [12,34]. Statistical analysis in healthy assumedly normal individuals from infancy to adulthood revealed a significant relationship between age and Ig concentration until certain ages [34]. In the case of IgM, no correlation was shown after 1 year of age, suggesting that adult concentration of IgM is normally reached and maintained by that time. In the case of IgG, adult concentration was reached by age of 3 years but in the case of IgA, insignificant difference was noted after 7 years [12] or 15 years [34] of age. Becaue of small sex difference of IgM only [34], it has become convenient in clinical practice to combine results for males and females.

Ethnic Differences in Black and White South African Children

Calculated geometric means and 95% confidence intervals for IgG, IgA, and IgM in white and black South African children (after Hobbs's table [34]) are shown graphically in Figure 2. Results were calculated as percentages of mean normal adult serum levels. Ranges of serum Ig concentrations in black South African children, grouped by age, were also determined by prospective assay, using a method of RID [77] with standards related to the international reference preparation 67/97. Samples used were excess serum after diagnostic tests had been carried out on patients with clinical diagnoses of illness for which Ig levels were very likely to be unaffected. Results were analysed in the same age ranges as those used for calculated values for white and black children. Assayed values were grouped together in defined age ranges according to clinical diagnosis. The data were also used as "control" for purposes of comparison of each category of patients, grouped on the

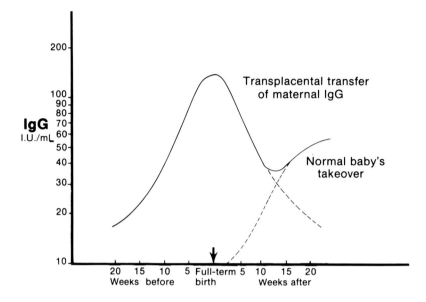

Fig. 1.   Serum immunoglobulin levels followed in premature infant born at 30 weeks' gestation contrasted with those of full-term babies (after Hobbs and Davis [32]).

basis of illness, with the "control". Figure 2 also shows ranges of assayed Igs in black children [79] together with calculated reference ranges. Similarly, results within reference ranges were obtained for white-children groups [76]. These studies revealed that interpretation of results are valid only when evaluated within reference ranges for the individual concerned. Results for boys and girls were combined, since only small differences occurred in IgM levels and mainly in the children over 1 year of age. Levels of all Igs in black children were much greater than ranges in corresponding age groups conventionally used for whites. Greater range in black children was particularly marked in the near absence of the physiologic fall in IgG level in the first few months of life: The black neonate starts off life with a greater median serum IgG level as a result of placental transfer from a greater median serum IgG level in black adult females. Median serum IgG in the first 3 months of a black infant's life falls to about 75% of the median value at birth, whereas in white infants it falls to about 50%. By 1 year, median serum IgG in black children returns to birth value, while white children, on average, take more than 3 years to accomplish the same increase. Further, black IgG levels in early adult life increase to 150% of the birth median value, whereas the white level increases to 135% [79]. Greater levels of all Igs in black children

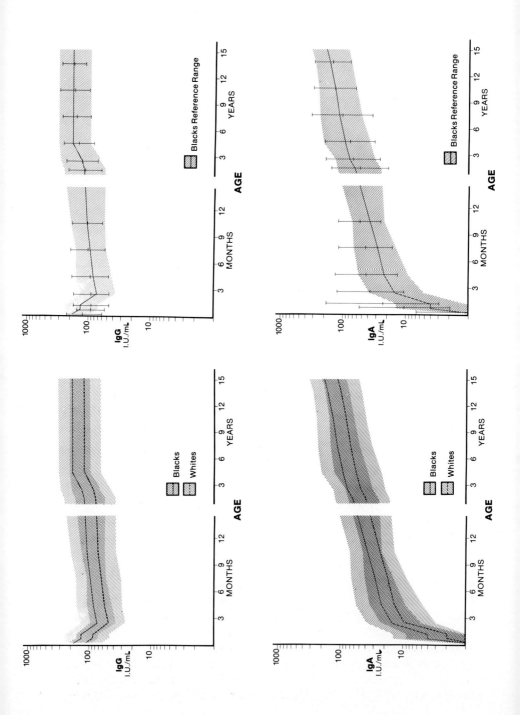

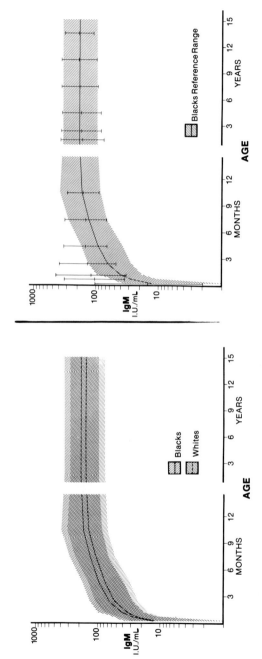

Fig. 2. Geometric means and 95% confidence intervals for serum immunoglobulins G, A, and M in black and white South African children (after Shulman and Gilich [79]). Results are graphically shown (left) in age ranges from birth to 15 years of age having been calculated (after Hobbs's tables [34]) from percentage mean normal adult levels expressed by Shulman et al. [80]. The vertical bars (right) indicate geometric means and 95% confidence intervals of assayed values for black children within the respective age ranges.

occurred in younger age groups than in whites, but having increased, the values tended to level off more rapidly [79], which contrasted with the slower rate of increase in white children, especially of IgA levels, where adult levels were only attained at 15 years of age [34,79]. Greater serum concentrations of Igs are said to occur in blacks mainly because of lower socioeconomic conditions, leading to more exposure to infections [79]. In the course of this study, minor variations of Ig levels were found in subjects in the same age ranges separated into different diagnostic categories. This was not unexpected since the material selected for study was drawn from patients in whom Ig levels were likely to be unaffected [79].

Ethnic Differences in Correlating Immunoglobulin Levels and Results of Electrophoresis

Physiological variation in serum Ig concentrations also has bearing on interpretation of serum electrophoretic patterns [78]. Important information can be gained by examining the electrophoretogram and the qualitative appearance of the bands. This is information that should be communicated to clinicians; depending on clinical and electrophoretic findings, analysis of certain serum specific proteins may be indicated [42]. Considerable variation in concentrations of the five electrophoretic protein bands on cellulose acetate was shown to occur in subjects of different racial and sex groups [78]. Of interest was a greater albumin concentration in blacks as compared with whites—a surprising finding due to better socioeconomic status of the latter group. Markedly greater concentrations of γ-globulin were also shown, which correlated with greater immunoglobulin levels that occur in blacks. While median γ-globulins (g/L with 95% confidence intervals) were 17.5 (11.7–26.2) in black males and 12.6 (9.0–17.7) in white males, median γ-globulins were 16.0 (11.6–22.6) in black females and 12.6 (8.0–18.2) in white females. All racial differences were very highly significant ($P < 0.002$). Additionally, there was a highly significant sex difference ($P < 0.005$) [78].

ETHNIC DIFFERENCES IN EXPRESSION OF IMMUNOGLOBULIN ABNORMALITIES

Multiple Myeloma in Black Populations

Although there are few studies detailing clinical and immunochemical features of immunocytoma from sub-Saharan Africa [38,57,73,82,96], the disease was considered uncommon in African black populations [18,72,91]. In North America, however, the incidence of multiple myeloma in the black population was reported to be greater than in the white population [55]. The black patient population was appreciably younger than the whites. After age

70 in males and age 60 in females, rates were higher for whites than for blacks. This relationship is one feature of the epidemiology of multiple myeloma which could not be explained on a diagnostic basis. In Jamaica, where the population is predominantly of West African descent, 101 cases of multiple myeloma in a 10-year period were described also with younger median age at diagnosis and low average survival [91]. In a report on the clinical and immunochemical presentations of immunocytoma in black and white South African patients [82], age-adjusted incidence rates for multiple myeloma in South African blacks were as high as those in the United States and Jamaica, contrasting with low incidence rates previously reported in Africa. Furthermore, it was noted that rates in Johannesburg blacks may have been underestimated, since some individuals may not seek conventional medical care, while there may also have been overestimation in whites due to nonresidents giving a Johannesburg address while receiving medical care in that district [82].

Multiple Myeloma and Primary Macroglobulinemia in South Africa

Age, sex, and race differences. Clinical and immunochemical presentations of myeloma and primary macroglobulinemia in 57 black and 84 white South African patients were described [82]. Distributions are summarized in Table II. Age frequency in white patients was similar to previously published series [33,55,66,104]. However, black patients with multiple myeloma and Waldenström's macroglobulinemia, on average, presented clinically 10 and 20 years, respectively, earlier than white patients. Median age in white patients with IgG and IgA myeloma (sexes combined since there was no age difference when comparing males and females) was 62 years each and with Bence Jones myeloma, 50 years. However, the median age for black patients with IgG and IgA myeloma (sexes combined) was 54 years each and with

TABLE II. Distribution of sex and race groups in immunochemical classes of 141 patients with multiple myeloma and primary macroglobulinemia Waldenström.

	Black	White
IgG myeloma	27 (48%)	47 (56%)
IgA myeloma	12 (21%)	9 (11%)
IgM myeloma	—	1 (1%)
IgD myeloma	—	1 (1%)
Bence Jones myeloma	10 (17%)	16 (19%)
Primary macroglobulinemia	8 (14%)	10 (12%)
Totals	57:	84:
	34 males	39 males
	23 females	45 females

Bence Jones myeloma, 49 years. Combining all the immunochemical classes in the two respective race groups, median age at clinical presentation in all white patients was ten years higher than that of all black patients (P < 0.02). Additionally, age incidences in South African black patients agree with results reported during the 15-year period 1960–1974 in a series of twenty black Nigerian myeloma patients [38]. In South Africa, white males presented at a significantly greater median age than black males (P < 0.02) as did white females when compared with black females (P < 0.01). There were equal sex incidences in the two respective race groups. In selected registers, calculated from world-standardized rates, there was a predominance of male cases of multiple myeloma with a percentage that has remained relatively constant for the time period covered [18].

Immunochemical studies. No significant difference in the various immunochemical classes of multiple myeloma was shown [82] despite greater serum Ig concentrations (especially IgA) described in the assumedly normal black population [80]. In black South African patients, distribution in immunochemical classes was similar to that in white South African patients [82] and to that previously reported in white patients in the United Kingdom [33]. Serum protein and immunochemical studies showed no significant difference in the mean concentrations for serum total protein, albumin, and M-components in patients (sexes combined) segregated into race groups, nor was there a sex difference within each race group. Median values for Ig other than those with immunochemical class of the M-protein were shown to be subnormal (Table III). Normal Igs were found suppressed to less than 20% of mean normal average levels in 0%, 38%, and 6% of black patients with IgG, IgA, and Bence Jones myeloma, respectively, and in 28%, 56%, and 44% of white patients, respectively [82]. This racial difference was significant (P < 0.01). Immune paresis, adjusted for reference ranges in appropriate control groups, was not as severe in black patients as in whites. While there was an impression of lower rates of complicating infections in blacks, the degrees of immune paresis still require correlation. Hyperviscosity was detected in seven white patients (IgG:3; IgA:2; IgM:2) and two black patients (IgM). Bence Jones proteinuria was detected in 44 (52%) white patients with myeloma and macroglobulinemia (κ/λ ratio of 3:2) and in 28 (49%) black patients (κ/λ ratio of 2:1); this difference in incidence is not significant. In white patients, Bence Jones proteinuria was detected in 46% of IgG, 25% of IgA; and in each of two patients with IgM and IgD myeloma, respectively, but not in any of the patients with macroglobulinemia. In black patients, Bence Jones proteinuria was detected in 70% of IgG and 41% of IgA myeloma, and in 29% of patients with macroglobulinemia, representing no significant difference between race groups. Combining myeloma results, Bence Jones proteinuria was detected in 56% of IgG and 37% of IgA myeloma and in 14% of patients with macroglobulinemia [82].

TABLE III. Results of Median (Lowest-Highest) Serum Immunoglobulins in Black and White Patients with Multiple Myeloma or Waldenström's Macroglobulinemia

		Number of cases	IgG (IU/mL)	IgA (IU/mL)	IgM (IU/mL)
IgG MM	(W)		25	30	
				(5–127)	(7–122)
	(B)	27	—	62	81
				(11–352)	(19–347)
				P < 0.001	P < 0.001
IgA MM	(W)	9	61	—	27
			(25–150)		(5–140)
	(B)	12	102	—	64
			(42–247)		(12–359)
			P < 0.05		P < 0.05
BJ MM	(W)	16	61	29	32
			(26–140)	(5–165)	(11–96)
	(B)	10	180	82	62
			(86–374)	(17–389)	(13–320)
			P < 0.001	P < 0.01	P < 0.05
MG	(W)	10	90	44	—
			(15–532)	(7–293)	
	(B)	8	206	74	
			(83–509)	(14–393)	
			P < 0.05	P.N.S.	

B = black; W = white; MM = multiple myeloma; MG = Waldenström's macroglobulinemia; BJ MM = Bence Jones myeloma (light chain disease).
P values were derived by Student's t-test on log-transformed data.

Complicated multiple myeloma. Significantly increased incidence in black patients of fracture of the thoracolumbar spine with vertebral collapse was noted in 21% of all black South African myeloma patients [82]. This finding agrees with the reported occurrence (25%) in patients in the Nigerian study [38]. Predisposing factors in South African black patients may relate to osteoporosis, secondary to hemosiderosis, which was described in increased incidence in this population [44], and to the presence of osteolytic bone lesions in persons who are mainly in the laboring class. A reported increased incidence of siderosis in black males, as compared to females [10], is also well correlated with increased incidence of fractured thoracolumbar spines in black males. While there was no difference in median concentrations of Bence Jones protein in urines of patients segregated into race groups, heavy Bence Jones proteinuria in black patients was frequently associated with more disastrous skeletal complications. This did not necessarily imply a more aggressive tumor, but may rather reflect differences imposed by occupation and socioeconomic restraint. Features of IgD myeloma [35] were seen in one white patient.

Comparison of Ethnic Differences of Multiple Myeloma in United States and South African Black and White Patients

In the United States multiple myeloma occurs more frequently in blacks than whites [107]. Age-adjusted incidence rates for the period 1973 to 1976 (1970 standard population) were 9.9 per 100,000 in blacks and 4.3 per 100,000 in whites [107]. During a 2-year period between 1973 and 1975, 29 black (19 male, 10 female) and 27 white (15 male, 12 female) South African patients were diagnosed in Johannesburg as having myeloma [8]. Age-adjusted incidence rates (world standard) per 100,000 were 7.47 in South African black males and 7.52 in American black males; 5.11 in South African black females and 5.17 in American black females [8]. These results suggest that the high rate for myeloma in blacks is not limited to America. Racial differences in immune response correlating with myeloma risk may have foundation in the observation of higher serum Ig levels in healthy native Africans and Afro-Americans than whites in the same areas [11,80]. Genetically determined racial differences in immune function have also been suggested in recent in vitro studies [26]. Greater incidence in United States black patients has been further confirmed [56]. Studies from Nigeria [20,21] and Uganda [105] point out a striking proportion of myeloma cases in younger age groups. These cases are found in areas where Burkitt's lymphoma is endemic, raising the possibility of common etiological factors. Further confirmation of younger median age for black African cases and a strong male preponderance have also been reported [38,67,93,96].

Multiple Myeloma in South America

Information concerning incidence of multiple myeloma in Central and South America is sparse, in large part due to lack of uniform case ascertainment. Only 18 cases were reported to the Colombian Registry between 1967 and 1971 out of a total population of approximately 77,000, with an age-standardized rate (world standard) in males of 1.1 per 100,000 [100]. Multiple myeloma in Sao Paulo, Brazil, comprises 3.4% of lymphoreticular tumors, with strong male preponderance and typical older age distribution [45]. A similar pattern (15% of all lymphomas, excluding leukemia) was reported from Peru, with 70 cases diagnosed between 1952 and 1970 [59]. An unusual racial breakdown of cases was reported from Cuba [51], with 59% in whites, 20% in blacks, and 20% in mestizos. Since whites do not constitute a majority of the population, differences in health care delivery may play a likely role. Chronic nasal infection with *Klebsiella rhinoscleromatis* (rhinoscleroma) predisposes to local plasmacytic infiltrate with potential for malignant transformation as plasma cell leukemia [2]. In El Salvador, a peculiar form of plasmacytoma has been reported as a possible consequence of long-standing rhinoscleroma [2], which relates to the suggestion in Africa of a link between chronic infection and multiple myeloma [108].

Multiple Myeloma in Western Europe

Risk estimates for myeloma in Western Europe (Sweden) [98] showed a high incidence, probably reflecting older age of the population investigated and special interest of the Scandinavian workers. Similar rates were also reported in white patients in England [50] but with an unexplained significant discrepancy in median age of clinical presentation: 70–80 years in Malmo versus 50–60 years in London. Results similar to the London report were found in three different North American series [3,27,85]. In Norway [86] multiple myeloma was reported as the most frequent form of lymphoreticular malignancy with higher rates in the rural population, which parallels a finding in the United States [41]. Based on small numbers of cases in Ireland [23] and Scotland [16], high rates were also suggested in these areas. Ethnic differences in the incidence of myeloma among whites in New York City have been described with higher rates in Jews, compared to Catholics and Protestants [62].

Multiple Myeloma in the Orient

Oriental populations have generally low rates of multiple myeloma. Cancer incidence rates available for the People's Republic of China during 1975 confirm a low rate for multiple myeloma [58]. A similar low percentage was reported from South Korea, where only 1.7% of a total of 601 cases of lymphoreticular malignancies were myeloma [39]. Comparison of mortality data in whites and blacks in the United States (1970–1975) to those in Japan (1969–1973) confirms a lower incidence of multiple myeloma at all ages among Japanese [9]. Age-specific rise after 50 years of age is also less steep in Japan, which contrasts with the pattern seen in the West. This may reflect differences in susceptibility or environmental exposures.

Trends in Multiple Myeloma Incidence and Mortality

Percentage increase in reported rates for myeloma in the United States was higher than for any other form of cancer [24] with upward trends greater among blacks than whites. This increased rate with time parallels the changes seen in European countries [86]. By comparison, rates of change for chronic lymphocytic leukemia and non-Hodgkin's lymphoma were approximately the same in both racial groups, while multiple myeloma showed a marked rise in whites and a dramatic increase in blacks [9]. Black males show most rapid rise in mortality over time but black females showed approximately equal rates of rise to white males and females [13]. A similar increase in mortality rates over calender time is also reported for a number of European countries showing marked increases between 1950 and 1962 [86]. Contrasting with these findings are the results of longitudinal studies of the relatively stable population of Olmstead County, Minnesota, with its northern European ethnic background and higher rates of multiple myeloma in persons from rural areas. The population is relatively homogeneous with regard to race, ethnic background and occupation, with blacks constituting an insignificant proportion. Yet, the incidence of myeloma has remained stable since 1945 [41]. It is still not clear whether the true incidence of multiple myeloma in different ethnic groups is changing with time.

Familial multiple myeloma has also been reported [47,49], but it is difficult to distinguish genetic from environmental factors. Benign monoclonal gammopathy has been described in families of myeloma cases and peptide maps of light chains from a mother with myeloma and her son with benign monoclonal gammopathy were found not to be identical, arguing that structural genes operative in M-protein light chain production in these relatives were different [28]. These data also suggest that familial M-proteins are produced by distinct plasma cell clones. Polyclonal Ig levels among close relatives of myeloma cases may be somewhat higher than those seen in the general population [65], but there was no significant difference in the incidence of monoclonal bands among family members or spouses compared to the population incidence.

Primary Macroglobulinemia

Primary macroglobulinemia of Waldenström is a rare malignancy in which plasmacytoid lymphocytes secrete Ig IgM. Many of the bizarre clinical manifestations of this disease arise because of unusual physicochemical properties of the "macroglobulin." In most surveys, macroglobulinemia occurs with a frequency one fourth that of multiple myeloma [1,37,92] with an annual prevalence rate of 0.53 per 100,000 [6]. Age distribution in macroglobulinemia is similar to myeloma, with nearly all cases diagnosed in persons over 60 years of age [52,84,98]. Younger age of presentation in blacks, reminiscent of the pattern observed for myeloma, was suggested in a study from South Africa [72], although based on an African population attenuated in the older age groups.

Benign Monoclonal Gammopathy and Solitary Myeloma

The prevalence of monoclonal Ig spikes, especially in older age groups, is relatively high and in an 11-year follow-up in the United States, the benign nature of the M-component was confirmed in most cases [4]. An overall prevalence rate of 1.25%, with a rate of 4.8% in the over 80-year age group, was identified [40]. This was further emphasized in Scandinavian reports that M-components are frequent and follow an age distribution which parallels multiple myeloma and Waldenström's macroglobulinemia [68,95]. Follow-up surveys in the United States and in Scandinavia indicated that about 10% of subjects with benign monoclonal spikes developed myeloma or related tumors [63,99]. A South African series of 168 immunocytoma patients (101 white; 67 black) with paraproteins, comprised 17 whites but no blacks who were diagnosed as having benign monoclonal gammopathy [82]. It was also noted that, in the same series, there were one white and ten black patients with solitary myeloma.

α-Heavy Chain Diseases

Of the heavy chain diseases, α-chain disease has mainly attracted attention on an ethnic basis. Primary small intestinal lymphoma with a distinct geographical distribution was first described in Arabs and subsequently in persons with low socioeconomic status in the Mediterranean area [74]. The condition has several noteworthy features, including steatorrhea and an associated heavy chain abnormality. Recently, the occurrence of this disease beyond the Mediterranean area has been recorded in South Africa [64,83]; Bangladesh, Greece, Libya, Pakistan, and Persia [17]; Nigeria [103]; and Columbia, Argentina, and Cambodia [75]. In view of the wide geographical distribution and the apparent rarity of this condition in Western countries, infection, possibly parasitic, may be the common factor in these patients, providing a stimulus for excess proliferation of intestinal IgA-synthesizing plasma cells [75]. A remarkable feature of all but one of the patients with α-chain disease so far described is the initial confinement of the abnormal plasma cells to the wall of the small intestine. In the one exceptional case of α-chain disease, only the lung appeared to be involved [90].

CONCLUSIONS

A variety of etiologic factors may contribute to concentration ranges of normal Igs and the development of their abnormalities. With monoclonal gammopathies being especially common in the elderly, age is a major risk factor. Ethnic difference is another important determinant and higher rate and earlier age of onset of myeloma in blacks may suggest inborn susceptibility, although environmental factors cannot be excluded. This correlates well with racial differences in baseline Ig levels in varying ethnic groups. For blacks, the relative frequency of myeloma is high after age 50, with relative deficit of other tumors. This contrasts with the pattern in Orientals, in whom undifferentiated forms of B-cell malignancy predominate over myeloma, suggesting an ethnically determined resistance to malignancies of mature B-cells. The role of chronic antigenic stimulation, perhaps by increasing the size of the clone of cells at risk, is provocative. Almost 20 years have elapsed since the reported link between rhinoscleroma and myeloma in El Salvador. Similarly of special interest is the occurrence in certain ethnic groups of Mediterranean lymphoma and α-chain disease, which has been attributed to chronic intestinal infection prevalent in the relative areas. There is also some support to the view that chronic antigenic exposure of the gut mucosa causes sustained stimulation of the IgA secreting system which is reflected by raised serum IgA levels. Additionally, there is the question of whether myeloma, especially in young persons, is more frequent in areas with a high incidence of Burkitt's lymphoma, where malarial infestation may be a co-factor in the etiology of both. Integration of epidemiologic, ethnic, and immunologic studies of monoclonal gammopathies and high-risk populations should provide new insights into the genesis of these conditions.

REFERENCES

1. Ameis A, Ko HS, Pruzanski WM: Components—a review of 1,242 cases. Can Med Assoc J 114:889, 1976.
2. Astacio JN, Noubleau V, Alfaro DA et al.: Plasmocitomas extramedulares de los tractos respiratorio supperior y gastro-intestinal. Relacion escleroma-plasmocitoma. Arch Col Med El Salvador 18:213, 1965.
3. Atkinson FRB: Multiple myelomata. Med Press 195:312, 327, 1937.
4. Axelsson U: An eleven-year follow-up on 64 subjects with M-components. Acta Med Scand 201:173, 1977.
5. Balduzzi PC, Vaughan JH, Greendyke RM: Immunoglobulin levels in sudden unexpected deaths of infants. J. Pediatr 72:689, 1968.
6. Benbassat J, Fluman N, Zlotnick A: Monoclonal immunoglobulin disorders: A report of 154 cases. Am J Med Sci 271:325, 1976.
7. Bence Jones H: Papers on chemical pathology: Prefaced by the Gulstonian Lectures read at the Royal College of Physicians, 1846. Lecture III. Lancet 2:88, 1847.
8. Blattner WA, Jacobson RJ, Shulman G: Multiple myeloma in South African blacks. Lancet 8122:928, 1979.
9. Blattner WA: Epidemiology of multiple myeloma and related plasma cell disorders: An analytic review. In Potter M (ed): "Multiple Myeloma and Related Disorders (Volume 2)." New York: Elsevier North-Holland, 1980, 1.
10. Bothwell TH, Isaacson C: Siderosis in the Bantu. Brit Med J 1:522, 1962.
11. Buckley CE III, Dorsey FC: Serum immunoglobulin levels throughout the life-span of healthy man. Ann Int Med 75:673, 1971.
12. Buckley RH, Dees SC, O'Fallon WM: Serum immunoglobulins: I. Levels in normal children and in uncomplicated childhood allergy. Pediatrics 41:600, 1968.
13. Burbank F: Patterns in cancer mortality in the United States: 1950–1967. Natl Cancer Inst Monogr 71:1, 1971.
14. Cohen S, McGregor IA, Carrington S: Gamma-globulin and acquired immunity to human malaria. Nature 192:733, 1961.
15. Dalrymple, J: On the microscopical character of "mollities ossium." Dublin Q J Med Sci 2:85, 1846.

16. Dawson AA, Ogston D: High incidence of myelomatosis in North-East Scotland. Scott Med J 18:75, 1973.
17. Doe WF, Henry K, Hobbs JR, et al. Five cases of alpha chain disease. Gut 13:947, 1972.
18. Doll R, Payne P, Waterhouse J (eds): Cancer incidence in five continents: A technical report. Publication of the International Union against Cancer. Heidelberg: Springer-Verlag, 1966.
19. Economidou O, Manousos D, Trichopoulos, et al. Serum immunoglobulins in a rural and an urban population of Greece with special reference to immunoglobulin A. J Clin Pathol 32:1140, 1979.
20. Edington GM: Tumours of lymphoreticular tissue including the Burkitt lymphoma but excluding leukaemia in Nigeria with special reference to the northern savanna. Niger Med J 8:75, 1978.
21. Edington GM, Hendrickse M: Incidence and frequency of lymphoreticular tumors in Ibadan and the western state of Nigeria. J Natl Cancer Inst 50:1623, 1973.
22. Editorial: Standards for immunoglobulins. Lancet 2:82, 1971.
23. Egan EL, O'Beirn DP, Grimes H: Multiple myeloma in the west of Ireland, presentation and frequency. Ir Med J 71:23, 1978.
24. Fraumeni JF Jr: Environmental and genetic determinants of cancer. J Envir Pathol Toxicol 1:19, 1977.
25. Fulginiti VA, Sieber OF Jr, Claman HN, Merrill D: Serum immunoglobulin measurements during the first year of life and in immunoglobulin-deficiency states. J Pediatr 68:723, 1966.
26. Ginsburg WW, Finkelman FD, Lipsky PE: Circulating and mitogen-induced immunoglobulin-secreting cells in human peripheral blood: Evaluation by a modified reverse hemolytic plaque assay. J Immunol 120:33, 1978.
27. Geschickter CF, Copeland MM: Multiple Myeloma. Arch Surg 16:807, 1928.
28. Grant JA, Blumenschein GR, Buckley CE III: Familial paraproteinemia. Arch Int Med 128:427, 1971.
29. Grundbacher FJ: Human X chromosome carries quantitative genes for immunoglobulin M. Science 176:311, 1972.
30. Hosty TA, Hollenbeck M, Shane S: Intercomparison of results obtained with five commercial diffusion plates supplied for quantitation of immunoglobulins. Clin Chem 19:524, 1973.
31. Hitzig WH: The blood protein picture in the healthy infant. Specific protein determinations with special reference to immunochemical methods. Helv Paediat Acta 16:46, 1961.
32. Hobbs JR, Davis JA: Serum γ-globulin levels and gestational age in premature babies. Lancet 1:757, 1967.
33. Hobbs, JR: Immunochemical classes of myelomatosis. Brit J Haematol 16:599, 1969.
34. Hobbs JR: Immunoglobulins in clinical chemistry. In Bodansky O, Latner AL (ed): "Advances in Clinical Chemistry (Volume 14)." New York: Academic Press, 1971, 263.
35. Hobbs JR, Corbett AA: Younger age of presentation and extraosseous tumour in IgD myelomatosis. Brit Med J 1:412, 1969.
36. Isaacson C, Seftel HC, Keeley KJ, Bothwell TH: Siderosis in the Bantu: The relationship between iron overload and cirrhosis. J Lab Clin Med 58:845, 1961.
37. Isobe T, Osserman EF: Pathologic conditions associated with plasma cell dyscrasias: A study of 806 cases. Ann NY Acad Sci 190:507, 1971.
38. Iyun A, Isaacs-Sodeye A: Multiple myeloma in Ibadan. A comparative Study. E Afr Med J 53:581, 1976.
39. Kim SI, Lee CK: Leukemia among Koreans—a statistical and hematological study of 601 cases of leukemia and allied conditions. In Hirayama T (ed): "Cancer in Asia." Baltimore, University Park Press, 1976 pp 229–37.

40. Kyle RA, Finkelstein S, Elveback LR et al.: Incidence of monoclonal proteins in a Minnesota community with a cluster of multiple myeloma. Blood 40:719, 1972.
41. Kyle RA, Nobrega FT, Kurland LT: Multiple myeloma in Olmsted County, Minnesota, 1945–1964. Blood 33:739, 1969.
42. Laurell CB: Electrophoresis, specific protein assays, or both in measurement of plasma proteins? Clin Chem 19:99, 1973.
43. Lichtman MA, Vaughn JH, Hames CG, McDonough JR: The distribution of serum immunoglobulins, anti-gamma G globulins ("rheumatoid factors") and antinuclear antibodies in White and Negro subjects in Evans County, Georgia. Arthritis Rheum 10:204, 1967.
44. Lynch SR, Berelowitz I, Seftel HC, et al.: Osteoporosis in Johannesburg Bantu Males. Its relationship to siderosis and ascorbic acid deficiency. Am J Clin Nutr 20:799, 1967.
45. Machado JC, Jamra M, Okuyama MH, et al.: Lymphoreticular tumors in Sao Paulo, Brazil. J Natl Cancer Inst 50:1651, 1973.
46. MacIntyre W: Case of mollities and fragilitas osseum accompanied with urine strongly charged with animal matter. Med Chir Trans 33:211, 1850.
47. Maldonado JE, Kyle RA: Familial myeloma. Report of eight families and a study of serum proteins in their relatives. Am J Med 57:875, 1974.
48. Mancini G, Carbonara AO, Heremans JF: Immunochemical quantitation of antigens by single radial immunodiffusion. Int J Immunochem 2:235, 1965.
49. Madema E, Wildervanck LS: La maladie de Kahler (myélomes multiples) chez deux soeurs. J Génét Hum (Geneve) 3:170, 1954.
50. Martin NH: The incidence of myelomatosis. Lancet 1:237, 1961.
51. Mas Martin JC: Study of 321 patients with multiple myeloma (Kahler's disease) in relation to age, race and sex in Cuba. Rev Cubana Med Trop 30:3, 1978.
52. McCallister BD, Bayrd ED, Harrison EG, et al.: Primary macroglobulinemia—review with a report on thirty-one cases and notes on the value of continuous chlorambucil therapy. Am J Med 43:394, 1967.
53. McFarlane H: Immunoglobulins in Nigeria. Lancet 2:445, 1966.
54. McFarlane H, Voller A: Studies on immunoglobulins of Nigerians. II. Immunoglobulins and malarial infections in Nigerians. J Trop Med Hyg 69:104, 1966.
55. McMahon B, Clark DW: The incidence of multiple myeloma. J Chron Dis 4:508, 1956.
56. McPhedran P, Heath CW Jr, Garcia J: Multiple myeloma incidence in metropolitan Atlanta, Georgia: Racial and seasonal variations. Blood 39:866, 1972.
57. Michaux JL: Les immunoglobulines des Bantous a l'etat normal et pathologique. Ann Soc Belg Med Trop 46:483, 1966.
58. Miller RW: Cancer epidemics in the People's Republic of China. J Natl Cancer Inst 60:1195, 1978.
59. Misad O, Brandon JG, Albujar P: Lymphoreticular tumors in Peru. J Natl Cancer Inst 50:1663, 1973.
60. Mohammed I, Tomkins AM, Greenwood BM: Normal immoglobulins in the tropics. Lancet 1:481, 1973.
61. Momma K: Immunochemical semiquantitative estimation of gamma-M-and gamma-A-immunoglobulins in healthy and diseased children. Part I. Immunoglobulin levels from the newborn period to adulthood. Acta Paediatr Jpn 7:1, 1965.
62. Newill VA: Distribution of cancer mortality among ethnic subgroups of the white population of New York City, 1953–1958, J Natl Cancer Inst 26:405, 1961.
63. Nørgaard O: Three cases of multiple myeloma in which the preclinical asymptomatic phases persisted throughout 15 to 24 years. Br J Cancer 25:417, 1971.
64. Novis BH, Bank S, Marks IN, et al.: Abnormal lymphoma presenting with malabsorption. Q J Med N.S. 40:521, 1971.

65. Odeberg H, Johansson BG, Berlin SO: Immunoglobulin analysis in families of myeloma patients. Acta Med Scand 196:361, 1974.
66. Osserman EF, Takatsuki K: Plasma cell myeloma: Gamma globulin synthesis and structure. Medicine 42:357, 1963.
67. Otieno LS, Ogada T: Multiple myeloma at Kenyatta National Hospital, 1973–1976. East Afr Med J 54:574, 1977.
68. Radl J, Sepers JM, Skvaril F, et al.: Immunoglobulin patterns in humans over 95 years of age. Clin Exp Immunol 22:84, 1975.
68a. Ritchie RF: Interpretation of serum protein values. In Ritzmann SE (ed.): "Physiology of Immunoglobulins: Diagnostic and Clinical Aspects." New York: Alan R. Liss, 1982, p 159.
69. Rowe DS: Concentration of serum-immunoglobulins in healthy young adult males estimated by assay against the international reference preparation. Lancet 2:1232, 1972.
70. Rowe DS, Anderson SG, Grab B: A research standard for human serum immunoglobulins IgG, IgA, and IgM. Bull WHO 42:535, 1970.
71. Rowe DS, McGregor IA, Smith SJ, et al.: Plasma immunoglobulin concentrations in a West African (Gambian) community and in a group of healthy British adults. Clin Exp Immun 3:63, 1968.
72. Sacher RA, Jacobson RJ, Derman D, et al.: Waldenström's macroglobulinemia in South African negroes. Trop Geogr Med 30:207, 1978.
73. Sankale M, Frament V, Diouf S: La maladie de Kahler dans un service de medicine generale a' Dakar. Medicine d' Afrique Noire 19:679, 1972.
74. Seligmann M, Danon F, Hurez D, et al.: Alpha chain disease: A new immunoglobulin abnormality. Science 162:1396, 1968.
75. Seligman M, Mihaesco E, Frangione B: Alpha chain disease. Ann NY Acad Sci 190:487, 1971.
76. Shulman G: Unpublished data.
77. Shulman G: Accuracy and precision in measurements of human serum immunoglobulins G, A, and M. S Afr J Med Sci 38:61, 1973.
78. Shulman G: The value of quantitative protein electrophoresis. South Afr Med J 50:2059, 1976.
79. Shulman G, Gilich GC: Serum immunoglobulins in black South African children. South Afr Med J 50:1465, 1976.
80. Shulman G, Gilich GC, Andrew MJA: Serum immunoglobulins G, A, and M in white and black adults on the Witwatersrand. South Afr Med J 49:1160, 1975.
81. Shulman G: Quality of commercially available controls in laser immunonephelometry. Ann Clin Biochem 17:178, 1982.
82. Shulman G, Jacobson RJ: Immunocytoma in black and white South Africans. Trop Geogr Med 32:112, 1980.
83. Shulman G, Lai York E, Grieve S: Alpha-chain disease in a non-Mediterranean climate. A case report. South Afr. Med. J. 49:2183, 1975.
84. Snapper I, Kahn A: "Myelomatosis—Fundamentals and Clinical Features." Baltimore: University Park Press, 1971.
85. Snapper I, Turner LB, Moscovitz HL: "Multiple Myeloma." New York: Grune and Stratton, Inc., 1953.
86. Stalsberg H: Lymphoreticular tumors in Norway and in other European countries. J Natl Cancer Inst 50:1685, 1973.
87. Stiehm ER, Fudenberg HH: Serum levels of immune globulins in health and disease: A Survey. Pediatrics 37:715, 1966.
88. Stiehm ER, Gold E: Immune globulin levels in the sudden death syndrome. Pediatrics 42:61, 1968.

89. Stoop JW, Zegers BJM, Sander PC, et al.: Serum immunoglobulin levels in healthy children and adults. Clin Exp Immunol 4:101, 1969.
90. Stoop JW, Ballieux RE, Hijmans W, et al.: Alpha chain disease with involvement of the respiratory tract in a Dutch child. Clin Exp Immunol 9:625, 1971.
91. Talerman A: Clinico-pathological study of multiple myeloma in Jamaica. Br J Cancer 23:285, 1969.
92. Tichy M, Hrncir Z, Mracek J, et al.: Immunochemical and clinical characteristics of series of 516 paraproteinemic patients. Neoplasma 25:477, 1978.
93. Traub N: Multiple myeloma at the University Teaching Hospital, Lusaka: A retrospective study. Med J Zambia 11:148, 1977.
94. Turner MW, Voller A: Studies on immunoglobulins of Nigerians. I. The immunoglobulin levels of a Nigerian population. J Trop Med Hyg 69:99, 1966.
95. Van Camp BG, Cole J, Peetermans ME: M-components in blood donors in Antwerp. (Eng Abstr) Acta Clin Belg 31:203, 1976.
96. Waldbaum B, Gelfand M: Myelomatosis in the Rhodesean African. Trop Geogr Med 26:26, 1974.
97. Waldenström J: Incipient myelomatosis or "essential" hyperglobulinemia with fibringen-openia—new syndrome? Acta Med Scand 117:216, 1944.
98. Waldenström J: Diseases associated with abnormal plasma proteins. Proc R Soc Med 53:789, 1960.
99. Waldenström J: The occurrence of benign, essential monoclonal (M type), non-macro-molecular hyperglobulinemia and its differential diagnosis. IV. Studies in the gammo-pathies. Acta Med Scand 176:345, 1964.
100. Waterhouse JA, Muir C, Correa P, et al: "Cancer Incidence in Five Continents, Volume III." Lyon: IARC Publication No 15, 1976.
101. Wells JV: Serum immunoglobulin levels in tropical splenomegaly syndrome in New Guinea. Clin Exp Immunol 3:943, 1968.
102. West CD, Hong R, Holland NH: Immunoglobulin levels from the newborn period to adulthood and in immunoglobulin deficiency states. J Clin Invest 41:2054, 1962.
103. Whicher JT: Ajdukiewicz A, Davies JD: Two cases of alpha chain disease from Nigeria. J Clin Pathol 30:678, 1977.
104. Williams RC Jr, Brunning RD, Wollheim FA: Light-chain disease. An abortive variant of multiple myeloma. Ann Intern Med 65:471, 1966.
105. Wright DH: Lymphoreticular neoplasms. In Stempleton AC (ed): "Recent Results in Cancer Research. Tumors in a Tropical Country." New York: Springer-Verlag, 1973, 270.
106. Yadav M, Shah FH: Normal plasma-immunoglobulin levels in Malaysians. Lancet 2:450, 1973.
107. Young JL, Asire AJ, Pollack ES: SEER program: Cancer Incidence and Mortality in the United States, 1973–1976. D.H.E.W. publication no. (NIH) 78-1837, 1978.
108. Michaux JL, Heremans JF: Thirty cases of monoclonal immunoglobulin disorders other than myeloma or macroglobulinemia. A classification of diseases associated with the production of monoclonal-type immunoglobulins. Am J Med 46:568, 1969.
109. Ritzmann SE: Immunoglobulin Abnormalities. In Ritzmann SE, Daniels JC: "Serum Protein Abnormalities: Diagnostic and Clinical Aspects," 2nd printing. New York: Alan R. Liss, Inc., 1982, pp 421–424.

Pathology of Immunoglobulins: Diagnostic and
Clinical Aspects, page 97
© 1982 Alan R. Liss, Inc., 150 Fifth Avenue, New York, NY 10011

Addendum

Serum IgG, IgA, IgM, and IgD Levels in Middle Eastern Populations

Samih Y. Alami, PhD, MD

Recently, supplementary data on serum immunoglobulin levels have been added by Alami, Zurayk, and Farah [1] for normal children and adults in Lebanese and other Arab Middle Eastern populations.

The extensive studies by these authors are based on the RID determination of serum IgG, A, M, and D levels in 1000 specimens obtained from normal and presumably healthy Middle Easterners. They represent the first systematic study of normal immunoglobulin levels, at various ages, of Middle East populations.

In general, their values compare with those of European and American investigators [2–6]. IgG and IgA levels follow similar trends, though this study reveals somewhat higher levels in the Middle Eastern population.

REFERENCES

1. Alami SY, Zurayk HC, Farah FS: Serum immunoglobulin levels in normal children and adults in the Lebanese and other Arab Middle Eastern populations. Leb Med J 31:1, 1980.
2. Gunvar S, Johansson O, Berg T: Immunoglobulin levels in healthy children. Acta Paediatrica Scandinavica 56:572, 1967.
3. Allansmith M, McClellan BH, Butterworth M, Maloney JR: The development of immunoglobulin levels in man. J Pediatr 72:276, 1968.
4. Stiehm ER, Fudenberg HH: Serum levels of immune globulins in health and disease. A survey. Pediatrics 37:715, 1966.
5. Stoop JW, Zegers JM, Sander PC, Ballieux RE: Serum immunoglobulin levels in healthy children and adults. Clin Exper Immunol 4:101, 1969.
6. Cejka T, Mood DW, Kim S: Immunoglobulin concentration in sera of normal children: Quantitation against an international reference preparation. Clin Chem 20:656, 1974.

Pathology of Immunoglobulins: Diagnostic and
Clinical Aspects, pages 99–107
© 1982 Alan R. Liss, Inc., 150 Fifth Avenue, New York, NY 10011

6

Cell Surface Proteins: Specific Receptor Sites

Jerry C. Daniels, MD, PhD

GENERAL CONCEPTS OF RECEPTORS

Responses to the multitude of extracellular signals coordinating human cell growth, development, and function begin at the cell surface. Examples of such extracellular signals include hormones, drugs, neurotransmitters, and antigens. Cell surface receptors that recognize these signals show high specificity in that a given stimulus usually triggers only a highly selective cellular response. Additionally, such receptors must be as diverse as the population of extracellular signals to be received. Thus, cell surface receptors exhibit dual requirements for specificity and diversity. Here, only a selection of receptors will be considered, which are either themselves protein in nature or are known to bind specific protein as the ligand. It has been postulated that, within the current model of the plasma membrane as a sea of lipid with boats of protein [1], receptors are at least in part protein in terms of structure [2].

Plasma membrane receptors are structures operationally defined as having the ability to interact specifically with a given ligand and to be saturated by that ligand, as demonstrated by competitive binding studies. This operational definition does not imply that a receptor is a single molecular species that remains intact upon disorganization of the plasma membrane. Semantic excesses in interpreting the receptor concept may lead either to simplistic approaches of receptor fractionation or to the total denial of the existence of receptors. The general problem of receptor purification is very complex [3].

Receptors must transform external environmental information into meaningful intracellular signals. Three functions have thus been envisioned for receptors: (1) recognition of a specific external stimulus, (2) transduction of a signal across the plasma membrane, and (3) induction of an intracellular response. Although few receptors have been in any way characterized at the molecular level, several reasonable assumptions concerning their common properties can be made. It is likely that receptors span the membrane and belong to the class of integral membrane components, probably proteinaceous. It is likely that receptors have discrete domains for the three aspects of their function: (1) Specific interaction of the recognition domain with external stimuli in the form of ligand molecules involves molecular complementarity typical of enzyme-substrate and antigen-antibody reactions. (2) Transduction of the extrinsic binding signal across the membrane involves conformational changes in the transducing domain, which could occur either consequent to ligand binding, causing changes in individual receptors, or to aggregation of identical receptors whose interaction with each other causes conformational changes. (3) The initiation functions of receptors can occur along any number of intracellular effector pathways, including the cytoskeleton, specific ion gates, ionic pumps, or cyclic nucleotides.

COMPLEMENT RECEPTORS

Complement (C) receptors on human cells are of two general types, the C3b and C3d types [4]. Receptors described for C4b are now thought to be identical to C3b receptors. A number of human cells possess these receptors at their surface, as shown in Table I. The presence of C receptors on B lymphocytes but not T lymphocytes is of practical importance in characterizing human lymphocyte classes [5]. An assay system is available for discriminating between the C3b receptor, which is also called the immune adherence receptor, and the C3d receptor [6]. By this technique, 20–40% of C receptor lymphocytes have only the immune adherence receptor and 10–25% only the C3d receptor. The two types of C receptors are antigenically distinct, cap independently, and have specificities for different regions of C4 or C3 molecules [4]. The immune adherence receptors on B lymphocytes are shared with erythrocytes, granulocytes, and monocytes and react with C4b or the C3c region of C3b. The C3d receptor is shared only with monocytes [7] and eosinophils [8], and reacts with either C3d or the C3d region of C3b.

In general, divalent cations are not required for binding to C receptors. Binding is optimal at 37°C and initial binding much reduced at 0°C. However, binding occurring at 37°C remains stable when decreased to 0°C. Cells killed by heat or metabolic poisons show near normal C receptor activity. C receptors are trypsin-sensitive, and this is useful in discriminating between binding by such receptors and by Fc receptors, which are trypsin-insensitive [9].

Receptors for C3b (immune adherence receptors) bind C3 following cleavage by C3 convertase or by C3 activator. The binding site on the C3b molecule may be located in the $\alpha_4\beta$ fragment (Table II). Binding can be inhibited by fluid phase C3b, C4b, and C3c, but not by C3d. On the other hand, receptors

TABLE I. Complement Receptors on Various Human Cells

Cell type	C3b receptor	C3d receptor
Erythrocytes	+	−
Platelets	−	−
Granulocytes	+	−
Eosinophils	−	+
Monocytes	+	±
Alveolar macrophages	+	±
T lymphocytes	−	−
B lymphocytes	+	+

TABLE II. Relationship Between C3 and Complement Receptors

Form of C3	Chain composition	Binds to receptor:	
		C3b	C3d
C3	$\alpha_1\ \alpha_2\ \alpha_3\ \alpha_4\ \beta$	−	−
C3a	α_1	−	−
C3b	$\alpha_2\ \alpha_3\ \alpha_4\ \beta$	+	+
C3b^i	$\alpha_3\ \alpha_4\ \beta$	+	+
C3c	$\alpha_4\ \beta$	+	−
C3d	α_3	−	+
C3b		+	−

for C3d are specific for the C3d fragment of C3 after cleavage by C3b inactivator. The binding site may be in the α_3 fragment (Table II), and therefore C3d remains on the erythrocyte surface following cleavage by the inactivator. Binding can be inhibited by fluid phase C3b and C3d, but not by C3c.

Receptors for C may be useful as markers for macrophage activation [9]. Normal macrophages bind, but do not ingest particles coated with C3b. On the other hand, activated macrophage bind and ingest opsonized particles by way of the C3b receptors. In the absence of IgG molecules, the fate of immune complexes depends on the state of activation of the macrophage.

SURFACE IMMUNOGLOBULINS ON B LYMPHOCYTES

Immunoglobulins (Igs) are the most thoroughly characterized cell surface receptors. The receptor Ig molecules associated with B lymphocytes are not found on T lymphocytes. They are virtually indistinguishable from the specific antibodies secreted by the same cell or its progeny [10]. The number of receptor Igs has been estimated to be between 5×10^4 and 2×10^5 molecules per lymphocyte.

Immunoglobulins M, D, G, and A have been identified by immunofluorescence as cell-surface receptors on B-lymphocyte membranes. Most lymphocytes appear to have receptor IgM and/or IgD. These molecules appear to be integral structural membrane proteins in that they can be isolated from membranes only by strong detergents. The C-terminal domain of the H chain appears to be anchored to the membrane because antibodies specific for the CH_2 domain of IgG molecules react with membrane-bound IgG, whereas antibodies specific for the CH_3 domain do not.[1]

Antisera directed against the idiotypic, allotypic, and isotypic moieties of the secreted Ig from individual clones of B lymphocytes also react with the corresponding membrane-bound Igs. These observations suggest that the V domains as well as the C domains of secreted and membrane Igs from a given B-lymphocyte are very similar, if not identical.

Using detergents, IgM, IgD, and IgG have been isolated from B-lymphocyte membranes. The sizes of the light (L) and heavy (H) chains are very similar in the membrane-bound and secreted Igs. To date, there is insufficient evidence to distinguish between the following four possibilities regarding the CH regions of membrane-bound and soluble Igs: 1) the CH regions may be identical; 2) they may differ only in their attached carbohydrate groups; 3) they may be different, although related, in amino acid sequence; 4) they may be identical except for a hydrophobic polypeptide belt attached to the CH homology unit.

Proof that membrane-bound Igs are receptors for antigen is still somewhat indirect. Anti-Igs block antigen binding to B lymphocytes. Antigen receptors and surface Igs can be induced to cocap by the addition of antigen, implying identity or near-identity. Finally, radiolabeled hapten-carrier binds to specific B lymphocytes, which, upon incubation *in vitro,* release into the tissue culture medium-labeled complexes equally precipitable by antibodies to either the hapten or to surface Igs. Each of these observations suggests, but does not prove, that the antigen receptors and membrane-associated Igs are the same molecules.

The role that surface Igs may play in triggering B-cell activation is still controversial. Several hypothetical models have been proposed.

There are preliminary indications, from x-ray diffraction and spectroscopic studies, that surface Igs may undergo molecular conformational changes upon binding antigen.

In summary, available evidence indicates that receptor Igs on B lymphocytes have properties expected of cell surface receptors for specific antigen.

---

[1]Ed. note: See also Hahn GS in Ritzmann SE (ed): "Physiology of Immunoglobulins: Diagnostic and Clinical Aspects" [36].

TABLE III. T-Lymphocyte Subset Distribution

Tissue	Total T lymphocytes		
	(%)	Tγ(%)	Tμ(%)
Thymus	98 ± 1	1 ± 1	3 ± 2
Tonsils	25 ± 5	6 ± 3	59 ± 7
Spleen	37 ± 5	45 ± 6	13 ± 3
Peripheral blood	70 ± 5	11 ± 1	56 ± 9
Cord blood	−	34 ± 2	51 ± 3
Lymph nodes	46 ± 3	< 1	56 ± 4

Igs probably evolved from more general recognition systems, which is compatible with a combined cellular-Ig complex within the immune system.

T-LYMPHOCYTE RECEPTORS FOR IMMUNOGLOBULIN Fc

A number of human cell types carry at their surface receptors for the Fc portion of Ig, which is exposed for binding availability upon formation of an antigen-antibody complex by the Ig [11]. These include monocytes, macrophages, granulocytes, null cells, T lymphocytes and probably, to a lesser degree, some B lymphocytes [12]. The T-lymphocyte Fc-binding receptors have become of considerable interest since the class of Ig Fc for which a given T-lymphocyte receptor shows specificity appears to reflect functional properties of that T lymphocyte [13].

Tγ Cells and T-Suppressor Function

A subset of T lymphocytes shows preferential binding of IgG, especially aggregated or complexed IgG, and have purported receptors for the Fc portion of IgG [14]. Such cells have been designated Tγ cells. They have a relatively low avidity for the substrate as shown by inhibition studies. This receptor appears to be trypsin-resistant [15]. By coating erythrocyte with IgG antibodies Tγ cells can be enumerated from an enriched T-lymphocyte fraction [16]. Normal values for peripheral blood are about 11 ± 1% [13], but differ for other lymphoid compartments (Table III).

Using a model of B-lymphocyte stimulation to antibody production by pokeweed mitogen (PWM), Tγ cells have been shown to exert a suppressor effect [17]. It has been suggested that this suppression occurs by decreasing the helper function of T-helper cells rather than by a direct inhibition of the responding B lymphocytes [13]. Soluble factors released by Tγ cells may substitute for the intact cells, suggesting further that the mechanism of suppression may be by means of a released substance [18].

Tμ Cells and T-Helper Function

A distinct lymphocyte subset carries membrane receptors for IgM, and such cells have been termed Tμ cells [19]. Such lymphocytes represent normally 56 ± 9% of the peripheral blood lymphocytes (Table III). These receptors are slow to bind, requiring up to 18 hours for optimal binding. Erythrocytes coated with IgM are used to enumerate Tμ cells.

Functionally, Tμ cells act as T-helper cells in the PWM stimulation of B lymphocytes to produce antibody *in vitro* [17]. This helper function appears to be in concert with helper activity of an adherent cell, probably a monocyte.

The nature and function of the residual non-Tγ-non-Tμ cells is unknown.

CLINICAL RELEVANCE OF CELLULAR PROTEIN RECEPTORS

Distinction Between T and B Lymphocytes

After separating mononuclear cells from peripheral blood by centrifuging the buffy coat through a density gradient, such as Ficoll-hypaque or bovine serum albumin, monocytes can be removed either by adherence or by the effect of a weak magnetic field on carbonyl iron-ingested phagocytes. The resulting cell mixture contains T, B, and null lymphocytes. Because T but not B or null lymphocytes carry a receptor for sheep erythrocytes, incubation of this mixture with fresh-washed sheep red blood cells will result in the formation of E-rosettes representing the T cells [20].

B lymphocytes, on the other hand, can be detected by so-called EAC-rosettes by virtue of their C receptors. The EAC complex is composed of erythrocytes, anti-erythrocyte antibodies, and C. Rosette formation through the C receptors reflects B lymphocytes. An alternative approach is by immunofluorescence directed against surface Igs. This is best accomplished by fluoresceinated anti-Fab$'_{(2)}$ antibodies [21].

Those lymphocytes showing neither T nor B cell surface characteristics are termed null lymphocytes. Although this population may contain cytotoxic killer (K cell) activity [22], the precise nature of null cells is still under debate [23].

The value of measuring T/B/null cell profiles has been shown in the differential diagnosis of leukemias, in evaluation of immunodeficiency disorders, and in monitoring immunosuppression in transplant patients or patients with autoimmune disease [10,18].

Classification of Lymphocyte Subsets

The finding that Tγ cells are rich in T-suppressor activity and Tμ cells are rich in T-helper activity [13] has been useful in examining T-suppressor status in autoimmunity, cancer, and transplantation immunology [13,24]. The decreased T-suppressor activity in patients with systemic lupus erythematosus [25] is paralleled by a diminution in the number of Tγ cells detectable in the peripheral blood [26]. This approach is proving useful in evaluating agents for their purported immunoregulatory activity [27–31]. Recently, the development of monoclonal antibodies of these receptors has provided a new dimension of enthusiasm for T-cell subtyping [32–34]. One representative set of reagents includes the following: OKT3 antibody reactive with all T cells; OKT4 antibody reactive primarily with T-helper cells; and OKT5 (or OKT8) antibody reactive primarily with T-suppressor cells [32]. In some laboratories, this monoclonal antibody approach, used principally as a direct or indirect immunofluorescence technique, will likely replace the rosette approach.

Detection of Soluble Immune Complexes

The fact that certain cells carry Fc receptors at their surface may be used to advantage in detecting the presence of circulating immune complexes, which can be trapped by virtue of their exposed Fc portion. This approach has been most widely used with a radiolabeled antiglobulin in conjunction with Fc-receptor-bearing cells in the form of longterm human lymphoblastoid cell lines, such as the Raji cell [35]. Immune complexes can be shown not only in autoimmune disorders, but also in cancer and during transplant rejection. The understanding of the role of immune complexes in disease processes should be greatly facilitated by the availability of such procedures.

REFERENCES

1. Singer SJ: Architecture and topography of biologic membranes. In Weissmann G, Claiborne R (eds): "Cell Membranes—Biochemistry, Cell Biology, and Biology." New York: H.P. Publishing Co., 1975, p 35.
2. Cuatrecasas P, Greaves MF (eds): "Receptors and Recognition." London: Chapman and Hall, Ltd., 1975.
3. Cuatrecasas P: Membrane receptors. Annu Rev Biochem 43:169–214, 1974.
4. Ross GD , Polley MJ: Specificity of human lymphocyte complement receptors. J Exp Med 141:1163–1180, 1975.
5. Shevach EM, Jaffe ES, Green I: Receptors for complement and immunoglobulin on human and animal lymphoid cells. Transplant Rev 140:1324–1335, 1973.
6. Ross GD, Polley MJ: Assay for the two different types of lymphocyte complement receptors. Scand J Immunol 5 (Suppl 5):99–111, 1976.
7. Bianco C, Nussenzweig V: Complement receptors. Contemp Top Mol Immunol 6:145–176, 1977.
8. Gupta S, Ross GD, Good RA, Siegal FP: Surface characteristics of human eosinophils. J Allergy Clin Immunol 57:189, 1976.
9. Bianco C: Plasma membrane receptors for complement. In Day NK, Good RA (eds): "Comprehensive Immunology Series, Vol. 2: Biological Amplification Systems in Immunology." New York: Plenum Press, 1977, pp 69–84.
10. Preud'Homme J-L, Seligmann M: Surface immunoglobulins on human lymphoid cells. Prog Clin Immunol 2:121–174, 1974.

11. Nussenzweig V: Receptors for immune complexes on lymphocytes. Adv Immunol 19:217–258, 1974.
12. Sandilands GP, Gray K, Reid F, Anderson JR: Demonstration of Fc receptors on the surface of B lymphocytes. Int Arch Allergy Appl Immunol 57:411–417, 1978.
13. Moretta L, Ferrarini M: Characterization of human T-cell subpopulations as defined by specific receptors for immunoglobulins. Contemp Top Immunobiol 8:19–52, 1978.
14. Ferrarini M, Moretta L, Abrile R, Durante ML: Receptors for IgG molecules on human lymphocytes forming spontaneous rosettes with sheep red cells. Eur J Immunol 5:70, 1975.
15. Gormus BJ, Woodson M, Kaplan ME: Heterogeneity of human lymphocyte Fc receptors. I. Differential susceptibility to proteolysis. Clin Exp Immunol 34:268–273, 1978.
16. Clements PJ, Levy J: Receptors for IgG (Fc receptors) on human lymphocytes: Reevaluation by multiple techniques. Clin Exp Immunol 34:281–287, 1978.
17. Moretta L, Webb SR, Grossi C, Lydyard P, Cooper M: Functional analysis of two human T cell subpopulations: Help and suppression of B cell response by T cells bearing receptors for IgM or IgG. J Exp Med 146:184, 1977.
18. Russell IJ, Tomasi TB: Mechanisms and abnormalities of immune regulation. Pathobiol Annu 8:1–33, 1978.
19. Moretta L, Ferrarini M, Durante ML, Mingari MC: Expression of a receptor for IgM by human T cells in vitro. Eur J Immunol 5:565, 1975.
20. Jondal M: SRBC rosette formation as a human T lymphocyte marker. Scand J Immunol 5(Suppl 5):69–76, 1976.
21. Winchester RJ, Fu SM: Lymphocyte surface membrane immunoglobulin. Scand J Immunol 5(Suppl 5):77–82, 1976.
22. Gormus BJ, Woodson M, Kaplan ME: Heterogeneity of human lymphocyte Fc receptors. II. Relationship to antibody-dependent cell-mediated cytotoxicity. Clin Exp Immunol 34:274–280, 1978.
23. Hokland P, Hokland M, Heron I: Two small lymphocyte subpopulations in human peripheral blood. II. Functional characterization in vitro. Int Arch Allergy Appl Immunol 57:514–520, 1978.
24. Gupta S, Good RA: Subpopulations of human lymphocytes. III. Distribution and quantitation in peripheral blood, cord blood, tonsils, bone marrow, thymus, lymph nodes, and spleen. Cell Immunol 36:263–270, 1978.
25. Sagawa A, Abdou NI: Suppressor-cell dysfunction in systemic lupus erythematosus: Cells involved and in vitro correction. J Clin Invest 62:789–796, 1978.
26. Koriyama K, Daniels JC: T lymphocyte subsets in systemic lupus erythematosus. Clin Res 26:714A, 1978.
27. Wybran J, Govaerts A: Levamisole and human lymphocyte surface markers. Clin Exp Immunol 27:319–321, 1977.
28. Michalevicz R, Many A, Ramot B, Trainin N: The in vitro effect of thymic humoral factor and levamisole on peripheral blood lymphocytes in systemic lupus erythematosus patients. Clin Exp Immunol 31:111–115, 1978.
29. Lavastida MT, Goldstein AL, Daniels JC: Thymosin administration in autoimmune disorders. Thymus: 2:287–295, 1981.
30. Koriyama K, Daniels JC: Effect of in vitro thymosin on T lymphocyte subpopulations in systemic lupus erythematosus (SLE). J Immunopharmacol 2:381–396, 1980.
31. Haynes BF, Fauci AS: The differential effect of in vivo hydrocortisone on the kinetics of subpopulations of human peripheral blood thymus-derived lymphocytes. J Clin Invest 61:703, 1978.

32. Reinherz EL, Kung PC, Goldstein G, Schlossman SF:Further characterization of the human inducer T cell subset defined by monoclonal antibody. J Immunol 123:2894–2896, 1979.
33. Reinherz EL, Kung PC, Goldstein G, Schlossman SF: A monoclonal antibody reactive with the human cytotoxic/suppressor T cell subset previously defined by a heteroserum termed TH_2. J Immunol 124:1301–1307, 1980.
34. Reinherz EL, Schlossman SF: Current concepts in immunology. Regulation of the immune response—inducer and suppressor T-lymphocyte subsets in human beings. New Eng J Med 303:370–373, 1980.
35. Theofilopoulos AN, Wilson CB, Dixon FJ: The Raji cell radioimmune assay for detecting immune complexes in human sera, J Clin Invest 57:169–182, 1976.
36. Hahn GS: Antibody Structure, Function, and Active Sites. In Ritzmann SE (ed): "Physiology of Immunoglobulins: Diagnostic and Clinical Aspects." New York: Alan R. Liss, Inc., 1982, pp 193–304.

CLINICAL ASPECTS OF IMMUNOGLOBULIN ABNORMALITIES

Pathology of Immunoglobulins: Diagnostic and
Clinical Aspects, pages 111-160
© 1982 Alan R. Liss, Inc., 150 Fifth Avenue, New York, NY 10011

7

Immunoglobulin Deficiencies

Walter H. Hitzig, MD

HISTORICAL REVIEW

Bruton's account of A-γ-globulinemia in 1952 [27] is generally considered the starting point of a new development: he clearly demonstrated that congenital absence of γ-globulin leads to increased susceptibility to infections. Investigators in Boston and Minneapolis confirmed and extended these findings [61,62,85]. These clinical observations provided a direct demonstration that the γ-globulin fraction contains specific antibodies; it is remarkable that this fact, although recognized almost a decade earlier, had been ignored by physicians at the practical level.

It soon became apparent, however, that lack of γ-globulin is not a condition essential for an insufficient antibody makeup of a patient. Barandun [13], consequently, introduced the term *Antibody Deficiency Syndrome* (ADS) in 1955, which proved of great value, in particular for the connotation of acquired deficiencies in the elderly. Imbalance of immunoglobulin (Ig) subgroups was subsequently described as a special form of ADS by Yount et al. [151].

Immune reactions involving an intimate cooperation between humoral antibodies and specific cellular reactions were recognized almost simultaneously in 1958, both by extensive clinical observations and animal experiments: Infants with severe combined immunodeficiency syndrome (SCID) [71,139], as well as animals subjected to thymectomy or total-body irradiation [36], yielded valuable basic information. The dualistic theory of the organization of the human immune system into T and B lymphocytes, with a hierarchic order of central and peripheral compartments, was deduced from these earlier observations [37], and proved to be one of the most productive hypotheses in immunology, which, with only minor modifications, is still serving an extremely useful purpose. The recognition by DiGeorge in 1968 [45] of children with congenital aplasia of the thymus and pure T-cell deficiency supplemented the prior descriptions of the selective lack of B cells and A-γ-globulinemia, as well as the clinical examples of deficiencies of both the T- and B-cell systems, resulting in the combined immunodeficiency syndrome (IDS).

The number and complexity of these rapidly accumulating observations called for attempts at a clinically applicable classification; a committee appointed by the WHO provided recommendations in 1968 [126], which were modified and updated in 1970 [50], 1974 [35], and 1978 [140]. These recommendations were essentially based on developmental aspects of immunologically active cells and their precursors. This principle, however, was not satisfactory for all observations, and, therefore, new aspects were introduced into the last classification, including metabolic disturbances, such as enzyme deficiencies [57,58,67]. These enzyme deficiencies associated with immune disorders point toward new avenues, such as deficiencies of adenosine deaminase (ADA) and of the vitamin B_{12} transport protein transcobalamine II [72]. It seems probable that in the future still other aspects will need to be included, such as chromosomal abnormalities (e.g., quantitative numerical aberrations and partial deletions, and qualitative disturbances reflected by the tendency for breaks or inadequate repairs).

These new considerations should aid in the characterization of the true primary causes of the above-mentioned arrests in immune cell differentiation and/or maturation. It will therefore be unavoidable to include some cellular aspects in the following discussion, although this volume is essentially concerned with protein abnormalities [15,16,55,83,102,121,134,136].

THE IMMUNODEFICIENCY SYNDROMES (IDS)

Congenital and hereditary, or primary, IDS are rare disorders, but as "experiments of nature" they have been of extraordinary scientific and didactic value. They are considered here in the context of the T- and B-cell immune concept. Basically, the same principles will be applied to the consideration of acquired IDS. The outlines of the WHO classification [140] will be followed throughout, but cellular aspects are deemphasized, whereas findings in the humoral compartment are described more extensively.

PRIMARY IMMUNODEFICIENCY SYNDROMES (PIDS)

Table I, reflecting the WHO classification [140], summarizes the various features of this group of PIDS.

Severe Combined Immunodeficiency (SCID) (Table II)

The most severe as well as the most frequent form of primary IDS is characterized by almost complete lack of both humoral and cellular immune

TABLE I. Classification of Primary Specific Immunodeficiencies

Designation	Usual phenotypic expression		Presumed level of basic cellular defect[a]	Known or presumed pathogenetic mechanism	Inheritance[b]	Main associated features
	Functional deficiencies	Cellular abnormalities				
1. Severe combined ID						
(a) Reticular dysgenesis	CMI[c], Ab[d], and phagocytes	↓ T, B, and phagocytes	HSC	Unknown	AR	—
(b) "Swiss type"	CMI and Ab	↓ T and B	LSC	Unknown	AR	—
(c) ADA deficiency	CMI and Ab	↓ T ± B	LSC or early T	Metabolic effects of ADA deficiency	AR	± Chondrocyte abnormalities
(d) With B lymphocytes	CMI and Ab	↓ T (B lymphocytes without or with normal isotype diversity)	Early T ± early B	Unknown	X-linked or AR	—
(e) Others						
2. Thymic hypoplasia (Di George syndrome)	CMI and impaired Ab	↓ T	Thymus	Embryopathy of 3rd and 4th pharyngeal pouch area	Usually not familial	(1) Hypoparathyroidism (2) Abnormal facies (3) Cardiovascular abnormalities
3. PNP deficiency	CMI ± Ab	↓ T	T	Metabolic effects of PNP deficiency	AR	Hypoplastic anaemia
4. ID with ataxia telangiectasia	CMI and Ab (partial)	↓ T and plasma cells (mainly IgA, IgE, ± IgG)	Early T and defective terminal differentiation of B lymphocytes	Unknown ? Faulty thymic epithelium ? DNA repair defect	AR	(1) Cerebellar ataxia (2) Telangiectasia (3) Ovarian dysgenesis (4) Chromosomal abnormalities

(Continued on next page)

TABLE I (Continued)

Designation	Usual phenotypic expression		Presumed level of basic cellular defect[a]	Known or presumed pathogenetic mechanism	Inheritance[b]	Main associated features
	Functional deficiencies	Cellular abnormalities				
5. ID with thymoma	Ab and impaired CMI (variable)	↓ pre-B and B ± ↓ T	HSC	Unknown	none	(1) Thymoma (2) Eosinopenia (3) Erythroblastopenia (4) Aplastic anaemia
6. X-linked Agammaglobulinaemia	Ab	↓ B	Pre-B	Unknown	X-linked	—
7. Transcobalamin II deficiency	Ab and phagocytosis	↓ Plasma cells	Failure of terminal differentiation of B lymphocytes	Metabolic effects of vitamin B_{12} deficiency	AR	(1) Pancytopenia with megaloblastic anaemia (2) Intestinal villous atrophy
8. Selective IgA deficiency	IgA Ab	↓ IgA plasma cells ± ↑ Bα lymphocytes ± ↓ T	Terminal differentiation of Bα lymphocytes impaired	(1) ? ↑ T_S (2) ? ↓ T_H (3) ? intrinsic B-cell defect	Unknown > AR > AD; frequent in families of patients with varied ID	(1) Occasional 18-chromosomal deletions (2) Anti-IgA antibodies
9. Selective deficiency of one other Ig class or subclass	Ab	↓ Plasma cells ± ↓ T	Unknown	Unknown ? ↑ T_S	Unknown	—
10. Secretory piece deficiency	Secretory IgA Ab	↓ Intestinal IgA plasma cells	Mucosal epithelial cell	Unknown	Unknown	—
11. Ig deficiencies with increased IgM	Ab	↓ IgG and IgA plasma cells, ↑ IgM plasma cells, ± ↑ B lymphocytes	Failure of terminal differentiation of Bγ and Bα lymphocytes	Unknown	X-linked or AR or unknown	—
12. Ig deficiencies with IgM production and without γ- and α-cells	Ab	Absent Bγ and Bα lymphocytes	Pre-B or B	Faulty isotype diversification	AR or unknown	—
13. Transient hypogammaglobulinaemia of infancy	Ab	↓ Plasma cells	Impaired terminal differentiation of B lymphocytes	? ↓ T help	Frequent in heterozygous individuals in families with various severe combined ID	—

14. Antibody deficiency with normal or hypergammaglobulinaemia	Impaired Ab for some antigens (mainly primary response)	↓ B	Pre-B or early B	? Reduced clonal size or diversity	AR in some	—
15. Kappa chain deficiency	Ab	↓ Bκ	Pre-B	Unknown	Unknown or familial	—
16. Wiskott-Aldrich syndrome	Ab to certain antigens (mainly polysaccharides and CMI (progressive)	↓ T and B (progressive)	Unknown	Unknown	X-linked	(1) Thrombocytopenia (2) Eczema
17. Varied ID (common and largely unclassified)						
(a) Predominant Ig deficiency	Ab ± CMI	± ↓ B	Pre-B or B in some	(1) intrinsic B-cell defect (2) Underproduction of B cells (3) ? ↑ T_S (4) ? ↓ T_H (5) Autoantibodies to B cells	Unknown or familial	—
(b) Predominant T-cell deficiency	CMI ± Ab	↓ T	Early T or T_H	(1) Unknown (2) Autoantibodies to T cells	Unknown or familial	—

↓ ↑ = Decrease or increase in level.
[a] HSC = haemopoietic stem cell; LSC = lymphopoietic stem cell.
[b] AR = autosomal recessive; AD = autosomal dominant.
[c] CMI = cell-mediated immunity.
[d] Ab = antibody.
From Torrigiani [140].

TABLE II. Severe Combined Immunodeficiency Syndrome (SCID)

Clinical features
  Polytopic severe infections since early infancy
  Malnutrition
  Pneumopathy
  Candidiasis
  Morbilliform rashes
  Death within first year of life
Laboratory characteristics
  Lymphocyte count diminished (rarely normal)
  Lymphocyte functions impaired
  Thymus absent or very small, not descended
  Immunoglobulins diminished (rarely normal)
  Antibody formation impaired
  Infecting agents: pathogenic as well as opportunistic bacteria, viruses, fungi
Heredity
  X-linked, recessive
  Autosomal recessive (ADA deficiency). Carriers detectable; prenatal diagnosis possible
  Sporadic = not inherited
Pathogenesis: varied, e.g., known enzymatic disturbances, inactive adenosine deaminase = ADA
  Graft versus host disease (mother versus fetus)
  Prenatal infection (rubella)
  Stem cell disease
Treatment
  Complete cure by grafting immunocytes (compatible bone marrow, thymus, fetal liver)

reactions [73]. The following alternative designations from previous descriptions should now be deleted: lymphocytophthisis [60], familial lymphopenia with A-γ-globulinemia [139], hereditary lymphoplasmocytic dysgenesis [78], thymic alymphoplasia [59], thymic dysplasia [104,150].

Heredity. The parents of patients with SCID are healthy and immunologically normal. The family history, however, may arouse suspicion: consanguinity of the parents, a disproportionate number of infant deaths, or a similar disease in siblings. Both autosomal recessive and X-chromosomal recessive transmission have been noted; in addition, sporadic cases occur. The heterozygotic carrier state can only be recognized in adenosine deaminase deficiency (see below), for which prenatal diagnosis, using fibroblast cultures from amniotic fluid, is feasible [67]. Finally, a nonhereditary prenatal cause may be provided by transplacental transmission of maternal lymphoid cells into the fetus with formation of an active clone leading to a graft-versus-host reaction [140] and subsequent destruction of the fetal immune system; a similar effect may be caused by prenatal rubella infections [129]. Increased chromosomal breaks were described in one case [84].

Clinical features

CASE FI.S. [78]

This girl was the sixth daughter of consanguineous parents (first cousins) (Fig. 1b). Three of her sisters had died previously, with essentially the same clinical picture, between 3 and 9 months of age. Although the diagnosis in this girl was made at birth from cord blood, she gradually developed all the classical signs of SCID: at 1 month she presented with oral thrush, which slowly progressed and later involved parts of the skin. Characteristic measles-like exanthemas, seen in most of these patients, have been attributed to this chronic fungal infection. Bacterial infections of the skin later caused multiple abscesses in this patient. At age 4 months, diarrhea started, which soon became intractable and led to severe malnutrition and failure to thrive. No pathogens were found in the stools (in other cases pathogenic *E. coli* or pyogenic germs as well as various fungi are encountered). Finally, at 5 months of age cough started, which became pertussis-like and difficult to treat. Pneumonia finally led to death at the age of 7 months.

Comments. This combination and course of infections is characteristic for SCID: polytopic inflammations due to pyogenic or opportunistic germs affect predominantly the integuments (skin and mucosae of gastrointestinal and pulmonary tracts) and cause lethal malnutrition or pneumopathy, often resulting in septicemia, sometimes with meningeal involvement, with high spiking fever and terminal marasmus.

Laboratory findings are quite characteristic, consisting of severe and usually persistent lymphocytopenia ($<1000/\mu L$, but usually $<100/\mu L$), complete lack of lymphocytic reactions, as evidenced by failure to respond to intradermal antigen injection, as well as *in vitro* stimulation to mitogens such as phytohemagglutinin (PHA) or to specific antigens. During the first few months of life, complete A-γ-globulinemia develops (after "consumption" of the transplacentally transmitted maternal IgG). Chest x-ray reveals absence of a thymus shadow. At autopsy the entire lymphatic system is extremely atrophic, the thymus is absent or reduced to a small trace, and is sometimes found in abnormal locations high in the neck region. Lymph nodes are barely discernable, the spleen is very small, and the Peyer's patches of the gut are absent. Accordingly, histological findings in the lymphatic system are quite characteristic [39], and consist of a predominance of reticulum cells and severe lymphocytopenia, lack of germinal centers and of Hassall's bodies in the thymus. Granulocytic reactions, however, are generally normal, with the exception of the most severe form of reticular dysgenesis, which also involves granulo- and monocytopenia [43].

The special form of IDS associated with adenosine deaminase (ADA) deficiency [2,58,67,73], manifests itself somewhat differently, since hypo-γ-globulinemia develops later in life and is less severe. Laboratory findings are characteristic and pathognomonic, consisting of ADA deficiency both in erythrocytes and lymphocytes.

A number of other subgroups of IDS have been described, but they have not been recognized as special forms by the WHO committee [140]. One

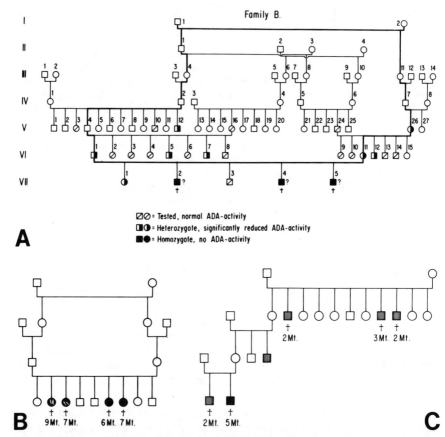

Fig. 1. Pedigree of families with severe combined immunodeficiency (SCID). A) Autosomal-recessive transmission in a family with ADA deficiency: The heterozygous carriers can be identified. B) Autosomal-recessive transmission in a family with normal ADA: identification of the heterozygous carriers is impossible. C) X-linked recessive transmission—SCID in males over three generations. The female carriers cannot be identified. B, C) Open symbols, normal individual; striped symbols, clinical findings of SCID but laboratory data are inadequate; solid symbols, typical clinical and laboratory findings of SCID. Mt = months of age at death.

such subgroup is the "Nezelof syndrome" [111], which may represent a variation of SCID with relatively high numbers of B lymphocytes. Combination of IDS with rare forms of malformations have been described. These include dysostoses leading to "short limbed dwarfism," and hair anomalies, such as the "cartilage hair hypoplasia." Attempts at further classifications (e.g., short-limbed dwarfism type I with combined IDS, type II with cellular IDS, type III with humoral IDS) remain purely descriptive and offer no further pathogenetic or etiologic insight [50a].

The clinical picture with the almost complete vanishment of the immunological system is merely the end result of different processes, two of which have been thoroughly investigated:

1) Failing differentiation of stem cells [34,53,73,135]: either the reservoir of undifferentiated hematopoietic stem cells fails to produce sufficient supplies, or the dominating controlling organs (i.e., thymus and bursa equivalent) are unable to modulate these stem cells to transform into effective T and B cells. It has been estimated that about one-third of observed cases are due to this mechanism; recent data, however, reduce this number to about one-tenth [53].

2) Deficient metabolic processes may inhibit differentiated T and B cells to mature or to further differentiate. This mechanism is well known for ADA deficiency [2,58,67]. The ubiquitous enzyme ADA degrades adenosine into inosine in a one-way reaction (Fig. 2). If inactive, adenosine and its metabolic products accumulate, especially adenosine monophosphate and hydroxy adenosine, which are both toxic to the lymphatic system if present in high concentrations. The lymphatic tissue, which is normal at birth, undergoes destruction or inactivation during the early postnatal period.

Therapy. Conventional therapy with antiinfectious agents only temporarily can combat acute bacterial infections. Replacement of Ig, even in large doses, is of little help, since the cellular immune mechanisms are also deficient [73]. However, the transplantation of compatible immunologic cells or organs has achieved spectacular and permanent reconstitution in numerous cases; in particular, the transplantation of bone marrow derived from compatible siblings has a success rate of more than 50% in patients with SCID [87]. Implantation of viable fetal organs, in particular fetal thymus and liver, or of thymic epithelium derived from immunologically healthy donors and cultured *in vitro* for 10 to 20 days, also leads to long-lasting although less predictable results, [8,31,32,65,73,81–83]. Even in this situation, at least partial HLA identity appears to be a prerequisite if Zinkernagel's [152,153] animal experiments bear a clinical analogy. Injection of various thymic factors and hormones can achieve temporary correction of immune reactions, but only as long as these agents are regularly administered [10,75,98,112,113,131,144].

Thymic Hypoplasia (Table III)

This sporadic disease has no hereditary basis but is due to arrested development of the third and fourth branchial arches and pouches during the 6th to 10th gestational weeks [45,100]. Accordingly, a combined malformation syndrome results, consisting of hypoplasia of the mandibles, ears, parathyroid glands, thymus, occasionally the thyroid gland, and of the aortic

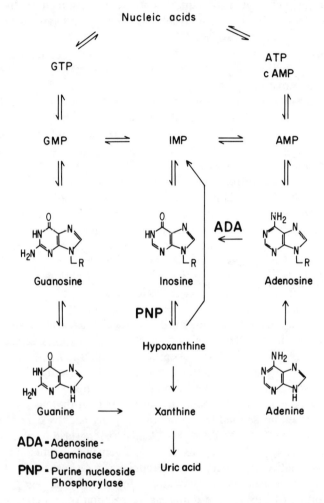

Fig. 2. Metabolism of purine-nucleotides: crucial steps for normal immunological functions are catalyzed by adenosin deaminase (ADA) and by purine nucleotide phosphorylase (PNP).

arch with complex cardiac anomalies. One family with apparently hereditary disease has been observed [133].

The clinical features of this syndrome are quite characteristic: the baby is born with the above-mentioned malformations. If untreated, severe generalized convulsions develop within the first week of life, which are the result of hypocalcemia due to hypoparathyroidism. If appropriately treated with calcium and parathyroid hormone, the patient survives this critical early

TABLE III. Immunodeficiency Syndrome with Thymic Aplasia (DiGeorge syndrome)

Clinical features
  Multiple malformations (variable):
    mandibular hypoplasia
    ear deformities
    cardiovascular anomalies
  Early signs: tetany, hypocalcemic convulsions during first week
  Late signs: multiple infections, end of first year
Laboratory characteristics
  Lymphocyte number normal
  Lymphocyte function impaired
  Immunoglobulin levels normal
  Antibody formation impaired
Heredity
  nonsporadic cases (one family described)
Pathogenesis
  Arrested development of third and fourth branchial pouches; leads to hypoplasia or
    aplasia of mandible, thymus, parathyroids, and aortic arch
Treatment
  Implantation of fetal thymus may restore immunological functions

phase, but after several months the patient develops the typical manifestations of IDS: lymphocytes are present in normal numbers but they fail to respond to antigenic and mitogenic stimulation, both *in vivo* (negative intracutaneous reactions) and *in vitro* (no response to PHA, pokeweed mitogen (PWM), or specific antigens). The concentrations of Ig are within normal ranges, but specific antibodies are completely lacking. This can be explained by faulty helper functions of T lymphocytes to instruct B lymphocytes for their appropriate responses. Although this part of the syndrome can be favorably influenced by injection of Ig preparations, the severe cellular defect often leads to early death.

Implantation of fetal thymus has led to immunological reconstitution in several patients [9]. This treatment, however, may be considered to be ethically objectionable, since it fails to correct the severe anatomical malformations. The incomplete or partial syndrome of thymic hypoplasia is much more frequently encountered than the complete form with the total absence of the thymus [100]. These patients may immunologically recover after 3 months and become practically normal.

Immunodeficiency Associated With Deficiency of Purine-Nucleoside-Phosphorylase (PNP)

PNP degrades inosine to hypoxanthine, in the metabolic sequence following the above-outlined ADA action [67,124] (Fig. 2). Its deficiency has been observed on a familial and sporadic basis [57]. The presenting manifestation is hypoplastic anemia of the Blackfan-Diamond type. In this context, the IDS presents only a secondary nonlife-threatening feature.

Immunodeficiency With Ataxia-Telangiectasia

The triad of cerebellar ataxia, mucosal and cutaneous telangiectasias, and increased susceptibility to infections is clinically characteristic (Table IV) [21,23,24]. Its common denominator has not yet been fully elucidated. Failure to form connective tissue with resultant telangiectasias of the skin and cerebellum has been suggested as the underlying abnormality, but this mechanism does not explain the thymic dysplasia. A different finding of basic importance involves the chromosomes with a characteristic tendency toward breakage and markedly reduced DNA repair [41].

Clinical findings. Patients are usually symptom-free during infancy and early childhood. The clinical triad [23] slowly develops during school age: the children's handwriting deteriorates, and their gait becomes unstable to such a degree that they may become confined to a wheelchair prior to puberty; their body posture resembles that of an aged patient with Parkinsonism. The speech becomes slurred and difficult to understand. The severe deterioration of body functions, however, is contrasted by the intelligence which remains intact, and with appropriate support, such patients can perform very well in school. Equally surprising is the fact that the psychological behavior remains well balanced. The neurological deterioration is usually arrested after an otherwise normal puberty, but soon thereafter, most patients develop progeria, possibly due to accelerated aging of connective and other tissues.

Infections predominantly affect the respiratory tract (85% sinopulmonary infections). However, an unknown percentage of patients, treated by neurologists, might be free of infections and of immunological problems.

The most frequent, albeit inconstant, laboratory finding is the lack of serum and secretory IgA. Local IgA deficiency explains the topical distribution of infections. In this situation, replacement therapy with injection of Ig preparations is inadequate. Recently, an additional deficiency of the IgG_2 subclass has been found in all 22 patients with ataxia-telangiectasia examined by Oxelius et al. [113a,b] (for details see below, section on selective IgA deficiency). α-Fetoprotein is greatly increased in serum.

Another characteristic feature is the high predilection for malignant tumors, mainly lymphomas, which occur in approximately 10% of these patients, during the first 20 years of life [51,88]. Impairment of the immunologic surveillance has been suggested as the underlying cause [29], however, the finding of numerous chromosomal breaks and of insufficient repair of DNA, possibly due to enzyme deficiencies, suggests that the frequency of mutations in such patients is much higher than in normal individuals [138]. This ten-

TABLE IV. Immunodeficiency Syndrome with Ataxia-Telangiectasia (AT)

Clinical features
  Cerebellar ataxia
    starts at preschool or school age
    progresses until puberty, then remains unchanged
    progeria-like premature aging
  Telangiectasias of skin (face) and mucosae (conjunctiva)
  Recurrent infections (especially sinupulmonary forms)
Laboratory characteristics: variable
    immunoglobulin changes, e.g., IgA low or absent in 80%, other Ig changes may occur
    lymphocyte functions impaired, especially T-lymphocytes
    α-fetoprotein in serum increased
    chromosomal breaks
    impaired DNA repair
    at autopsy, thymic dysplasia and cerebellar atrophy
Heredity
  Autosomal recessive. Carriers not detectable
Pathogenesis: unknown
  Connective tissue anomaly may lead to degeneration of cerebellum and thymus
  Impaired DNA repair may predispose to malignancies
Treatment
  None

dency toward chromosomal breakage could explain the markedly abnormal reaction to irradiation with roentgen or γ-rays [41]. The response to cytostatic agents is probably also abnormal.

Immunodeficiency Syndrome With Thymoma

Tumors of the thymus may lead to reversible IDS, usually presenting as a typical ADS [86]. Histological examination reveals a strikingly abnormal B lymphocyte system consisting of a paucity or absence of plasma cells in the peripheral lymphatic tissues and a lack of germinal centers. Specific antibodies are not formed after appropriate antigenic stimulation. These seemingly contradictory findings could not be reconciled previously, but they may now be interpreted as an impairment of the T- and B-cell cooperation [36,63]. On the other hand, frequently autoantibodies are formed, often with specificity for striated muscles. Their presence sometimes, but not always, coincides with the development of myasthenia gravis. These clinical manifestations occur relatively late in life (25 to 77 years, mean 50 years). This fact together with a lack of familial incidence, argues against a primary cause and suggests an acquired disorder. The size of the thymic tumors differs between 42 and 2050 g. After complete surgical removal of the tumor, the IDS regresses—in a few instances, completely. In a few instances, malignant tumors have developed, mostly of the lymphatic system.

Infantile Sex-Linked A-γ-globulinemia

This classical example of IDS was the first clearly delineated form of IDS. It is defined as X-chromosomally transmitted deficiency of B lymphocytes that fail to mature into plasma cells. From infancy, the affected boys are unable to synthesize Ig of any class and they develop no protective antibodies. Without treatment, these patients die during the first years of life of polytopic recurring infections [27,28,61,62,85].

Clinical features. The initial report by Bruton [27] presents such a succinct outline (Table V) of this disease entity that it might be quoted here:

A hitherto unrecognized entity manifested by complete absence of γ-globulin with otherwise normal serum proteins and recurrent pneumococcal sepsis is described in an 8-year-old male. The patient appears to be normal in other respects. . . . He was unable to produce antibody for the pneumococcus; a positive Schick test persisted in spite of numerous attempts to reverse it with diphtheria toxoid. No antibody could be demonstrated following administration of typhoid vaccine in the usual manner, and his serum was negative for complement-fixing antibodies of epidemic parotitis after he experienced a typical clinical picture of that disease.

γ-Globulin could be demonstrated in his serum after concentrated immune human serum globulin was administered subcutaneously, and its gradual disappearance could be followed. . . . Concurrently, and following the administration of human globulin (3.2 g γ-globulin) at monthly intervals, he has been free of pneumococcal sepsis for more than a year, whereas he had experienced clinical sepsis at least 19 times in the previous 4 years. . . . It is postulated that the patient's antibody mechanism has been altered so that he is no longer able to synthesize and/or to hold antibody to a specific organism.

Hereditary transmission by the sex-linked mode was added to this otherwise perfect description [85]. Today, we consider the following points to be important: the disease is rare—an incidence of 1 in 1 million to 13 in 1 million population has been calculated [132]. Earlier estimates are unreliable since they include also cases with SCID [61]. Although the sex-linked hereditary transmission is clear-cut in some large families, it is, however, not always apparent. Unfortunately, the healthy female carriers cannot yet be reliably identified, in spite of numerous such attempts. This failure might be a clue for a rather complex pathogenesis involving possibly an organisator gene for the overall Ig synthesis, or hyperactivity of a repressor gene that impedes the organisator gene [36,63,142,143].

The number of B cells in the peripheral blood is usually markedly decreased, but in a few patients normal numbers of B cells have been encountered. This situation may be analogous to the induction of A-γ-globulinemia in animal experiments, by destruction of the bursa of Fabricius in freshly hatched birds. However, even the most thorough investigation of patients has not provided any definite clue for the localization of a bursa equivalent in man. In the rare patient with normal B-cell numbers, the pathogenesis of A-γ-globulinemia is probably different; further differentiation of

TABLE V. Congenital A-γ-globulinemia, X-linked

Clinical features
    Recurring polytopic severe infections
    Lymphatic tissue atrophic (tonsils, lymph nodes)
    First signs during preschool or school age, rarely during infancy
    Death during first year of life if no treatment
Laboratory characteristics
    Immunoglobulins markedly diminished ($\ll$ 10% of normal values)
    Lymphocyte count normal
    Lymphocyte functions normal
    B lymphocytes absent, rarely normal
    Antibodies and antibody formation absent
    Histology of lymphatic tissue
        generalized atrophy
        no germinal centers
        no plasma cells
    Infectious agents: bacterial, encapsulated pathogens
Heredity
    X-linked recessive
    Carriers not detectable
Pathogenesis
    Maturation arrest of pre-B lymphocytes
    Anomaly of regulator gene for Ig synthesis?
Treatment
    Immunoglobulin substitution every 2–6 weeks leads to complete remission

the B cells into plasma cells is most likely blocked. One patient, with lack of Clq [91], and transient A-γ-globulinemia associated with vitamin B_{12} deficiency, will be further discussed [76].

Diagnosis. The typical history of recurring polytopic infections leads to the suspicion of an underlying ADS. This diagnosis can be confirmed by serum protein electrophoresis which shows complete lack of the entire γ-globulin fraction (Fig. 3). Supplementary determination of Ig classes always shows IgG below 20 mg/dL and often below the limits of detectability. Likewise, IgM and IgA are extremely low. Of course, previous injections of γ-globulin, or administration of plasma or other blood products may result in Ig levels spuriously above the patient's baseline concentrations.

The absence of specific antibodies can easily be ascertained by the determination of "natural antibodies," such as isohemagglutinins, or of antistreptolysin titers, or the streptozyme test, which will be negative. Since children usually have been immunized previously, specific antibodies against diphtheria and tetanus may be determined; the titers are usually negative in

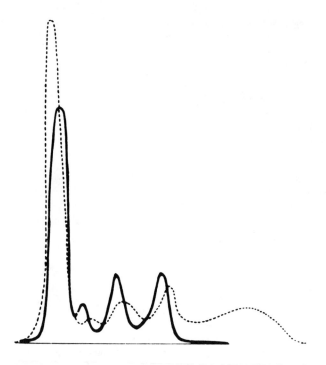

Fig. 3. Electrophoresis of serum from 7-year old boy with congenital A-γ-globulinemia: solid line. Normal control for comparison: dotted line.

	Total protein	Albumin	α_1	α_2	β	γ-Globulin
Control	71 g/L	42	3	6	9	11
Patient	52	26	5	9	11	<0.1

such patients. For confirmation, these immunizations can be repeated one to three times, with expected negative antibody responses.

A morphological clue for the atrophy of the lymphatic system is the complete absence of tonsils on inspection, and the lack of adenoid tissue on lateral skull x-rays. Additional tests are of little practical importance: the blood count and differential (CBC) are essentially normal, and the lymphocyte number is not decreased. Functional tests of lymphocytes *in vivo* and *in vitro* show normal response patterns to mitogenic or antigenic stimulation; and finally, in the past it has been shown that allogeneic skin transplants are rejected normally.

TABLE VI. Immunoglobulins for Therapy

A) Indications			Dosage
1. Prophylaxis for			
— viral diseases, e.g., measles			1–10 mg/kg
— toxins, e.g., tetanus			0.01–0.1 mg/kg
— erythrocyte antigens (RhD)			0.001–0.01 mg/kg
2. Substitution for antibody deficiency every 4 (2–6) weeks			100–200 mg/kg
B) Preparations	Contain	Route	T/2
Plasma/blood	IgG,IgM,IgA	IV	1–3 weeks
Standard γ-globulin			
16.5%[a]	IgG	IM	2–3 weeks
IV γ-globulin	IgG	IV	½–1 week
Older preparations 5%	IgG	IV	½–1 week
Newer preparations			
lyophilized	IgG	IV	3 weeks

Specific preparations rich in antibodies against tetanus, vaccinia, varicella, etc., are available

C) Side effects

Clinical features: during or immediately after injection rapid emergence of
— shock with hypotension and cyanosis
— respiratory symptoms: cough, dyspnea, asthma
— skin signs, urticaria, rapidly changing rashes

Etiology and pathogenesis:
1. Anticomplementary reactions: immunoglobulin-aggregates immediately activate the complement cascade
2. Phlogistic reactions: infused antibodies opsonize bacteria which are rapidly phagocytized and thus provoke an inflammatory reaction
3. Kinin-produced reactions due to vasoactive kallikrein-like substances in the preparation
4. Anaphylactic reactions by antibodies vs. IgA, formed in patients with isolated IgA deficiency

[a]Ed. Note: In order to convert the γ-globulin concentration of this liquid preparation into mL/kg, it is necessary to multiply the suggested mg/kg dose by a factor of 6; e.g., a 10-kg infant requiring 0.1 g/kg γ-globulin solution should receive 10 kg × 0.1 g/kg × 6 (dilution factor) = 6 mL.

Therapy. In an extension of the therapeutic approach to A-γ-globulinemia, the efficacy of γ-globulin substitution therapy has been clearly demonstrated (Table VI): if Ig preparations containing specific antibodies are injected in sufficient amounts, the patients remain practically free of infections. Intramuscular injection of commercial γ-globulin concentrates (16.5%) at a dose of 0.1–0.2 g γ-globulin/kg body weight (approximately 0.6–1.2 mL/kg body weight), repeated every 3 weeks, are given with satisfactory results. However, the large volumes required cause considerable discomfort to the patient, which often lasts several days. A certain amount of the injected Ig is locally degraded by proteolytic enzymes and it never reaches the circultaion.

Attempts have been made to avoid these drawbacks by developing Ig preparations that can be administered intravenously. This is feasible by the administration of plasma. The i.v. route of administration of γ-globulin concentrates, however, leads to severe, even life-threatening complications [68,70,77,106]. These side effects occur predominantly in severely hypogammaglobulinemic patients, i.e., those who need this therapy most. The pathogenesis of these complications has recently been clarified [111a]:

Anticomplementary reactions. γ-Globulin aggregates in the preparation rapidly activate the complement cascade leading to a deleterious release of biologically active substances, i.e., autacoids.[1] They produce dramatic shocklike manifestations of respiratory distress (cough, dyspnea, asthma) and skin lesions (including rapidly changing urticaria). During bouts of shaking chills the temperature may rise quickly to 40°C. Recently, modified and more careful manufacturing techniques have yielded γ-globulin preparations which are practically free of IgG aggregates; these newer γ-globulin preparations are tolerated well when given intravenously [154].

Phlogogenic reactions. A slow rise of body temperature occurs within 1 to 6 hours after the intravenous infusion of the γ-globulin preparation. The rapid opsonization of microorganisms and their subsequent phagocytosis seems to explain this phenomenon.

Kinin-generated reactions. Rapidly occurring vascular changes and urticarial rashes may be produced by kinins which are not removed from the γ-globulin preparation by the manufacturing process.

Anaphylactic reactions. They have been observed in IgA-deficient patients after repeated treatment with IgA-containing preparations. These patients are able to produce antibodies against IgA, which are responsible for these reactions.

With intravenous γ-globulins, higher IgG serum concentrations are achieved, since the IgG remains in the circulation for longer periods of time; the T/2 of about 20 days is comparable with that of native IgG. This fact, therefore, allows the sustenance of a higher baseline concentration (i.e., IgG value prior to the next injection). The dose is calculated on an individual basis, taking into account the patient's serum immunoglobulin concentration and the blood volume. This new technical approach to γ-globulin substitution has substantially improved the effectiveness and safety of the management of severely hypo-γ-globulinemic patients (see also Table VI for indications of γ-globulin therapy).

---

[1]Ed. note: Autacoids is a collective term for mediators and modulators of inflammation such as histamine, prostaglandins of the E and A series, and the β-mimetic catecholamines [155].

Prognosis. During the earlier time periods, all patients with this γ-globulin deficiency died of overwhelming infections, usually within the first years of life. With appropriate antibiotic treatment, they survived but suffered from recurrent bacterial infections. During recent years, however, substitution therapy with γ-globulin has kept most patients free of severe infections, and enabled them to lead practically normal lives. A new syndrome of *late manifestation,* however, has emerged in the guise of rheumatoid arthritis. This complication, however, can be avoided by effective γ-globulin treatment; it is, therefore, not caused by the disease itself, but probably by its infectious episodes. More severe and usually lethal complications are due to chronic ECHO virus infections that manifest themselves by myositis and encephalitis. These patients could possibly be protected by treatment with specific antibodies to ECHO viruses [8a]. Gastrointestinal disease is infrequently encountered, which may occasionally pose major clinical problems. Several causative agents have been identified, such as Lamblia Giardia, Coccidia, and intraepithelial bacteria [8a,111a].

Deficiency of Transcobalamin II

Vitamin B_{12} (cobalamine) in the circulation is bound to specific proteins, the transcobalamins (TC) [74]. One of these, the TC II, is of vital importance since the congenital deficiency [72] leads within the first weeks of life—after an apparently normal intrauterine development—to rapidly progressing abnormalities of hematopoiesis (macrocytic anemia, pancytopenia), of the gastrointestinal tract (vomiting, diarrhea, atrophy of mucosal membranes), and of immune reactions (A-γ-globulinemia, phagocytic dysfunctions). Injection of pharmacological doses of vitamin B_{12} (1–2 mg daily intramuscularly) results in dramatic clinical improvement and rapid normalization of the pancytopenia. The pathogenetic basis of these abnormalities is most likely the inability of vitamin B_{12}-deficient cells to divide, which, in turn, leads to deleterious consequences, especially in the rapidly proliferating tissues (i.e., bone marrow, enteric mucosa, immune system).

In a patient suffering from IDS associated with TC II deficiency, humoral immunodeficiency prevailed [76]: although B lymphocytes were present in sufficient numbers in the peripheral blood of this patient, the level of Ig was markedly reduced, and no antibody formation could be elicited in spite of intensive antigenic stimulation. There appeared, however, some effect on the immunocompetent cells: after adequate vitamin B_{12} treatment not only a spontaneous rise of serum γ-globulin concentration was noted, but also a vigorous degree of specific antibody formation occurred within a few days following one single antigenic stimulation. This antibody reaction was of the secondary type, i.e., antibodies were predominantly of the IgG class. Therefore, B-cell differentiation takes place even in the vitamin B_{12}-deficient state, but clonal expansion of antigenically primed plasma cells appears blocked. The latter effect, however, can rapidly be overcome as a result of "lubrication" of the intracellular "machinery" by the supplied vitamin B_{12}. With continued vitamin B_{12} therapy, the Ig concentrations and antibody functions have remained normal. The patient, however, continued to suffer from recurring severe pulmonary infections; several episodes of life-threatening bouts of fibrinoplastic bronchitis and pulmonary infections occurred. Some phagocytic functions were abnormal; in particular, the in vitro killing of staphylococcus aureus was greatly reduced [16,89,136]. Infusion of plasma saturated with vitamin B_{12} (in order to provide the patient with the essential TC II) led to the normalization of granulocytic functions and an increase of intracellular B_{12} metabolites. Incidentally, the oral administration of tetrahydrofolic acid (leucovorin factor) also normalized all granulocytic functions [125] in this patient.

Selective IgA Deficiency

Selective IgA deficiency is considered to be the most frequent IDS [7,30,83,130]. This statement is based on older studies and systematic assays of serum IgA in healthy blood donors; 0.2% of these were found to be IgA-deficient [11]. Some doubt, however, has recently arisen from diagnostic uncertainties: the application of the strict definition of IgA deficiency—namely, requiring the demonstration of no detectable IgA in serum and mucosal secretions—greatly reduces the frequency of this syndrome. An alternative and less strict definition of selective IgA deficiency only requires that patients have <5 mg/dL of serum IgA, irrespective of secretory IgA levels. If, however, secretory IgA is also taken into account, then many of the so called IgA-deficient individuals are shown to actually produce IgA. In addition, transitory IgA deficiencies have been found on follow-up studies, which also were neglected by the earlier studies. This less demanding definition of selective IgA deficiency probably accounts, in large measure, for the marked differences of clinical manifestations reported, ranging from completely asymptomatic states to severely disabling disorders.

Recently, a combined deficiency of IgA and IgG_2 has been described as a new clinical and biochemical entity: these patients suffer from frequent sinopulmonary infections, presumably because of a lack of antibodies of IgG_2 subclass, against bacterial polysaccharide capsules, which are important virulence factors for Haemophilus influenzae type b and pneumococci. The IgG_2-deficient individuals are usually unable to produce antibodies against such subtypes [111a,113a,113b].

Pathogenesis. Selective IgA deficiency has been described in patients with anomalies, such as chromosomal aberrations and ataxia-telangiectasia, as well as syndromes due to prenatal viral infections; it has also been reported in seemingly normal individuals [68]. This syndrome, therefore, may be considered to represent one end result of different factors. The frequent involvement of chromosome 18 (partial deletion of the long arm, deletion of the short arm, ring formation and trisomy), has led to the presumption of the existence of a regulator gene for IgA synthesis at that location. The structural gene for IgA can be excluded in this position, however, since in all appropriately investigated cases, B cells carrying IgA on the membrane surface have been found. The C α-locus has been assigned for the large IGH-cluster on chromosome 14, which codes for the constant regions of all Ig classes. Therefore, only inhibition of maturation into plasma cells, or of IgA release from mature plasma cells, needs to be considered. Stimulation of *in vitro*-cultured patients' lymphocytes by poke weed mitogen (PWM) provokes maturation into plasma cells and activation of the excretion mechanism. The possibility of an overwhelming suppressor mechanism due to T-suppressor cells or inadequate promotion by T-helper cells must also be considered [63,143] as possible pathogenetic mechanisms.

Clinical features. The clinical spectrum encompasses the entire range from complete absence of symptoms and signs, on the one hand, to severe disease manifestations, on the other [30,83,130].

Four outstanding features of selective IgA deficiency are frequently encountered:

Respiratory infections. Frequently, recurrent or chronic otitis media, sinusitis, tonsillitis, pharyngitis, and pneumonia are encountered. Lack of IgA might not be the only Ig deficiency, since in a number of patients an additional deficiency of IgE has been documented, and this combined IgA and IgE deficiency, might be responsible for these clinical manifestations. A precarious balance between IgA and IgE levels appears important for the protection of mucosal surfaces (see below, *Atopy*). The above-mentioned combined IgA-IgG$_2$ deficiency may be of even greater importance in this respect [113a].

Atopy. Atopy presenting with allergic rhinitis, asthma, urticaria, and eczema is found with inordinate frequency in patients with selective IgA deficiency. Such patients may have high or excessive concentrations of IgE, which could partly account for their clinical manifestations. The increased production of IgE might be a primary (hereditary?) phenomenon, or an (secondary) attempt to compensate for the increased mucosal permeability by foreign antigens due to the lack of secretory IgA.

The "IgA-deficient sprue syndrome." This disorder is well delineated; it consists of gastrointestinal signs, including abdominal pain, vomiting, diarrhea with malabsorption and steatorrhea [40]. On biopsy, the mucosa is flat and without villi, and in histological sections the submucosa contains a normal number of plasma cells, which, however do not produce IgA. Gluten-free diet occasionally leads to some clinical improvement, but the IgA deficiency persists. The pathogenesis of the syndrome is uncertain, but anomalies in the gut flora or autoimmune phenomena have been implicated. Ammann and Hong [7] have demonstrated autoantibodies with specificity for the basal membranes of the gastrointestinal epithelium.

Autoimmune diseases. An inordinate incidence of autoimmune diseases is encountered in selective IgA deficiency [7,30]. They include rheumatoid arthritis, lupus erythematosus, dermatomyositis, thyroiditis, pernicious anemia, chronic active hepatitis, Sjogren's syndrome, thrombocytopenic purpura, hemolytic anemia, Crohn's disease, ulcerative colitis, and pulmonary idiopathic hemosiderosis. The lack of the protective function of the secretory IgA system may enable antigens to penetrate the mucosal surfaces and reach the circulation where they could stimulate immunological responses. Long beyond infancy, these patients may still absorb "unprocessed" milk proteins and, as a consequence, produce high titers of precipitating antibodies against cow's milk proteins that cross-react with host tissues, thus acting as "auto-antibodies."

Diagnosis. Strict criteria for the assay of Ig concentrations, in particular of IgA, must be fulfilled, which was not necessarily the case in the older literature. IEP analysis of serum is not sufficiently sensitive for this purpose. Acceptable methods must be sensitive enough to detect concentrations of at least 1–2 mg/dL; such methods include immunonephelometry or electroimmunodiffusion. It is essential that both IgA and secretory component be measured in secretions. Secretions best suited for these assays are tears. Additional Ig globulin anomalies, including those of IgG and its subclasses, IgM, and IgE must also be ruled out.

Therapy. Until recently, there existed considerable controversy about the treatment of selective IgA deficiency; newer data, however, have largely resolved this dilemma: the obvious treatment is the substitution of the lacking IgA, which is technically feasible by administering plasma, serum, or IgA concentrates. This approach is now obsolete for two reasons:

1) Careful studies with labeled IgA have shown that intravenously administered IgA molecules never appear on mucosal surfaces. It is now known that only IgA produced locally is secreted across the mucosal epithelial cells.

2) In patients with selective IgA deficiency who received multiple blood tranfusions, formation of isoantibodies against the missing IgA protein is frequently observed. If such patients again receive IgA-containing preparations, they may suffer from severe anaphylactic reactions.

Administration of IgA, thus, is not only useless, but it can be harmful. It has been suggested to administer only IgA-free Ig preparations to IgA-deficient patients. (Therefore, such patients should never receive IgA concentrates, or even the ordinary γ-globulin preparations, because they inevitably contain some IgA.) In any event, IgA-containing preparations should be administered only under close supervision by an experienced physician who would be prepared to recognize and manage anaphylactic reactions. In contrast to this cautious therapeutic approach, Ig-replacement therapy is recommended for patients with the combined IgA-IgG$_2$-deficiency syndrome complicated by infection [113a]; marked clinical improvement has been noted.

Treatment of symptomatic IgA-deficient individuals consists largely of a symptomatic approach, i.e., antibiotics for acute respiratory infections and appropriate diet for intestinal complications. Fortunately, in many patients other immune mechanisms substitute for the missing IgA; in particular, IgM or even IgG may be linked to the secretory piece, thus allowing them to be secreted onto the mucosal surfaces as "secretory IgM" or "secretory IgG." Such patients may, therefore, improve and experience fewer infections with progressing age.

Finally, patients with allergic manifestations should be treated in the customary way: avoidance of exposure to antigens, administration of disodium cromoglycine prior to an expected antigen exposure, and administration of antihistamines after exposure to pathogenic antigens.

Selective Deficiency of Ig-Classes or Subclasses

A few cases of hypo-γ-globulinemia with increased susceptibility to infections are due to isolated deficiencies of single classes or subclasses of Ig [33,107,108] resulting from lack of synthesis. Such deficiencies may be genetically determined, as was demonstrated in a patient with A-γ-globulinemia who was doubly heterozygous for such a deficiency, while both his parents were singly heterozygous and clinically healthy [151].

Deficiency of Secretory Piece

The clinical manifestations of secretory-piece deficiency in all mucosal epithelia is similar to that of IgA deficiency, i.e., the patients suffer from gastrointestinal and respiratory infections [92,137].

Immunodeficiency Syndrome With Sex Linked Hyper-IgM

These male patients present with normal or decreased IgG and IgA but greatly increased IgM concentrations, as well as persistent or periodic granulocytopenia [47,95,120,141]. When the first cases with this Ig imbalance were described, the anomaly was termed dysgammaglobulinemia type I by American, and dysgammaglobulinemia type II by European authors [122]. This obfuscation was one of the reasons to obviate the term *dysgammaglobulinemia*.

Etiology and pathogenesis. Phylogenetically and ontogenetically IgM-producing cells are the first to appear on the scene [48]. The cause of this Ig deficiency in these patients can, therefore, be characterized as one of faulty differentiation of IgG- and IgA-producing plasma cells. However, surface Ig of the IgG and IgA classes are found on B cells, and therefore only a failing clonal expansion of these cells must be assumed [34]. On the other hand, the presence of autoantibodies of IgM class with specificity against homologous IgG in such patients suggests a different etiology, namely, autoimmunization. Similarly, autoantibodies against the patient's own blood cells could explain the frequently observed neutropenia. Still another hypothesis postulates a mutation of the operator gene for the regulation of Ig synthesis, analogously to the hereditary persistence of fetal hemoglobin in man or a similar disorder in mice.

Clinical findings. Severe polytopic and recurring bacterial infections are the hallmark in afflicted boys; they usually start toward the end of the first year of life and include skin abscesses, mucosal ulcerations, respiratory infections with pneumonia, lymphadenitis, and septicemia. The tonsils might be extremely hypertrophic. Occasionally, hepatosplenomegaly develops. In a few patients, glomerulonephritis and in others, excessive wart formation may be observed (Table VII).

Laboratory findings. Constant or transitory granulocytopenia aggravates such infections. It is sometimes combined with hemolytic or aplastic anemia, or with thrombocytopenia. Serum IgM concentrations are often more than ten times normal, whereas IgG and IgA levels are slightly to markedly diminished. Monoclonal Igs were not found in the patients tested for such abnormalities. Antibody formation after immunization with phage φX 174 was essentially normal during the primary phase (IgM) but deficient during the secondary response (IgG) [145]. B cells in the peripheral blood predom-

TABLE VII. Immunodeficiency Syndrome with Hyper-IgM, X-linked

Clinical features
  Recurrent polytopic infections, oral ulcers
  Beginning at preschool or school age
  Death at school age
Laboratory features
  Polymorphonuclear leukocyte (PMN) count decreased (neutropenia)
  Lymphocyte count normal
  Immunoglobulin changes: IgM ↑ (up to ten times normal values)
                       IgG ↓ IgA ↓ (variable)
Heredity
  X-linked, recessive
  Carriers not detectable
Pathogenesis
  Autoantibody formation of IgM class against IgG and PMN leukocytes?
Treatment
  Temporary improvement by immunoglobulin substitution

inantly carry IgM membrane markers. Germinal centers in lymph nodes and in tonsils were absent. T-lymphocyte deficiency could not be proved, and antibody-dependent cytotoxicity was normal.

Therapy. Continuous substitution by Ig preparations is recommended. In one of our own cases, the injection of γ-globulin regularly induced a decrease of the IgM concentration and a rapid rise of the neutrophil count. After 2 years, the γ-globulin requirement increased and its efficiency decreased. If autoantibodies should be proved to be responsible for this phenomenon, then immunosuppressive treatment might have to be considered. In view of the invariably poor prognosis, experimental therapeutic approaches seem justified, in particular, attempts at bone marrow transplantation.

Immunoglobulin Deficiency With Selective IgM Production

These patients are capable of mounting primary immune responses with the formation of IgM antibodies. IgM, however, is not replaced by IgG after repeated immunization, but each time a primary response recurs. Apparently, the switch from IgM to IgG formation does not occur, and higher IgG and IgA levels are not formed. Since these patients apparently have no immunological memory, the disease has been termed "immunologic amnesia" [93].

Transitory Infantile Hypo-γ-globulinemia

The newborn child is supplied with a considerable amount of maternal IgG [52,110]. These antibodies provide an excellent protection during the first few months of life, while they are being progressively catabolized. The child's own increasing Ig and specific antibody production gradually replaces passive by active immunization. Since the T/2 of IgG is about 2 to 3 weeks, its concentration approaches zero levels between 6 and 12 months after birth. This is in accordance with clinical experience, as reflected by the fact that infants are protected against measles for 6 to 12 months.

Normally, the newborn's own immune system is stimulated immediately after birth by its bacterial colonization. The IgM concentration can reach very high values, approaching those of adult levels, within a few days after birth [5]. IgG production starts more slowly, but for serum IgA, it takes many years to reach adult normal values.[2] The resultant IgG concentrations, from the superimposition of decreasing maternal IgG and the infant's increasing IgG, reaches a nadir ("trough" value) between the third to sixth month of life. Again, there exists a correlate, and according to clinical experience, infants are most susceptible to infections during this time period.

---

[2]Ed. note: See also Ritzmann SE, Fisher CL, Nakamura RM in Ritzmann SE, Daniels JC (eds): "Serum Protein Abnormalities: Diagnostic and Clinical Aspects," 2nd printing [157].

IgD does not traverse the placenta, and its increase in serum during the first year of life is slow. In contrast, IgE, which also does not cross the placental barrier, can be found very early in life, especially in conjunction with a clinical allergic diathesis; in healthy children, IgE concentrations increase slowly during the first years of life.

Prenatal activation of *Ig synthesis* may occur during fetal life as a response to intensive antigenic stimulation [5]. This affects primarily the IgM system; increase of IgM to levels of more than 20 mg/dL is accordingly a rather reliable but indirect indicator for prenatal infection, and the determination of IgM immediately after birth has been recommended as a screening procedure.[3] To reliably exclude postnatal stimulation, the blood must be collected before the age of 48 hours. Increase of IgA in cord blood is usually considered as a sign of admixture of maternal blood (maternofetal transfusion). Some investigators using very sensitive techniques, however, consider the rise of IgA in cord blood also as a sign of prenatal infection.

Physiologic hypo-γ-globulinemia may be defined as the range of normal values determined in a collective group of full-term, healthy infants. We recommend the use of "percentile curves" instead of standard deviations [68,117].

Pathological hypo-γ-globulinemia occurs in three well-defined situations:

1) In *premature babies,* the transplacental acquisition of the maternal IgG, normally starting around the 20th gestational week, is interrupted in its rising limb by the untimely birthdate [79,117]. Accordingly, the degree of hypo-γ-globulinemia is closely correlated with that of prematurity. The postnatal decrease of IgG is similar to that in full-term babies, but obviously the minimum reached after several weeks is considerably lower than that in normal babies; indeed, it might subsequently decrease to dangerously low hypo-γ-globulinemic levels. This unfavorable development is enhanced by two additional factors: more extensive dilution of the acquired supplies of maternal γ-globulin due to a relatively larger increase of the blood volume; and the delay of the child's own Ig synthesis. It has, therefore, been necessary to establish normal values for premature babies of different gestational ages (see normal values in [68] and [117]).

2) *Hypo-γ-globulinemia of the mother* inevitably leads to the same deficiency in the newborn infant. Such cases, although rare, directly demonstrate the exclusive transplacental acquisition of IgG in the newborn infant [68].

3) *Delayed "maturation" of Ig synthesis* can also lead to severe hypo-γ-globulinemia. These children are often free of symptoms; in particular they may not develop infections, and the low or very low Ig concentrations are

---

[3]Ed. note: See also Introduction to this volume and Ritzmann SE in Ritzmann SE, Daniels JC (eds): "Serum Protein Abnormalities: Diagnostic and Clinical Aspects," 2nd printing [158].

discovered only by chance. An analogy with germ-free or gnotobiotic conditions in animals might partially explain its pathogenesis: lack of antigenic stimulation leads to hypoplasia of the lymphatic system and to hypo-γ-globulinemia. Our limit of the "normal" with the 10th percentile is probably arbitrary, but at least it appears clear-cut [68]. By systematic longitudinal monitoring of the Ig concentrations, we usually see that each infection leads to a rise of the Ig concentration. In rare cases, however, very severe hypo-γ-globulinemia has been observed during many months or even years. The etiology is varied: some of these children have continuous protein loss, in particular through the gut (i.e., protein-losing gastroenteropathy), and they therefore belong to the group of acquired IDS combined with general hypoproteinemia. In another group, however, hypo-γ-globulinemia is isolated, without obvious cause. In these, decreased rate of Ig synthesis, therefore, seems the most obvious explanation. In some of these patients, hypo-γ-globulinemia is combined with neutropenia; if they are treated with γ-globulin substitution, the neutrophil count usually normalizes within a few days. We have occasionally seen a permanent normalization after three to four γ-globulin injections, given at intervals of 3 weeks. In patients with frequent infections, an alternative hypothesis assumes that the insufficiently produced γ-globulin is continuously used up by the infectious process, and that therefore normal γ-globulin values cannot be attained. It is true that these children in particular benefit from γ-globulin substitution, which helps them to overcome this situation of imbalance.

Immunodeficiency Syndrome With Normo- and Hyperimmunoglobulinemia

This condition has been extensively studied by Barandun [13]. It is observed in patients of all age groups. They are able to synthesize Ig in normal or even increased amounts, but their response to antigenic stimulation, by formation of specific antibodies, is insufficient. This group of patients is certainly heterogeneous, and earlier descriptions should be reviewed critically since some patients have been included who were subsequently recognized as suffering from chronic granulomatous disease [16,80,89]. Furthermore, selective deficiencies of single Ig classes or subclasses must be considered, since this deficiency may lead to increased formation of other subclasses.

Light Chain Deficiencies[4]

The normal ratio of the κ- and λ-light (L) chains of about 65% to 35% (or κ/λ ratio $= 1.8 \pm 1.3$) may be persistently disturbed due to a congenital or inherited imbalance of synthesis [14]. These patients may have normal

---

[4]Ed. note: See also Chapter 2.

concentrations of total γ-globulin or decreased individual Ig classes (e.g., IgG and IgE [19,20]). In two patients (father and son) gastrointestinal infections were prevailing, leading to a syndrome resembling celiac disease [14]. In addition, vitamin B_{12} deficiency with pernicious anemia was temporarily observed, which manifested itself at the age of 28 years and responded immediately to vitamin B_{12} treatment. Monoclonal Igs were not found. Cytoplasmic immunofluorescence studies on peripheral B lymphocytes stimulated by PWM showed transformation into IgM-containing lymphoblasts which were capable of forming both κ- and λ-L chains *in vitro*. The reason why either κ- or λ-L-chain synthesizing plasma cell clones fail to develop *in vivo* remains unknown. Analyses of the Inv genetic markers revealed no evidence for a structural gene defect, and the authors therefore assumed an abnormality of as yet unknown regulatory mechanisms. They also stressed the correlation with a severe intrinsic factor deficiency associated with pernicious anemia, which has also been described by several investigators [18,76]. A possible correlation with a deficient vitamin B_{12} transport mechanism has been mentioned [74]. Such mechanisms warrant a systematic investigation.

IDS With Thrombocytopenia and Eczema (Wiskott-Aldrich Syndrome)

The clinical triad of thrombocytopenic purpura, eczema, and increased susceptibility to infections, known as Wiskott-Aldrich syndrome (WAS) (Table VIII), follows an X-chromosomal recessive mode of inheritance [3,148]. One hypothesis for the common denominator assumes a central role of the macrophage [22]: increased phagocytosis of thrombocytes in the bone marrow by macrophages with abnormal α-granules could account for thrombocytopenia, and for insufficient localization, uptake, or concentration of antigenic material. In contrast, the effector cells (B and T lymphocytes) and their cell products (Ig, mediators of delayed hypersensitivity reactions) are essentially normal, but they remain inactive, since no signal to initiate the efferent phase of the immune response reaches them. In fact, patients dying early of WAS do not present any morphological anomalies of the lymphatic organs (thymus, lymph nodes, spleen, and gut-associated lymphatic system).

Clinical manifestations. A sex-linked inheritance mode is obvious from the numerous pedigrees studied [3,17,22,148] (Table VIII). Mothers who are the hemizygous carriers are clinically healthy. Most of the patients developed their first disease manifestations during early infancy, occasionally even during the newborn period, consisting of hemorrhagic diathesis involving the skin, mucosal surfaces of the nose and the gastrointestinal tract; thrombocytes are already low, and they usually persist at subnormal levels throughout life. Typical eczema also develops during the first 3 months of life and it usually persists albeit with changing severity. The complications

TABLE VIII. Immunodeficiency Syndrome with Eczema and Thrombocytopenia (Wiskott-Aldrich Syndrome)

Clinical features
  Hemorrhagic diathesis since infancy
  Eczema, multiple atopic manifestations
  Recurring polytopic severe infections
  Death during early childhood
  Rarely milder manifestations
Laboratory characteristics
  Thrombocytopenia, megakaryocytopenia
  Immunoglobulins: IgM ↓ in 70%, IgE ↑
  Antibody formation partly impaired
  Lymphocyte count and functions normal?
Heredity
  X-linked recessive
  Carriers detectable by abnormal thrombocyte function
Pathogenesis: unknown
  Macrophage insufficiency? Immune reaction disturbed at its afferent limb
Treatment
  Reconstitution by bone marrow transplant

by bleeding produce a rather typical setting and often create additional problems, which again are potentiated by the patient's tendency to scratch the skin due to the intense pruritus. Somewhat later, usually during the second half of the first year, polytopic infections begin and quite often become predominant: superinfections of the eczematous skin, infections of the respiratory tract, septicemia, meningitis, etc. Bacterial infections are frequent, but in addition, skin and mucosal surfaces are affected by fungi and viruses, in particular the herpes simplex type. Acute allergic symptoms have been found in certain families, especially severe asthma or spastic bronchitis.

Death usually occurs during the first years of life, due to a multiple combination of skin lesions, infections, hemorrhages, and impaired defense mechanisms. Conventional treatment has only slightly changed this gloomy prognosis. Alternative treatment modes are therefore needed. A second important cause of death are malignancies, mostly of the lymphatic system, which have been observed in 10% to 15% of the patients surviving only a few years [88].

Laboratory findings. Thrombocytopenia is the predominant blood abnormality. The thrombocytes present are very small, and morphologically abnormal under the electron microscope. Their capacity to aggregate *in vitro* is decreased [127]. Hypochromic microcytic anemia may develop as a consequence of recurring blood loss. Transitory hemolytic anemia with a positive antiglobulin Coombs' test has also been observed. The leukocyte count is increased as a result of infections. Eosinophilia is usually present; it may be excessive and persist during infectious episodes [56].

Serum proteins do not provide pathognomonic information: during infections, intensive signs of the acute phase reaction are present. Ig values do not reflect the severely lowered resistance to infections [22]: they are essentially normal, and only IgM is diminished in 50% to 60%, and accordingly, isohemagglutinins and antibacterial antibodies against polysaccharide antigens of pneumococci and polysaccharide antigens can be low or absent. The concentration of IgG is usually within the normal range, and the other Igs (IgA, IgD, and IgE) are usually normal or increased. The rate of synthesis of all Igs has been found to be increased two- to fivefold; the normal or decreased Ig concentrations in blood, especially of IgM, result from a similar or even more rapid rate of catabolism in the reticuloendothelial system. The number of B and T lymphocytes in the peripheral blood is normal, but with increasing age, progressive deficiency of T lymphocytes has been encountered, and the initially normal absolute lymphocyte count may decrease progressively. Stimulation of lymphocytes by mitogens in vitro usually elicits normal results within the first years of life, but then they slowly decrease. The assumed deficiency within the afferent limb of the immune reaction has not been demonstrated in all cases, and there is no concensus about the evaluating techniques. Levin et al. [98] described the lack of certain IgG receptors on the cell surface of monocytes, but their statement that patients with Ig-deficient monocytes would respond favorably to treatment with transfer factor has not been uniformly confirmed.

Marked differences in the expression of the clinical triad have been observed, with an apparent hereditary determinant: in one of our families studied, 3 boys died early in life of extremely severe respiratory infections with asthmatic complications [56], whereas in another sibship with 14 affected boys, the manifestations were unusually mild, and 6 boys survived into adult life, with rare bleeding episodes, rather mild and treatable skin disease, and not excessively frequent infections that responded to the usual treatment [44]. Until recently, apparently healthy carriers of the genetic trait could not be diagnosed. An insufficient platelet response after metabolic stress with diagnostic significance has now been reported [127].

Therapy. Our attempts at treatment of the WAS are limited to symptomatic approaches [83]: platelet transfusions have changed the immediate outlook for many patients since they usually result in the amelioration of the hemorrhagic episodes. It has been recommended to use only irradiated blood (3,000 rads) in order to avoid graft-versus-host reactions due to inadvertently transfused incompatible lymphocytes. Splenectomy appears useless for the control of thrombocytopenia, and even contraindicated, since it increases the susceptibility to infections. Local treatment of eczema in the usual manner can improve this condition, but is often ineffective. In these cases the local application of steroid-containing ointments may be helpful, but it should be restricted to small areas. Systemic cortisone treatment is generally ineffective and should be restricted to short treatment periods. Percutaneous protein loss may lead to hypoproteinemia, which rarely may cause edema; in such cases plasma transfusions may be indicated, but its etiological treatment by curing the skin lesions should, however, first be attempted. Injection of γ-globulin is ineffectual; furthermore, subcutaneous or intramuscular injections are dangerous because of the thrombocytopenia.

As a specific immunological treatment, the injection of transfer factor has been recommended, and it was found to be useful in an international, controlled study based on 30 patients [131]. More critical considerations of this area during the last few years, however, have cast some doubt on the validity of these results. At present, transfer factor injections appear not to change the prognosis [69,75].

In a few patients, bone marrow transplantation has been attempted, and two patients have been immunologically corrected [114]. Since this is the only treatment mode with potential cure, it should be considered in all patients, and efforts to find a compatible donor are indicated.

Variable Immunodeficiency Syndromes

At present, many patients with IDS cannot be allocated to any of the above-mentioned categories. It has, therefore, been recommended to group them together under the general heading of "variable immunodeficiency syndromes, largely unclassified," until other disease entities can be differentiated. Some of these patients have previously been described as suffering from "dysgammaglobulinemia," or "forme fruste" of one of the above-mentioned categories. Both assumptions, however, seem quite improbable since in many patients the Ig anomalies are inconstant; and, therefore, causes others than abnormalities of Ig synthesis or metabolism might be responsible. It is, therefore, premature to propose a new classification for these patients, but a systematic investigation and analysis of the results of as many patients as possible is required, which will, it is hoped, allow the definition of new pathogenetic mechanisms and/or congenital deficiencies.

With the present techniques, it is possible to quantitate the number and functions of T and B cells, and to allocate some of the failures to one of these groups. However, apparently too-simplistic previous views had to be corrected, since intimate interactions between T and B cells were subsequently recognized [36,63]. Hypo-γ-globulinemia with low or normal B-cell numbers was shown to be in many cases due to hyperactivity of suppressor T cells [94,142,143], a pathogenetic mechanism which is now clearly demonstrable *in vitro*. Doubts have, however, arisen whether such sophisticated *in vitro* systems may create artifacts, thus leading to spurious assumptions.

Other possible mechanisms that have been considered include the following: lack of B lymphocytes; B lymphocytes that are present but do not respond adequately to polyclonal activators; B lymphocytes that are able to synthesize but unable to secrete antibodies because they may lack receptors for Epstein-Barr virus; secretion of specific antibodies from B cells may be suppressed by *in vivo* inhibitors.

Similar hypotheses can be offered for T-cell deficiencies that might be suppressed by autoantibodies, but much less is known in this field than for the B lymphocytes. Peculiar combinations may or may not represent new syndromes, as, for instance, the IDS with albinism [64].

Without doubt there exists a fertile area for rewarding investigative work, and important new findings may be expected in this field during the forthcoming years.

"Duncan's syndrome" is a well-defined familial X-linked disease entity documented in an extensive pedigree [119]. The basic feature is an abnormal response to Epstein-Barr virus, which in male family members provokes variegated pathologic changes: persistent mononucleosis, polyclonal and monoclonal hyper-γ-globulinemia, A-γ-globulinemia, lymphoma, leukemia, and lymphoproliferative disease. It should be added to the WHO classification as a separate paragraph.

MALIGNANT DISEASE IN PATIENTS WITH IMMUNODEFICIENCY SYNDROMES

Systematic observations in patients with different IDS have revealed an excessive incidence of malignancies [51]; in particular, patients with ataxia-telangiectasia, WAS, and congenital A-γ-globulinemia are affected by malignancies in 10% to 15% of the cases, which translates to 1,000 to 10,000 times the frequency in a normal, age-matched pediatric population. Cases collected worldwide in a registry (Minneapolis, MN) have further confirmed this fact by documenting 267 cases until 1978 [88,130a].

At first, these findings seemed to confirm Burnet's hypothesis of immunologic surveillance [29], which states that immune mechanisms have primarily evolved to protect the body against its own mutant cells with neoplastic potential, which are thereby recognized and eliminated. Closer investigation and newer facts, however, have cast serious doubt on the validity of this hypothesis in its original form [105,115]. It has already been mentioned that in ataxia-telangiectasia the normal DNA repair mechanism is profoundly deficient, and that chromosomal breaks and somatic mutations occur much more frequently than in normal individuals [138]. A similar anomaly is present in several other disease states, such as Fanconi's anemia, Bloom's syndrome, and xeroderma pigmentosum. In these patients, malignant tumors are found with an excessive frequency in spite of a normal immune system. Furthermore, it has been noted that the tumors in patients with the IDS arise predominantly from the lymphoreticular system itself. It is, therefore, more probable that the primary disease of this cell line is expressed both in the failure to respond (i.e., deficiency) and in uncontrolled proliferation (i.e., malignancy).

The Epstein-Barr virus (EBV) promotes proliferation of lymphoid cells and can even trigger malignant transformation. Patients with the X-linked familial "Duncan's syndrome" are apparently extremely susceptible to this agent [119].

CONGENITAL DEFICIENCIES OF THE COMPLEMENT SYSTEM

The high degree of perfection in the chemical analyses of the complement (C) system has elucidated the molecular understanding of its physiological mode of action [38,109,118]. Parallel with such progress in the knowledge of the physiology of the system, a number of congenital C deficiencies has been identified and correlated with the corresponding clinical findings. This is now a well-delineated area. For the exact diagnosis of the C abnormalities, a well-equipped, experienced, and highly specialized laboratory is needed. Particularly interesting are the hereditary disturbances, most of which provide classical clinical examples for the geneticists.

The nomenclature of C factors has been unified and is now generally accepted [146]: complement factors are abbreviated by "C" with their corresponding numbers (C_1, C_2, C_3, etc.). To express the genetic locus, this sequence is inverted, (i.e., the gene for C_2 is called 2C gene, etc.) The deficient gene is designated by $C°$ (i.e., the gene for C_2 deficiency is written as $2C°$). A healthy heterozygote individual would present the genetic setting of 2C–2C and normal C_2 plasma levels. The deficient homozygote with almost complete absence of plasma C_2 has the genetic formula $2C°$-$2C°$, and the *heterozygote* with intermediate C_2 concentrations (i.e., about 50% of the normal level) is reflected by the formula $2C$-$2C°$. There are two recognized causes of C-factor deficiency: the inability to synthesize the C factor and the synthesis of normal quantities of a functionally deficient C factor. Another group of C disturbances is due to the hereditary lack of an inhibitor, which leads to uncontrolled reactions of the C cascade with uncontrolled production of kinins. In general, it can be stated that deficiencies of single C components are mostly connected with increased susceptibility to infections due to disturbed phagocytic mechanisms or to slowly progressing inflammatory processes, whereas the deficiencies of inhibitors produce life-threatening acute situations. Deficiencies of the activators early in the C cascade (i.e., C_1, C_4, and C_2) are predominantly correlated with rheumatoid or anaphylactoid inflammations or with vasculitis and connective tissue diseases.

TABLE IX. Congenital Deficiencies of the Complement System

Deficient factor	Associated disease	Reference
C_1q	A-γ-globulinemia	[91]
	Infections, skin ulcerations	[101]
C_1r	Chronic glomerulonephritis, systemic lupus erythematosus (SLE)	[42]
C_1	SLE-like syndrome	[118]
C_2	SLE-like syndrome	[4,96]
C_3	Bacterial infections	[6,12]
C_4	SLE-like syndrome	[66]
C_5	Familial Leiner's syndrome	[103]
C_6	Raynaud's syndrome	[97]
	Recurring gonococcal and meningococcal infections	[99]
C_7	Raynaud's syndrome, telangiectasia	[25]
C_8	Gonococcal infections	[116]
C_1S-inhibitor	Hereditary angioneurotic edema (HANE)	[90]
C_3b inactivator	Recurring bacterial infections	[1]

The observations on single-factor C deficiencies are listed in Table IX. Most of these syndromes are very rare and therefore need no further consideration here. A few examples may suffice.

C_2 deficiency is the most frequently encountered C abnormality [4,96]. Many afflicted individuals remain asymptomatic if they are able to activate C_3 by the alternative C pathway. Others, however, display severe disease manifestations, such as membranous glomerulonephritis, systemic lupus erythematosus, anaphylactoid purpura, and chronic dermatomyositis.

Deficiency of C_3. C_3 is functionally the pivotal and quantitatively the most important C factor; its deficiency is associated with recurring severe polytopic infections [6,12]. In spite of the presence of specific antibodies, the bacteria are not opsonized and therefore are not prepared for the normal phagocytosis. Treatment by infusion of fresh plasma leads to rapid, albeit transitory, improvement.

Deficiencies of factors C_4 to C_8 are complicated by disturbed phagocytosis or lupus erythematosus-like syndromes. Deficiency of C_9 is not associated with obvious and specific disease manifestations [156].

Deficiencies of inhibitors. Of particular importance is the deficiency of the C_1 esterase inhibitor (C$\bar{1}$s): patients with this deficiency present with the picture of hereditary angioneurotic edema (HANE) or hereditary Quincke edema [46,49,54,90,109]. C_1 esterase initiates the activation of the classical pathway of the C cascade. Normally, this process is inhibited very early by inactivation of the active enzyme. If this fails, excessive amounts of C are continuously cleaved, thus leading to degradation products, in particular to the vasoactive peptides C_3a and C_5a, which increase vascular permeability and produce urticaria and edema. The attacks are self-limited since they consume all available C, but each attack is life-threatening to the patient because of laryngeal edema with the danger of suffocation.

Therapeutic recommendations to administer fresh plasma are contraindicated: this supplies new C factors, which will reactivate the edema-producing process and eventually increase and renew the danger to the patient. Instead, ε-amino-caproic acid, in particular in its cyclic form tranexamic acid, which possess antifibrinolytic potentials, effectively interrupts this activation process [49,128]. Even more important is the activation of C_1s inhibitor synthesis by ethinyltestosterone or its derivative Danazol. With this treatment, virtually all patients remain free of new attacks [54].

Quite differently, deficiency of C_3a inactivator leads to increased utilization of C_3 with secondary C_3 deficiency [1]. Accordingly, the clinical manifestations are similar to those of congenital C_3 deficiency.

ACQUIRED IMMUNODEFICIENCY SYNDROMES

In practice, acquired IDS are certainly much more frequently encountered than the very rare congenital deficiencies. In spite of this fact, the acquired IDS are not discussed extensively here since they are less uniform and of less didactic importance. Although there are no generally accepted recommendations for their classification, the WHO recommendations on immunodeficiencies [140] will be followed whenever possible.

Acquired Idiopathic IDS

In this group of IDS, the clinical signs as described for the congenital diseases appear at any age without detectable underlying cause.

Acquired Idiopathic Antibody Deficiency Syndrome[5]

The isolated humoral deficiency has been described by Barandun in 1955 and more extensively in 1959 [13]. The clinical manifestations in such patients are akin to those described for boys with congenital A-γ-globulinemia.

Nothing is known about the frequency of the disease. In the large pedigree described by Wollheim [149], many late manifestations of hypo-γ-globulinemia do, however, suggest a genetic mode of transmission.

The diagnosis can simply be made by SPE, which discloses a marked degree of hypo-γ-globulinemia.[6] Specific determinations of IgG and IgM

[5]Ed note: See also newly recognized Acquired Immunodeficiency Syndrome (AIDS) [161,162].

[6]Ed. note: See also Ritzmann SE, Daniels JC; and Ritzmann SE; in Ritzmann SE and Daniels JC (eds): "Serum Protein Abnormalities: Diagnostic and Clinical Aspects," 2nd printing [159,160].

reveal levels usually decreased to <1/10 of normal. According to the definition by the British Research Council, diminution of the γ-globulin concentration to <2 g/L is considered to reflect severe hypo-γ-globulinemia, and to <1 g/L, A-γ-globulinemia [132]. By definition, specific antibody responses are lacking. According to Wedgwood et al [145], the congenital cases of hypo-γ-globulinemia can be distinguished from the acquired forms by different reactions to the antigen phage φX 174.

Acquired Idiopathic Combined IDS

In rare cases, the full picture as described for hereditary SCID has been observed with onset at any time during adult life. In the future, investigation of enzyme activities, in particular of ADA, are warranted in such cases.

Acquired Symptomatic IDS

In these cases, a well-defined underlying disease exists, which can explain the immunologic deficiencies. Therefore, a search for such causes is imperative; however, the clinical manifestations are superimposable on those of the corresponding congenital disease.

The leading immunologic feature is depression of the B-cell system with resulting lack of humoral antibodies. The following underlying diseases are known:

Neoplasms of the lymphoreticular tissue.[7] The normal maturation of B lymphocytes advances through at least six well-defined stages [123]. In each of these, clonal degeneration or blockade may occur (Fig. 4), which leads to excessive proliferation of one single-cell species with the attendant crowding out of the other stages and, as a final consequence, to suppression of the normal maturation processes. The clinical manifestations are quite different depending upon the stages of the maturation arrests, as shown in Table X. Two special situations may be mentioned:

In *chronic lymphocytic leukemia (CLL)*, a relatively immature B_2 lymphocyte proliferates in the lymphatic system and appears in the peripheral blood. Lymphocytosis, increases of the lymphatic organs, and A-γ-globulinemia are the consequences. If the *clonal degeneration takes place at a later stage of maturation,* more mature plasma cells proliferate within the bone marrow and in the lymphatic system. They may produce monoclonal immunoglobulins in excessive amounts, which may be easily detected by electrophoresis and identified by IEP or analogous techniques. These Igs contain only one Ig class and only one L chain type (e.g., IgA-λ). The synthesis of normal Ig is often depressed: in spite of the excessive total production, little normal Ig and few specific antibodies are synthesized. Many

[7]Ed. note: See also Chapter 8 and [160].

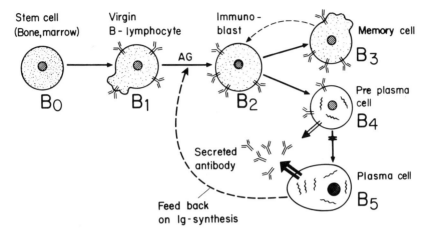

Fig. 4. B-lymphocyte system, steps of differentiation [126]: The stem cell (Bo) acquiring membrane-bound Ig becomes a pre-B-cell (B_1) which by antigen is primed (B_2, immunoblast). Memory cells (B_3) keep the antigenic information, and plasma cells (B_5) produce and secrete specific antibodies, which neutralize the corresponding antigen, and thus brake exaggerated B_1-stimulation by feedback. Arrest of differentiation and malignant degeneration may occur at each level.

TABLE X. B-Lymphocyte Malignancies

Stage of arrested differentiation and clonal formation	Membrane-bound Ig	Serum Ig	Disease
B_1	+ +	↓ ↓	Chronic lymphocytic leukemia (CLL)
B_2	+ + or $\mu \gg \gamma$	Normal	Burkitt's lymphoma, histiocytic lymphosarcoma
B_2–B_3	+ +	↓ or normal	CLL
B_4	+	↑ ↑ monoclonal	CLL with monoclonal Ig
B_4	+ μ	↑ ↑ monoclonal IgM	Macroglobulinemia (Waldenström)
B_5	—	↑ ↑ monoclonal IgG, IgA, or others	Multiple myeloma

side effects of this monoclonal cell proliferation occur, which often lead to characteristic clinical manifestations, e.g. bone destruction by activation of osteoclasts and/or by a specific "calcium mobilizing factor," or secondary effects due to special properties of the monoclonal proteins, e.g., hyperviscosity, coagulation defects, etc.

Secondary IDS With Autoantibody Formation

Impairment of the normal immune reactions can be accompanied by formation of autoantibodies [102]. This seemingly paradoxical situation is a well-documented fact; it is most probably due to a lack of regulation and control of Ig formation [83,94,134].

IDS With Protein Loss[8]

Continuous loss of plasma proteins exceeding the normal degradation by metabolism and by utilization stimulates the rate of synthesis which might compensate for the total protein loss and consumption and keep the plasma levels normal. Imbalance from excessive losses, however, results in hypoproteinemia. Loss of Ig can be in the form of a general "bulk loss" or of a disproportionate nature, the latter depending upon factors such as molecular weight of the proteins lost. If the loss exceeds the synthetic capacity, antibody deficiency ensues. Protein loss and associated manifestations greatly depend on the location of the disease process and its pathogenesis. The lymphoreticular system may be stimulated or even overstimulated, and accordingly, its histological features vary markedly. After antigenic stimulation, the production of antibodies is possible and may even be increased, but their half-life in the circulation is greatly reduced, and therefore their serum concentrations are decreased. Attempts at substitution by injection of γ-globulin or plasma has met with little success as long as the primary cause of protein loss is not ameliorated.

Depending upon the location of the protein loss, four different forms of this syndrome are recognized [68]:

Renal protein loss.[9] The amount and quality of the protein loss are determined by the nature of the renal disease. The bulk of urinary proteins is derived from plasma, from which they escape through "leaky" glomerular capillaries into the primary urinary ultrafiltrate. If this amount exceeds the tubular reabsorption capacity, proteins appear in the urine. A close correlation exists between the type and quantity of proteinuria and the histological findings in the kidney, as can be shown by differential protein clearance determinations [68]. β_2-microglobulin (β_2M) is of particular interest [26], since its glomerular filtration rate is inversely related to its plasma concentration, and its urinary excretion allows the direct measurement of the tubular reabsorption capacity.

A typical example is the *nephrotic syndrome with minimal glomerular changes*. The glomerular filtrating rate is normal, and large quantities of

[8]Ed. note: See also [160].

[9]Ed. note: See also chapter on urinary proteins in Volume 3, this series.

low and of medium molecular weight proteins are lost into the ultrafiltrate. As a consequence, plasma albumin and γ-globulin concentrations are diminished, but retention of high molecular weight proteins, such as α_2-macroglobulin, β-lipoprotein, and IgM, all migrating in the electrophoretic fractions of the α_2- and β-globulins [Fig. 5A], are increased; β_2M is lost into the urine, its serum concentration is therefore lowered, and its quantity in the urine is greatly increased. IgG and IgA may be very low in the serum, but IgM is high. In spite of this hypo-γ-globulinemia, antibody production may be perfectly normal; in fact, clinical manifestations of hypo-γ-globulinemia, such as severe infections, are relatively rare, but if they occur, they are often of a hyperacute course. Another example is chronic glomerulonephritis: the degree of protein loss diminishes in accordance with the reduction of glomerular filtration rate in progressive diseases; accordingly,

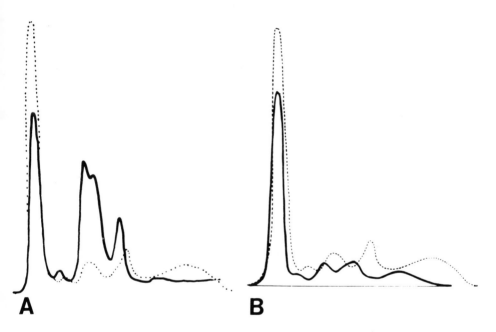

Fig. 5. Serum protein electrophoresis patterns from patients with protein loss. Solid line, patient's serum; dotted line, normal control serum. A) Renal protein loss syndrome (nephrotic syndrome). B) Exudative enteropathy (intestinal lymphangiectasia).

	Total protein	Albumin	α_1	α_2	β	γ-Globulin
Normal control	71 g/L	42	3	6	9	11
Renal protein loss (A)	38	13	3	16	6	0.1
Enteric protein loss (B)	45	23	2	4	6	9

hypoproteinemia is corrected, but β_2M in serum rises correspondingly to the level of creatinine, and its urinary excretion decreases [147]. Antibody deficiency is not a feature in this situation and may only appear with pronounced uremia. Finally, determination of serum β_2M has been recommended as a reliable parameter of pending rejection of kidney transplants [26].

Enteric protein loss. Hypertrophic and ulcerating diseases of the gastrointestinal tract may lead to exudation of large amounts of plasma proteins into the gut lumen. Of the synonyms used, "exudative enteropathy" is applied here. The major difficulty that delayed the recognition and delineation of the pathogenesis of this hypoproteinemic syndrome is the fact of a normal digestion mechanism of the human plasma proteins secreted into the gut. Protein loss can now be measured by intravenous injection of ^{51}Cr-tagged albumin[10] and detection of the label in stools. Numerous factors leading to this end result (Table XI) must be identified by standard gastroenterological examinations. The effect of protein loss on the composition of the serum proteins is almost uniform since all proteins are decreased to a comparable extent, irrespective of serum molecular weights (Fig. 5B). This includes the three Igs G, A, and M. If the lymphatic system is also involved, as in intestinal lymphangiectasia, blood lymphocytes are equally lost, resulting in lymphocytopenia, which is, however, rarely as severe as that seen in combined immunodeficiency syndrome.

Cutaneous protein loss. Extensive exudation through the skin is observed in severe eczema, after destruction of large parts of the skin by trauma, thermal burns, or other injuries. Again, generalized hypoproteinemia ensues, since all plasma proteins are lost at comparable rates, and the three major Ig classes are equally diminished.

Exudative protein loss syndromes. Rapid exudation into body cavities (e.g., pleuropneumonia, pulmonary edema, ascites, edema) may lead to extensive fluid and protein loss from the vascular compartment. Hypovoluminemia may first obscure the real extent of protein loss, which can only be estimated accurately after adequate therapy of shock with infusion of sufficient amounts of fluid and plasma. All three main Ig classes are initially equally decreased, but IgM is the first to recover.

Immunodeficiency in Protozoal and Helminthic Infections[11]

In experimental animals depression of immune responses to heterologous antigens has been observed in hosts infected with protozoa and helminthic parasites [140]. A few studies in humans have shown an analogous situation;

[10]Ed. note: Unfortunately, this is no longer available commercially.

[11]Ed. note: See also chapter on immunoglobulin abnormalities associated with parasitic infections in Volume 4, this series.

TABLE XI. Exudative Enteropathy, Etiology

Gut epithelium impaired
  Necrotizing enteritis and colitis
  Hyperplastic gastritis
  Regional enteritis (Crohn)
  Celiac disease
  Intestinal stenoses
  Polyposis or diverticulosis of the colon
  tumors, in particular carcinoma of the stomach
  Postirradiation syndrome
Lymphatic system impaired
  Malformation, lymphangiectasia
  Lymphatic fistula
  Lymphatic blockage by inflammation, tumor, trauma
Distant disease
  Cardiac insufficiency
  Nephrotic syndrome

for instance, antibody responses to toxoids and to cell-mediated reactions *in vivo* and *in vitro* were found to be depressed in patients infected with tropical parasites (e.g., plasmodium falciparum, trypanosoma gambiense, and Leishmania Donovani). The causes of this immune depression are not fully understood, and they may be multiple and complex. The following factors are of importance, and their predominance may vary from patient to patient:

1) *Nonspecific suppressor cells* have been found in the spleens of trypanosoma-infected mice. They can suppress the responses of normal spleen cells to both T- and B-cell mitogens.

2) *Defective macrophages* are unable to process the antigen and/or to present it to lymphocytes.

3) *Parasite-induced mitogens* continue to stimulate the lymphocytes. This may lead to progressive depletion of antigen-sensitive B cells, and to a failure of humoral responses to heterologous antigens.

4) *Parasite-derived lymphocytotoxic factors* extracted from the larvae of certain nematodes can agglutinate and subsequently kill lymph node cells.

5) *Parasite-derived lymphocyte-suppressive factors* lower the stimulability of lymphocytes *in vitro*. They act on both T and B cells.

6) *Alteration in host physiology or nutrition*[12] may indirectly depress the entire immune system, for instance, by triggering increased output of corticosteroid hormones. Clinical studies on these topics are needed, since their correlations play a major role for large populations in the developing countries.

---

[12]Ed. note: See also chapter on malnutrition and protein abnormalities in Volume 4, this series.

Immunodeficiency Associated With Bacterial Infections

Depression of T-cell reactions by bacterial infections is known to occur, in particular, in leprosy, tuberculosis, and syphilis.

Immunodeficiencies in Viral Infections

The transient depression of T-cell reactivity after viral infections is one of the classical observations in immunology: von Pirquet observed anergy to tuberculin and exacerbation of tuberculosis after measles infections. Such mechanisms are important in persistent viral infections (possibly in subacute sclerosing panencephalitis (SSPE), chronic hepatitis B, etc.) and after congenital infections (e.g., cytomegalovirus, rubella).

IDS and Malnutrition[13]

Chronic infection and affection of the gastrointesitnal tract may lead to malabsorption. If long-standing, it may induce malnutrition, which in itself is a factor decreasing resistance to infections. In developing countries this vicious cycle is usually extremely difficult to break.

The pathogenesis of IDS is certainly complex, and several factors have been discussed. The role of local immunity is not yet sufficiently appreciated: destruction of the gut epithelium removes the site of synthesis of secretory piece which is an integral part of the mucosal IgA defense system. Even if numerous plasma cells in the submucosa produce abundant amounts of IgA, this is probably not secreted onto the mucosal surfaces.

REFERENCES

1. Abramson N, Alper CA, Lachmann PJ, Rosen FS, Jandel JH: Deficiency of C3 inactivator in man. J Immunol 107:19–27, 1971.
2. Ackeret C, Plüss HJ, Hitzig WH: Hereditary severe combined immunodeficiency and adenosine deaminase deficiency. Pediatr Res 10:67–70, 1976.
3. Aldrich RA, Steinberg AG, Campbell DC: Pedigree demonstrating a sex-linked recessive condition characterized by draining ears, eczematoid dermatitis and bloody diarrhea. Pediatrics 13:133, 1954.
4. Agnello V, DeBraco MME, Kunkel HG: Hereditary C2 deficiency with some manifestations of systemic lupus erythematosus. J Immunol 108:837–840, 1972.
5. Allansmith MR, McClellan BH, Butterworth M: Individual patterns of immunoglobulin development in ten infants. J Pediatr 75:1231, 1969.
6. Alper CA, Colten HR, Rosen FS, Rabson AR, Macnab GM, Gear JSS: Homozygous deficiency of C3 in a patient with repeated infections. Lancet II:1179, 1972.

---

[13]Ed. Note: See also chapter on malnutrition and protein abnormalities in Volume 4, this series.

7. Ammann AJ, Hong R: Selective IgA deficiency: presentation of 30 cases and a review of the literature. Medicine 50:223–236, 1971.

8. Ammann AJ, Wara DW, Salmon S, Perkins H: Thymus transplantation: permanent reconstitution of cellular immunity in a patient with sex-linked combined immunodeficiency. N Engl J Med 289:5–9, 1973.

8a. Asherson GL, Webster ADB: "Diagnosis and Treatment of Immunodeficiency Diseases." Oxford, London, Edinburgh, Melbourne: Blackwell Scientific Publ, 1980.

9. August CS, Berkel AI, Levey RH, Rosen FS: Establishment of immunological competence in a child with congenital thymic aplasia by a graft of fetal thymus. Lancet I:1080–1083, 1970.

10. Bach J-F, Dardenne M, Pleau J-M: Biochemical characterisation of a serum thymic factor. Nature 266:55–57, 1977.

11. Bachmann R: Studies on the serum γ1A-globulin level. III. The frequency of A-γA-Globulinemia. Scand J Clin Lab Invest 17:316, 1965.

12. Ballow M, Shira JE, Harden L, Yang SY, Day NK: Complete absence of the third component of complement in man. J Clin Invest 56:703, 1975.

13. Barandun S, Cottier H, Hässig A, Riva G: "Das Antikörpermangelsyndrom." Basel: Schwabe, 1959.

14. Barandun S, Morell A, Skvaril F, Oberdorfer A: Deficiency of κ- or λ-type immunoglobulins. Blood 47:79–89, 1976.

15. Bellanti JA: "Immunology." Philadelplphia, London, Toronto: WB Saunders, 1971.

16. Bellanti JA, Dayton DH: "The Phagocytic Cell in Host Resistance." New York: Raven Press, 1975.

17. Belohradsky BH, Griscelli C, Fudenberg HH, Marget W: Das Wiskott-Aldrich Syndrom. In Frick P, et al (eds): "Ergebnisse der Inneren Medizin und Kinderheilkunde." Vol 41. Heidelberg: Berlin, Springer, 1978, pp 85–184.

18. Bernier GM, Hines JD: Immunological heterogeneity of autoantibodies in patients with pernicious anemia. N Engl J Med 277:1386–91, 1967.

19. Bernier GM: Adult hypogammaglobulinemia. Analysis of 100 cases. Am J Med 36:618, 1964.

20. Bernier GM, Gunderman JR, Ruymann FB: Kappa-chain deficiency. Blood 40:795–805, 1972.

21. Biggar WD, Good RA: Immunodeficiency in ataxia-telangiectasia. Birth Defects 11:271–276, 1975.

22. Blaese RM, Strober W, Waldmann TA: Immunodeficiency in the Wiskott-Aldrich syndrome. Birth Defects 11:250–254, 1975.

23. Boder E: Ataxia-teleangiectasia: Some historic, clinical and pathologic observations. Birth Defects 11:255–270, 1975.

24. Boder E, Sedgwick RP: Ataxia-teleangectasia. A familial syndrome of progressive cerebellar ataxia, oculocutaneous telangiectasia and frequent pulmonary infection. Pediatrics 21:526, 1958.

25. Boyer JT, Gall EP, Normann ME, Nilsson UR, Zimmermann TS: Hereditary deficiency of the seventh component of complement. J Clin Invest 56:905–913, 1975.

26. Braumann H, Etienne J, Dupont E, van Geertruyden J, Vereerstraeten P, Toussaint Ch: Plasma β2-microglobulin in kidney transplant patients. Acta Clin Belg 31:38–43, 1976.

27. Bruton OC: Agammaglobulinemia. Pediatrics 9:722, 1952.

28. Bruton OC, Apt L, Gitlin D, Janeway Ch A: Absence of serum gamma globulin. Am J Dis Child 84:632, 1952.

29. Burnet FM: Immunological surveillance in neoplasia. Transplant Rev 7:3–25, 1971.
30. Buckley RH: Clinical and immunologic features of selective IgA deficiency. In Bergsma D, Good RA, Finstad I (eds): "Immunodeficiency in Men and Animals." Sunderland, MA: Sinauer, 1975.
31. Buckley RH: Immunoreconstitution. Pediatr Clin North Am 24:313, 1977.
32. Buckley RH, Whisnant JK, Schiff RI, Gilbertsen RB, Huang AT, Platt MS: Correction of severe combined immunodeficiency by fetal liver cells. N Engl J Med 294:1076–1081, 1976.
33. Catty D, Drew R, Seger R: Transmission of IgG subclasses to the human foetus. In Hemmings WA (ed): "Protein Transmission through Living Membranes." Amsterdam: Elsevier/North-Holland Biomedical Press, 1979.
34. Cooper MD, Burrows PD, Lawton AR: Molecular and cellular aspects of clonal diversification. In Gelfand EW, Dosch HM (eds): "Biological Basis of Immunodeficiency." New York: Raven Press, 1980, pp 57–69
35. Cooper MD, Faulk WP, Fudenberg HH, Good RA, Hitzig W, Kunkel HG, Roitt IM, Rosen FS, Seligmann M, Soothill JF, Wedgwood RJ: Primary immunodeficiency diseases in man. Clin Immunol Immunopathol 2:416–445, 1974.
36. Cooper M, Lawton A: Development of T and B cells and their functional interaction. In Bergsma D (ed): "Immunodeficiency in Man and Animals." Sunderland, MA: Sinauer, 1975.
37. Cooper MD, Perey DY, Peterson RDA, Gabrielsen AE, Good RA: The two-component-concept of the lymphoid system. In Bergsma D, Good RA (eds): "Immunologic Deficiency in Man." Birth Defects 4:7, 1968
38. Cooper NR, Polley MJ, Müller-Eberhard HJ: Biology of complement. In Samter M (ed): "Immunological Diseases." 3rd ed. Boston: Little, Brown, 1978.
39. Cottier H: Zur Histopathologie des Antikörpermangelsyndroms. Trans 6th Congr Eur Soc Haematol Copenhagen. Basel, New York: S Karger, 1957.
40. Crabbé PA, Heremans JF: Lack of γ A-globulin in serum of patients with steatorrhea. Gut 7:119, 1966.
41. Cunliffe P, Mann J, Cameron A, Roberts U, Ward H: Radiosensitivity in ataxia-telean-giectasia. Br J Radiol 48:374–376, 1975.
42. Day NK, Geiger H, Stroud R, DeBracco M, Moncada D, Windhorst D, Good RA: C1r deficiency: An inborn error associated with cutaneous and renal disease. J Clin Invest 51:1102, 1972.
43. DeVaal OM, Seynehaeve V: Reticular dysgenesis. Lancet II:1123–1125, 1959.
44. Diemer I: Wiskott-Aldrich-Syndrom: Genetische Heterogeneität in einer grossen Schweizer Sippe Diss Med Zürich, 1975.
45. DiGeorge AM: Congenital absence of the thymus and its immunologic consequences: Concurrence with congenital hypoparathyroidism. In Bergsma D, Good RA (eds): "Immunologic Deficiency Diseases in Man." Birth Defects 4:116, 1968.
46. Donaldson VH, Evans RR: A biochemical abnormality in hereditary angioneurotic edema. Absence of serum inhibitor of Cl-esterase. Am J Med 35:37–44, 1973.
47. Feldmann G, Koziner B, Talamo R, Bloch KJ: Familial variable immunodeficiency: Autosomal dominant pattern of inheritance with variable expression of the defect(s). J Pediatr 87:534–549, 1975.
48. Finstad J, Good R: Phylogenetic studies of adaptive immune response in the lower vertebrates. In Smith R, Miescher P, Good R (Eds): "Phylogeny of Immunity." Gainesville: University of Florida Press, 1966.
49. Frank MM, Gelfand JA, Atkinson JP: Hereditary angioedema: The clinical syndrome and its management. Ann Intern Med 84:580–593, 1976.

50. Fudenberg HH, Good RA, Hitzig W, Kunkel HG, Roitt IM, Rosen FS, Rowe DS, Seligmann M, Soothill JR: Classification of the primary immune deficiencies. WHO recommendation. N Engl J Med 283:656, 1970.

50a. Fudenberg HH, Stites DP, Caldwell JL, Wells JV: "Basic and Clinical Immunology." 3rd ed. Los Altos, CA: Lange, 1980.

51. Gatti RA, Good RA: Occurrence of malignancy in immunodeficiency diseases. Cancer 28:89–98, 1971.

52. Geiger H, Hoffmann P: Quantitative immunologische Bestimmung von 16 verschiedenen Serumproteinen bei 260 normalen, 0–15 Jahre alten Kindern Z Kinderheilk 109:22–40, 1970.

53. Gelfand EW, Dosch H-M, Shore A, Limatibul S, Lee JWW: Role of the thymus in human T cell differentiation. In Gelfand EW, Dosch H-M (eds): "Biological Basis of Immunodeficiency." New York: Raven Press, 1980, pp 39–56.

54. Gelfand JA, Sherins RJ, Alling DW, Frank MM: Treatment of hereditary angioedema with Danazol. N Engl J Med 295:1444–1448, 1976.

55. Gell P, Coombs R, Lachmann P: "Clinical Aspects of Immunology." 3rd ed. Oxford: Blackwell, 1975.

56. Gelzer J, Gasser C: Wiskott-Aldrich-Syndrom. Helv Paediatr Acta 16:17, 1961.

57. Giblett ER, Ammann AJ, Sandmann R, Wara DW, Diamond LK: Nucleoside-phosphorylase deficiency in a child with severely defective T-cell immunity and normal B-cell immunity. Lancet I:1010–1013, 1975.

58. Giblett ER, Anderson JE, Cohen F, Pollara B, Meuwissen HJ: Adenosine-deaminase deficiency in two patients with severely impaired cellular immunity. Lancet II:1067–1069, 1972.

59. Gitlin D, Craig JM: The thymus and other lymphoid tissues in congenital agammaglobulinemia. 1. Thymic alymphoplasia and lymphocytic hypoplasia and their relation to infection. Pediatrics 32:517, 1963.

60. Glanzmann E, Riniker P: Essentielle Lymphocytophthise. Ein neues Krankheitsbild aus der Säuglingspathologie. Ann Paediatr (Basel) 175:1, 1950.

61. Good RA: Studies on Agammaglobulinemia. II. Failure of plasma cell formation in the bone marrow and lymph nodes of patients with agammaglobulinemia. J Lab Clin Med 46:167, 1955.

62. Good RA: Agammaglobulinemia: An experimental study. Am J Dis Child 88:625, 1954.

63. Goodwin JS, Williams RC: Suppressor Cells. A recent conceptual epidemic. J Clin Lab Immunol 2:89–91, 1979.

64. Griscelli C, Durandy A, Guy-Grand D, Daguillard F, Herzog C, Prunieras M: A syndrome associating partial albinism and immunodeficiency. Am J Med 65:691–702, 1978.

65. Haneberg B, Frøland SS, Einne PH, Bakke T, Thunold S, Moe PJ, Tønder O, Solberg CO, Solheim BG, Dalen A: Fetal thymus transplantations in severe combined immunodeficiency. Scand J Immunol 5:917–924, 1976.

66. Hauptmann G, Grosshans E, Heid E, Mayer S, Basset A: Acute lupus erythematosus with total absence of the C4 fraction of complement. Nouv Presse Med 3:881, 1974.

67. Hirschhorn R: Defects of purine metabolism in immunodeficiency diseases. In Schwartz RS: "Progress in Clinical Immunology." 1977, pp 67–83.

68. Hitzig WH: "Plasmaproteine. Pathophysiologie und Klinik." Berlin, Heidelberg, New York: Springer, 1977.

69. Hitzig WH: Transfer factor: Characterization and clinical application. A critical review. In Doria G, Eshkol A (eds): "The Immune System: Functions and Therapy of Dysfunction." London, New York, Toronto, Sydney, San Francisco: Academic Press, 1980, pp 227–239.

70. Hitzig WH: Therapeutische Anwendung von Immunglobulinen bei Kindern. (Uebersicht). Blut 40:215–224, 1980.
71. Hitzig WH, Birò Z, Bosch H, Huser HJ: Agammaglobulinämie und Alymphozytose mit Schwund des lymphatischen Gewebes. Helv Paediatr Acta 13:551, 1958.
72. Hitzig WH, Döhmann U, Plüss HJ, Vischer D: Hereditary Transcobalamin II Deficiency: Clinical Findings in a new family. J Pediatr 85:622–628, 1974.
73. Hitzig WH, Dooren LJ, Vossen JM: Severe combined immunodeficiency disease. Springer Seminars in Immunopathology 1:283–298, 1978.
74. Hitzig WH, Fràter-Schröder M, Seger R: Clinical diseases related to deficiencies of vitamin B12 transport proteins. In Zagalak B, Friedrich W (eds): "Vitamin B12." Berlin, New York: Gruyter, 1979.
75. Hitzig WH, Grob PJ: Therapeutic uses of transfer factor. In Schwartz RS (ed): "Progress in Clinical Immunology." Vol 2. New York, London: Grune & Stratton, Inc., 1974, pp 69–100.
76. Hitzig WH, Kenny AB: The role of vitamin B12 and its transport globulins in the production of antibodies. Clin Exp Immunol 20:105–111, 1975.
77. Hitzig WH, Müntener U: Conventional immunoglobulin therapy. Birth Defects: Orig Article Ser 11:339–342, 1975.
78. Hitzig WH, Willi H: Hereditäre lympho-plasmocytäre Dysgenesie ("Alymphocytose mit Agammaglobulinämie") Schweiz Med Wochenschr 91:1625, 1961.
79. Hobbs JR, Davis JA: Serum γG-Globulin levels and gestational age in premature babies. Lancet I:757–759, 1967.
80. Holmes B, Quie PG, Windhorst DB, Good RA: Fetal granulomatous disease of childhood. An inborn abnormality of phagocytic function. Lancet I:1225, 1966.
81. Hong R, Schulte-Wissermann H, Horowitz S, Borzy M, Finlay J: Cultured thymic epithelium (CTE) in severe combined immunodeficiency. Transplant Proc 10:201–202, 1978.
82. Horowitz SD: Fetal thymus and liver transplantation in immunodeficiency. In "Human Health and Disease Biological Handbook." Washington, DC: Federation of the Am Soc Exp Biol Med, 1977.
83. Horowitz SD, Hong R: The pathogenesis and treatment of immunodeficiency. In "Allergy." Vol 10. Basel: Karger, 1977.
84. Jacobs JC, Blanc WA, DePapoa A, Heird WC, McGilvray E, Miller OJ, Morse JH, Rosser RD, Schullinger JN, Walzer RD: Complement deficiency and chromosomal breaks in a case of Swiss-type agammaglobulinaemia. Lancet I:499, 1968.
85. Janeway CA, Apt L, Gitlin D: Agammaglobulinemia. Trans Assoc Am Physicians 66:200, 1953.
86. Jeunet FS, Good RA: Thymoma, Immunologic Deficiencies and Hematological Abnormalities. In Bergsma D, Good RA (eds): "Immunologic Deficiency Diseases in Man." Birth Defects 4:192, 1968.
87. Kenny AB, Hitzig WH: Bone marrow transplantation for severe combined immunodeficiency disease. Reported from 1968–77. Eur J Pediatr 131:155–177, 1979.
88. Kersey JH, Spector BD, Good RA: Primary immunodeficiency and malignancy. Birth Defects 11:289–298, 1975.
89. Klebanoff S, Clark R: "The Neutrophil." Amsterdam: North-Holland, 1978.
90. Kohler PF: Hereditary angioedema (HAE) and familial systemic lupus erythematosus (SLE) in identical twin boys. J Immunol 111:307, 1973.
91. Kohler PF, Müller-Eberhard HJ: Complement-immunoglobulin relation deficiency of Clq associated with impaired immunoglobulin G synthesis. Science 163:474–475, 1969.
92. Krakauer R, Zinneman HH, Hong R: Deficiency of secretory Ig-A and intestinal mal-

absorption. Am J Gastroenterology 64:319–323, 1975.

93. Kretschmer R, Janeway CA, Rosen FS: Immunologic Amnesia. Pediatr Res 2:7–16, 1968.

94. Kwan S-P, Scharff MD: Regulation of Synthesis, Assembly, and Secretion of Immunoglobulins. In Gelfand EW, Dosch H-M (eds): "Biological Basis of Immunodeficiency." New York: Raven Press, 1980, pp 177–188.

95. Kyong CU, Virella G, Fudenberg HH, Darby CP: X-linked immunodeficiency with increased IgM: Clinical, ethnic, and immunologic heterogeneity. Pediatr Res 12:1024–1026, 1978.

96. Leddy JP, Griggs RC, Klemperer MR, Frank MM: Hereditary complement (C2) deficiency with dermatomyositis. Am J Med 58:83, 1975.

97. Leddy JP, Frank MM, Gaither T, Baum J, Klemperer MR: Hereditary deficiency of the sixth component of complement in man. I. Immunochemical, biologic and family studies. J Clin Invest 53:544, 1974.

98. Levin AS, Spitler LE, Stites DP, Fudenberg HH: Wiskott-Aldrich syndrome. A genetically determined cellular immunologic deficiency: Clinical and laboratory responses to therapy with transfer factor. Proc Natl Acad Sci 67:821–828, 1970.

99. Lim D, Gewurz A, Lint TF, Ghaze M, Sepheri B: Absence of the sixth component of complement in a patient with repeated episodes of meningococcal meningitis. J Pediatr 89:42, 1976.

100. Lischner HW, Huff DS: T-cell deficiency in partial DiGeorge Syndrome. Birth Defects 9:16–21, 1975.

101. Loos M, Thesen R, Berkel AI: The role of C1q in the internal activation of the first component of complement (C1): Studies in serum of a selective C1q deficient patient. Seventh international complement workshop. J Immunol 120:1783, 1978.

102. Miescher PA, Müller-Eberhard H: "Textbook of Immunopathology." 2 vols. New York, London: Grune & Stratton, 1968.

103. Miller ME, Koblenzer PJ: Leiner's disease and deficiency of C2. J Pediatr 80:879, 1972.

104. Miller ME, Schieken RM: Thymic dysplasia. A separable entity from "Swiss agammaglobulinemia." Am J Med Sci 253:741, 1967.

105. Möller G, Möller E: The concept of immunological surveillance against neoplasia. Transplant Rev 28:3–15, 1976.

106. Morell A, Skvaril F: Struktur und biologische Eigenschaften von Immunglobulinen und γ-Globulin-Präparaten. II. Eigenschaften von γ-Globulin-Präparaten. Schweiz. Med Wochenschr 110:80–85, 1980.

107. Morell A, Skvaril F, Hitzig WH, Barandun S: IgG subclasses: Development of the serum concentrations in "normal" infants and children. J Pediatr 80:960, 1972.

108. Morell A, Skvaril F, Radl J, Dooren LJ, Barandun S: IgG-subclass abnormalities in primary immunodeficiency diseases. Birth Defects 11:108–111, 1975.

109. Müller-Eberhard HJ: Complement. Ann Rev Biochem 45:697, 1975.

110. Muralt Gde: Immunoglobulins in the human fetus and newborn. In Stave U (ed): "Physiology of the Perinatal Period." New York: Meredith Corp., 1970, p 323.

111. Nézelof Ch: Thymic dysplasia with normal immunoglobulins and immunologic deficiency: Pure alymphocytosis. In Bergsma D, Good RA (eds): "Immunologic Deficiency Diseases in Man." Birth Defects 4:104, 1968.

111a. Nydegger UE (ed): "Immunohemotherapy. A guide to immunoglobulin prophylaxis and therapy." London and New York: Academic Press, 1981.

112. O'Reilly RJ, Pahwa R, Dupont B, Good RA: Severe combined immunodeficiency: Transplantation approaches for patients lacking an HLA genotypically identical sibling. Transplant Proc 10:187–199, 1978.

113. O'Reilly RJ, Pahwa R, Sorell M, Kapoor N, Kapadia A, Kirkpatrick D, Pollack M, Dupont B, Incefy G, Iwata T, Good RA: Transplantation of foetal liver and thymus in patients with severe combined immunodeficiencies. In Doria G, Eshkol A (eds): "The immune system: Functions and therapy of dysfunction." London, New York, Toronto, Sydney, San Francisco: Academic Press, 1980 pp 241–253.

113a. Oxelius VA, Laurell AB, Lindquist B, Golebiowska H, Axelsson U, Bjorkander J, Hanson LA: Ig subclasses in selective IgA deficiency: importance of IgG_2-IgA deficiency. N Engl J Med 304:1476–7, 1981.

113b. Oxelius VA, Berkel AI, Hanson LA: IgG_2 deficiency in ataxia-telangiectasia. N Engl J Med 306:515–517, 1982.

114. Parkman R, Rappaport J, Geha R, Belli J, Cassady R, Levey R, Nathan DG, Rosen FS: Complete correction of the Wiskott-Aldrich syndrome by allogeneic bone-marrow transplantation. N Engl J Med 298:921–927, 1978.

115. Penn I: Second Malignant Neoplasms associated with Immunosuppressive Medications. Cancer 37:1024–1032, 1976.

116. Peterson BH, Graham JA, Brooks GF: Human deficiency of the 8th component of complement: The requirement of C8 for serum Neisseria gonorrheae bactericidal activity. J Clin Invest 57:283–290, 1976.

117. Pilgrim U, Fontanellaz HP, Evers G, Hitzig WH: Normal values of immunoglobulins in premature and in full-term infants, calculated as percentiles. Helv Paediatr Acta 30:212–234, 1975.

118. Pondman KW, Stoop JW, Cormane RH, Hanneman AJ: Abnormal Cl in a patient with systemic lupus erythematosus. J Immunol 101:811, 1968.

119. Purtilo DT, Riordan JA, Deflorio D, Yang JPS, Sun P, Vawter G: Immunological disorders and malignancies in five young brothers. Arch Dis Child 52:310–313, 1977.

120. Rieger CHL, Moohr JW, Rothberg RM: Correction of neutropenia associated with dysgammaglobulinemia. Pediatrics 54:508–611, 1974.

121. Rosen FS: Immunodeficiency. In Benacerraf B (ed): "Immunogenetics and Immunodeficiency." Lancaster: MTP, 1975, pp 230–257.

122. Rosen FS, Kevy SV, Merler E, Janeway Ch A, Gitlin D: Recurrent bacterial infections and dysgammaglobulinemia: deficiency of 7S gamma-globulins in the presence of elevated 19S gamma-globulins. Report of 2 cases. Pediatrics 28:182, 1961.

123. Salmon SE, Seligmann M: B-cell neoplasia in man. Lancet II:1230–1233, 1974.

124. Seegmiller JE, Thompson L, Bluestein H, Willis R, Matsumoto S, Carson D: Nucleotide and nucleoside metabolism and lymphocyte function. In Gelfand EW, Dosch H-M (eds): "Biological Basis of Immunodeficiency." New York: Raven Press, 1980, pp 251–268.

125. Seger R, Fràter-Schröder M, Hitzig WH, Wildfeuer A, Linnell JC: Granulocyte dysfunction in transcobalamin II deficiency responding to leucovorin or hydroxocobalaminplasma transfusion. J inherit metab Dis 3:3–9, 1980.

126. Seligmann M, Fudenberg HH, Good RA: A proposed classification of primary immunologic deficiencies. Am J Med 45:817, 1968.

127. Shapiro RS, Perry GS III, Krivitt W, Gerrard JM, White JG, Kersey JH: Wiskott-Aldrich syndrome: Detection of carrier state of metabolic stress of platelets. Lancet I:121–123, 1978.

128. Sheffer AL, Austen KF, Rosen FS: Tranexamic acid therapy in hereditary angioneurotic edema. N Engl J Med 287:452–454, 1972.

129. Soothill JF, Chandra RK, Dudgeon JA: Some relationships between serum immunoglobulin deficiencies and infection in utero and in the early weeks of life. J Pediatr 75:1257, 1969.

130. South MA, Cooper MD, Wollheim FA, Good RA: The IgA system. II. The clinical

significance of IgA deficiency: Studies in patients with agammaglobulinemia and ataxia-telangiectasia. Am J Med 44:168–178, 1968.

130a. Spector BD, Perry III GS, Kersey JH: Genetically determined immunodeficiency diseases (GDID) and malignancy: Report from the Immunodeficiency-Cancer Registry. Clin Immunol Immunopathol 11:12–29, 1978.

131. Spitler LE, Levin AS, Fudenberg HH: Transfer factor. II. Results of therapy. In Bergsma D, Good R, Finstad J, Paul B (eds): "Immunodeficiency in Man and Animals." Sunderland, MA: Sinauer, 1975, pp 449–456.

132. Squire JR: Hypogammaglobulinaemia in Great Britain. Acta Haematol 24:99, 1960.

133. Steele RW, Limas C, Thurman GB, Schuelein M, Bauer H, Bellanti JA: Familial thymic aplasia. N Engl J Med 287:787–791, 1972.

134. Stiehm ER, Fulginiti VA: "Immunologic Disorders in Infants and Children." Philadelphia, London, Toronto: WB Saunders Company, 1973.

135. Stites D: Ontogeny of cellular immunity in man. In Bergsma D (ed): "Immunodeficiency in Man and Animals." Sunderland, MA: Sinauer, 1975

136. Stossel TP: Phagocytosis: Recognition and ingestion. Semin Haematol 12:83–116, 1975.

137. Strober W, Krakauer R, Klaeveman HL, Reynolds HY, Nelson DI: Secretory component deficiency. A disorder of the IgA immune system. N Engl J Med 294:351–356, 1976.

138. Taylor A, Metcalfe J, Oxford J, Harnden D: Is chromatid-type damage in ataxia teleangiectasia after irradiation at G_0 a consequence of defective repair? Nature 260:441–443, 1976.

139. Tobler R, Cottier H: Familiäre Lymphopenie mit Agammaglobulinämie und schwerer Moniliasis. Die "essentielle Lymphocytophthise" als besondere Form der frühkindlichen Agammaglobulinämie. Helv Paediatr Acta 13:313, 1958.

140. Torrigiani G: Classification of immunodeficiency syndromes. WHO Technical Reports, 1978

141. Vanderhoof JA, Rich KC, Stiehm ER, Ament ME: Esophageal ulcers in immunodeficiency with elevated levels of IgM and neutropenia. Am J Dis Child 131:551–552, 1977.

142. Waldmann TA, Broder S, Blaese RM, Durm M, Blackman M, Strober W: Role of suppressor T cells in pathogenesis of common variable hypogammaglobulinaemia. Lancet II:609–613, 1974.

143. Waldmann TA, Broder, S, Blaese RM, Durm M, Goldmann C, Muul L: Role of Suppressor Cells in Human Disease. In Gelfand EW, Dosch H-M (eds): "Biological Basis of Immunodeficiency." New York: Raven Press, 1980, pp 223–239.

144. Wara DW, Ammann AJ: Thymosin treatment of children with primary immunodeficiency disease. Transplant Proc 10:203–209, 1978.

145. Wedgwood RJ, Ochs HD, Davis SD: The recognition and classification of immunodeficiency diseases with bacteriophage φX174. Birth Def 11:311, 1975.

146. WHO: Nomenclature of complement. Immunochemistry 7:137–142, 1970.

147. Wibell LB: Studies on β2-microglobulin in patients and normal subjects. Acta Clin Belg 31(suppl 8): 14–26, 1976.

148. Wiskott A: Familiärer, angeborener Morbus Werlhofii? Mschr Kinderhk 68:212–216, 1937.

149. Wollheim F: Inherited "acquired" hypogammaglobulinaemia. Lancet I:316, 1961.

150. Yakovac WC: Thymic dysplasia in congenital agammaglobulinemia. J Pediatr 63:699, 1963.

151. Yount WJ, Hong R, Seligmann M, Good R, Kunkel HG: Imbalances of gamma globulin subgroups and gene defects in patients with primary hypogammaglobulinemia. J Clin Invest 49:1957, 1970.

152. Zinkernagel RM: Thymus function and reconstitution of immunodeficiency. N Engl J

Med 298:222, 1978.

153. Zinkernagel RM: Role of the thymus and lymphohemopoietic stem cells in determining T cells' restriction-specificity and responsiveness: Implications for the reconstitution of immunodeficiency. In Gelfand EW, Dosch H-M (eds): "Biological Basis of Immunodeficiency." New York: Raven Press, 1980, pp 283–291.

154. Hanson LA, Bjorkander J, Wadsworth C, Bake B: Intravenous immunoglobulins in antibody deficiency syndromes. Lancet I:396, 1982.

155. Melmon KL, Rocklin RE, Rosenkranz RP: Autacoids as modulators of the inflammatory and immune response. Am J Med 71:100–106, 1981.

156. Lint TF, Zeitz HJ, Gewurz H: Inherited deficiency of the 9th component of complement in man. J Immunol 125:2252–2257, 1980.

157. Ritzmann SE, Fischer CL, Nakamura RM: Quantitative immunochemical procedures. In Ritzmann SE, Daniels JC (eds): "Serum Protein Abnormalities: Diagnostic and Clinical Aspects," 2nd printing. New York: Alan R Liss, Inc., 1982, pp 61–84.

158. Ritzmann SE: Immunoglobulin abnormalities. In Ritzmann SE, Daniels JC (eds): "Serum Protein Abnormalities: Diagnostic and Clinical Aspects," 2nd printing. New York: Alan R Liss, Inc., 1982, pp 376–382 ("TORCH syndrome").

159. Ritzmann SE, Daniels JC: Serum protein electrophoresis and total serum proteins. In Ritzmann SE, Daniels JC (eds): "Serum Protein Abnormalities: Diagnostic and Clinical Aspects," 2nd printing. New York: Alan R Liss, Inc., 1982, pp 3–25.

160. Ritzmann SE: Immunoglobulin abnormalities. In Ritzmann SE, Daniels JC (eds): "Serum Protein Abnormalities: Diagnostic and Clinical Aspects," 2nd printing. New York: Alan R Liss, Inc., 1982, pp 351–485.

161. Gottlieb MS, Schraff R, Schanker HM et al: Pneumocystis carinii pneumonia and mucosal candidiases in previously healthy homosexual men. Evidence of a newly acquired cellular immunodeficiency. NEJM 305:1425–1431, 1981.

162. Siegal FP, Lopez C, Hammer GS et al: Severe acquired immunodeficiency in male homosexuals, manifested by chronic perianal ulcerative herpes simplex lesions. NEJM 305:1439–1444, 1981.

Pathology of Immunoglobulins: Diagnostic and
Clinical Aspects, pages 161–236
© 1982 Alan R. Liss, Inc., 150 Fifth Avenue, New York, NY 10011

8

Monoclonal Gammopathies: Clinical Aspects

Marvin J. Stone, MD

INTRODUCTION

The monoclonal gammopathies (MG) (plasma-cell dyscrasias) provide an excellent example of the interdependent relationship between basic science and clinical medicine critical to the advancement of knowledge in both disciplines. The proteins excreted in the urine of patients with multiple myeloma were originally studied by Dr. Henry Bence Jones over 130 years ago [1]. During the next century, many investigators attempted to characterize Bence Jones proteins (BJPs). Though their chemical nature remained an enigma, the identification of BJPs became a key diagnostic finding for clinicians. The demonstration of these unusual proteins in the urine indicated a diagnosis of multiple myeloma (MM) and was said to occur in approximately half the patients with this disorder.

In 1959, the classic studies of Porter [2] and Edelman [3] ushered in the modern era of immunochemistry. These investigators showed that antibody γ-globulin molecules could be proteolytically cleaved into large functionally distinct fragments (Fab and Fc), or dissociated into polypeptide chains of different size (light and heavy). These landmark discoveries, together with the availability of large quantities of homogeneous immunoglobulins (Igs) from patients with multiple myeloma and related disorders, have resulted in an explosive increase in knowledge of normal Ig structure, function, and genetics. The recent conceptual and methodologic advances in immunology have, in turn, provided new insights, definitions, and improved diagnostic techniques for patients with myeloma-type disorders. Any discussion of the clinical features of these diseases must, therefore, begin with a brief consideration of Ig properties.[1]

---

[1]Ed. note: See also [486].

NORMAL AND MONOCLONAL IMMUNOGLOBULINS

Normal Igs are produced via the proliferation and differentiation of antigen-reactive B lymphocytes into plasma cells. These heterogeneous (polyclonal) Igs possess antibody activity and are the effectors of humoral immune responses. Monoclonal Igs are structurally homogeneous molecules; those which display identifiable antigen-binding activity are also functionally homogeneous.

The principal features of Ig structure (Fig. 1) can be summarized as follows [4–8]:

1) All Igs have a common fundamental four-chain structure consisting of two *light* (L) polypeptide chains (mol wt about 23,000 daltons) linked by disulfide bonds to two *heavy* (H) chains (mol wt about 50,000–70,000 daltons).

2) All Igs contain a "hinge" region in the area of the interheavy chain disulfide bridges that is uniquely susceptible to proteolytic enzymes (e.g., papain, pepsin, trypsin); brief exposure to such enzymes results in cleavage of

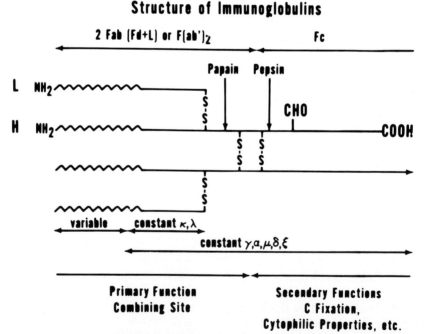

Fig. 1. Schematic diagram of immunoglobulin molecules and localization of structures responsible for primary and secondary functions of antibodies. H = heavy chain; L = light chain; CHO = carbohydrate. (From Spiegelberg [4].)

the molecule into large fragments that are functionally distinct. The amino-terminal (N-terminal) part of the H chain, together with the entire L chain, is termed the Fab fragment, which contains a single antigen-binding site. The carboxyl-terminal (C-terminal) portions of H chains make up the Fc fragment, a region of the molecule in which the amino acid sequence tends to be constant and thus contains many of the features common to individual immunoglobulin classes. The hinge region in the middle of the molecule also may act as a swivel point, allowing for limited flexibility of the Fab regions on combination with antigen.

3) The five human Ig *classes* (IgG, IgA, IgM, IgD, and IgE) are defined by structural differences in their H chains (γ, α, μ, δ, and ε, respectively). These may be delineated by the use of appropriate antisera specific for each chain.

4) The two L chain types (κ and λ) are common to all the H chain classes. Normally, the serum (or urine) κ:λ ratio is about 2:1, but any single Ig molecule is symmetric, i.e., it bears either κ- or λ-L chains.

5) The amino-terminal (variable) portions of both H (V_H) and L (V_L) chains contribute to the antibody site. Amino acid sequence, x-ray crystallography, and affinity-labeling studies all suggest that three short "hypervariable" regions are present in V_L and V_H, which appear to form the actual combining site for antigen; these hypervariable regions on each Fab fragment are brought into close proximity in the three-dimensional structure of Ig molecules and are in contact with bound antigen. Computer analysis shows similar hypervariable regions on all L chains and H chains for which sequence data are available. It appears that in all Igs, there is one combining site per Fab. Antibody specificity is determined by the amino acid sequence (and thus the genetic code) of the variable portions of each chain. It follows, therefore, that antibodies having different specificities differ in primary structure (i.e., amino acid sequence). Such structural and functional diversity is unique to this family of proteins; the precise mechanism for its generation is unclear [489]. Individual specificity (idiotypy) refers to the fact that each Ig molecule bears unique antigenic determinants; these are located on the V regions. It should be pointed out that most commercially available antisera are directed to determinants on the constant regions of H and L chains; these reagents usually do not recognize the variable regions.

6) Structural and functional subunits (domains, homology regions) have been recognized within each intact H and L polypeptide chain. These domains (Fig. 2) are characterized by the following features: a) length of 110 to 120 amino acid residues; b) the presence of an intrachain disulfide loop linking about 60 residues; and c) homology in amino acid sequence.

Domains differ in such biologically important properties as antigen-binding, complement-fixation, and cytophilic properties. Although L chains have only two domains (V_L and C_L), H-chain classes differ in length and in the number of domains in the constant region. All L and H chains have a homologous structure. It seems likely that the individual domains of each chain evolved with different mutation rates from a common primordial gene. Hence, individual domains rather than whole chains should be compared with respect to function and evolution. Chemical and x-ray diffraction studies suggest that the domains are compact units connected by somewhat flexible segments of polypeptide chains that are accessible to solvent and enzymes. Ig domains also have been recognized to be homologous with β_2-microglobulin, a polypeptide chain (mol wt ~ 11,800 daltons) which is believed to be a subunit of HLA histocompatibility antigens.

7) A small (mol wt ~ 15,000 daltons) non-Ig polypeptide component is found in polymeric Igs (IgM and IgA). This J (joining) chain appears to be required for polymerization of these molecules [9]. It is synthesized by the same plasma cell that produces the Ig molecule to which it is bound and is probably added on just before release from the cell. The J chain is bound by disulfide bridges to the Fc portion of the H chain. Only one J chain is present on each polymer of IgA or pentameric IgM. J chains are not present in normal IgG or monomeric IgA, but have been described in the malignant monoclonal gammopathies [381].

In addition to the five major classes of human Igs, *subclasses* or *isotypes* with unique H-chain antigenic determinants have been identified [10]. Thus

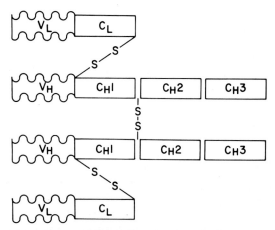

Fig. 2. Homology regions in immunoglobulins. The abbreviations V_L and V_H denote the variable regions of light and heavy chains, respectively, and C_L and C_H the constant regions. The μ- and ε-heavy chains have a fourth constant domain (C_H4) (From Putnam [6].)

TABLE I. Properties of Human Immunoglobulins

	IgG$_1$	IgG$_2$	IgG$_3$	IgG$_4$	IgA	IgM	IgD	IgE
Serum concentration (mg/ml)	5–12	2–6	0.5–1	0.2–1	0–2.5	0.5–1.5	0–0.4	0–0.002
Electrophoretic mobility	γ	γ-β	γ	γ-β	β	β-γ	γ-β	γ-β
Svedberg coefficient	6.6S	6.6S	6.6S	6.6S	7S[a]	18S	6.5S	7.9S
Heavy chains	γ$_1$	γ$_2$	γ$_3$	γ$_4$	α	μ	δ	ε
Light chains (κ/λ ratio)	2 : 1	1 : 1	1 : 1	5 : 1	1 : 1	3 : 1	1 : 4	
Half-life (days)	23	23	8	23	6	5	3	2
% Intravascular	45	45	45	45	42	76	75	
Placental transfer	+	+	+	+	0	0	0	0
Complement fixation[b]	+ +	+	+ +	0	0	+	0	0
PCA reactivity[c]	+	0	+	+	0	0	0	0
P-K reactivity[d]	0	0	0	0	0	0	0	+
Macrophage binding	+	±	+	±	0	0	0	0

[a]Some IgA molecules 9S, 11S, and 13S.
[b]Classic complement pathway.
[c]Passive cutaneous anaphylaxis.
[d]Prausnitz-Küstner.
From Stone [11] with permission.

normal IgG contains four subclasses (IgG$_1$, IgG$_2$, IgG$_3$, and IgG$_4$), and IgA contains two subclasses (IgA$_1$ and IgA$_2$).[2] Similar class heterogeneity may exist for IgM, IgD, and IgE. Subclasses have also been recognized in each of the two types of L chains. The properties and biologic activities of human Igs are summarized in Table I [11].

IgG accounts for approximately 75% of the Igs in normal serum. IgG is also the only class which is transferred across the placenta and in which catabolic rate is influenced by the serum level [12].

IgA is the principal Ig present in secretions (gastrointestinal and respiratory tracts, urine, colostrum, and tears) and thus serves as a "first line of defense" to many invading organisms [13,382]. In glandular secretions, secretory IgA (SIgA) is present as a dimer attached by disulfide bonds to a glycoprotein (mol wt ~ 60,000–80,000 daltons) called the "secretory piece"; the latter is synthesized in mucosal epithelial cells and enhances the resistance of IgA to digestion by proteolytic enzymes [9]. SIgA has a sedimentation coefficient of 11S (mol wt ~ 390,000 daltons) and displays both antibacterial and antiviral activity.

IgM (macroglobulin) is predominantly intravascular and is associated with several distinct antibody activities. The initial antibodies detected after primary immunization are usually of the IgM class, with a later switch occurring to IgG. Isohemagglutinins, cold agglutinins, Wasserman antibodies, rheu-

[2]Ed. note: See also [486].

matoid factors, and antibodies against the somatic O antigen of gram-negative bacteria are typically, but not exclusively, IgM antibodies. The heterophile antibody of infectious mononucleosis also belongs to the IgM class. Considerable data support the fact that IgM is the first Ig to appear both phylogenetically and ontogenetically [5].

The precise role of IgD is unclear, but it appears to function primarily as a receptor Ig. Surface IgD molecules have been identified, along with IgM, on B lymphocytes from normal individuals, as well as on those from patients with chronic lymphocytic leukemia and macroglobulinemia [14,15]. IgD may serve a "triggering" function for blast transformation after antigen makes contact with an appropriate B lymphocyte.

IgE mediates immediate-type hypersensitivity (type I); combination of antigen (allergen) with cell-fixed IgE antibody leads to the release of multiple vasoactive molecules responsible for many manifestations of the allergic (reaginic) response [16]. Serum IgE levels are frequently elevated in patients with extrinsic asthma, hay fever, and parasitic infestations.

L Chains and Bence Jones Proteins (BJPs)

As noted previously, the peculiar protein excreted in the urine of some patients with MM was originally described by Doctor Henry Bence Jones, a London physician, in the midnineteenth century [1]. Bence Jones found that the urine of a patient with myeloma precipitated when heated, cleared when boiled, but reprecipitated when cooled; he concluded that this unusual protein was the "hydrated deutoxide of albumin."

In 1962, Edelman and Gally [17] demonstrated that the L chains prepared from a serum IgG myeloma protein had identical properties (molecular weight, electrophoretic, thermosolubility, and spectrofluorometric) as those of the BJP isolated from the same patient's urine. Subsequently, the same investigators showed that free monoclonal L chains (BJP) exist as both monomers (mol wt $\sim$ 23,000 daltons) and dimers (mol wt $\sim$ 46,000 daltons). Type κ-chains exist mainly as monomers; type λ-chains occur predominately as covalently-linked dimers. The classic reversible thermal solubility property as well as "amyloidogenic" characteristics are associated with the variable (V_L) half of the molecule [18].

BJPs are synthesized *de novo* and are not degradation products of the complete Ig in the serum. A slight excess of light chains is produced normally, and small amounts of free polyclonal κ- and λ-chains (up to 40 mg/24 h) are present in the urine of normal subjects. Both free polyclonal L chains and monoclonal BJP are catabolized by the proximal renal tubular cells [18].

Genetic Markers (Allotypes) and Allelic Exclusion

As is true of other serum proteins, Ig chains exhibit various genetic markers (allotypes). These serologically-detected inherited antigenic determinants are due to specific amino acid substitutions in the constant regions of the polypeptide chains. Examples include the various Gm markers on γ-H chains and the Km marker on κ-chains [19]. Studies on Ig allotypic markers have shown that in heterozygotes, only one of the two alternative markers is expressed by each mature plasma cell. Thus no single cell will make antibody molecules of more than one allotype. Because structural genes for Igs are not sex-linked, these genes were the first example of allelic exclusion of autosomal chromosomes in humans. The mechanism of this intriguing immunogenetic phenomenon is unclear [383].

In summary, Igs differ from other proteins in their variability, heterogeneity, genetic control, and specific antibody properties. Much of our current knowledge about normal Ig structure, genetics, synthesis, and metabolism has been established by the study of monoclonal (myeloma-type) Igs; they have been invaluable in these investigations because of their availability in large amounts and their homogeneous nature. At the clinical level, identification and characterization of these proteins are critical to diagnosis and management of patients in whom they are found. These and other advances attributable to the study of myeloma-type Igs are listed in Table II. In addition, the recent advent of "hybridoma" technology permits the production of virtually unlimited amounts of monoclonal antibodies having predefined specificity.

THE CONCEPT OF PLASMA-CELL DYSCRASIAS

During the past 15 years, electrophoretic and immunoelectrophoretic analyses of serum and urine proteins have become available in most hospital and clinical laboratories. The widespread application of these techniques has made it clear that homogeneous or monoclonal Ig molecules (M-proteins) are found in the serums of many individuals other than patients with classic MM or macroglobulinemia. As noted, such M-proteins are structurally similar to typical antibody molecules. In most instances, detailed investigation of these "paraproteins" has failed to generate convincing evidence of abnormality [20]. The recognition that serum M-components are present in many conditions other than myeloma or macroglobulinemia prompted Osserman to formulate the concept of "plasma-cell dyscrasias," defined as follows: A group of clinically and immunochemically diverse disorders characterized by the disproportionate proliferation of one clone of cells normally engaged in Ig synthesis and secretion, and the presence of a structurally and electrophoretically homogeneous (monoclonal) Ig or polypeptide subunit in serum or urine. The disorders vary from asymptomatic and apparently stable conditions to progressive, overtly neoplastic disorders such as multiple myeloma. The classification of plasma cell dyscrasias (PCDs) is given in Table III. Both clinical and immunochemical criteria must be used to diagnose these disorders [21–23].

The etiology of the PCDs is unknown; both genetic and environmental factors have been implicated [20–24,384,385]. Most of the monoclonal Igs

(M-components) synthesized by plasma cells are not qualitatively abnormal; rather, they appear to be the normal products of a single clone of cells that has undergone intense proliferation. Some of these M-proteins show antibody activity, most frequently directed toward autoantigens, bacterial antigens, or haptens (see Monoclonal Igs as Antibodies). Serum levels of normal Igs are commonly reduced in these disorders.

The structural features of Ig molecules and delineation of the major Ig classes have been discussed. Normal production of antibody Igs is polyclonal and heterogeneous, with individual clones of plasma cells producing the different Igs (IgG, IgM, IgA, IgD, or IgE) (Fig. 3). In general, each plasma-

TABLE II. Results, Research Tools, and Practical Applications Derived from Basic Research on Bence Jones Proteins, Myeloma Globulins, and Macroglobulins

1. Clinical test for Bence Jones proteinuria in the diagnosis of multiple myeloma: modification of the heat test.
2. Elucidation of the aberration of protein synthesis in multiple myeloma, macroglobulinemia, and related diseases.
3. Identification of κ and λ light chains in normal immunoglobulins: quantitation of normal immunoglobulins.
4. Classification of normal "γ-globulin" into IgG, IgA, IgM, IgD and IgE: quantitation of normal abundance.
5. Principles of structure of antibodies.
6. Amino acid sequence diversity of antibodies and immunoglobulins: theories of genetic control of antibody biosynthesis.
7. Modules for X-ray analysis of antibody binding sites.
8. Antisera for detection and quantitation of Ig types in hypergammaglobulinemia in many diseases and in hereditary hypogammaglobulinemia and agammaglobulinemias.
9. Antisera for routine quantitation of Ig types in plasma proteins by automated immunoprecipitation.
10. Antisera for cellular localization of antibodies.
11. Antisera for detection of surface receptors on immunocytes for study of antibody biosynthesis.
12. Immunogenetics—discovery of genetic differences in immunoglobulins of possible value in transfusion reactions and organ transplantation.
13. Immunogenetics—applications to population genetics, forensic medicine, and evolution of immunoglobulins.
14. Discovery of normal IgE and its function as the skin-sensitizing antibody: quantitative radioimmunoassay (RIA) and radioallergosorbent test (RAST).
15. Identification of Bence Jones protein as the paramyloid protein causing primary amyloidosis.
16. Nature of antibody-mediated autoimmune reactions. e.g., rheumatoid factor IgM as the antibody to IgG.
17. Binding site of complement: conformational changes.
18. Cellular system for study of mutation and clonal variation.
19. Subcellular study of protein biosynthesis and mutation.
20. Animal and cellular models for clonal restriction and cellular differentiation.

From Putnam [6] with permission.

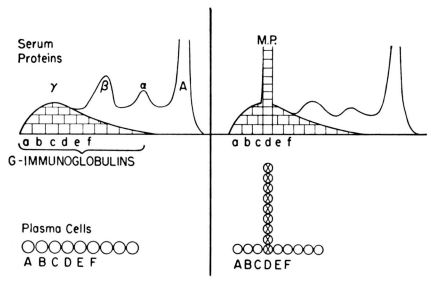

Fig. 3.   Schematic representation of normal (left panel) and monoclonal (right panel) marrow plasma-cell proliferation. Upper portions of each panel show resulting serum protein electrophoretic (SPE) patterns. Note the homogeneous, monoclonal protein (M.P.) component in the SPE pattern on right. (From Osserman [21].)

TABLE III. Plasma-Cell Dyscrasias

Clinically Overt (Symptomatic) Forms
    Multiple myeloma (IgG, light chain disease, IgA, IgD, IgE, nonsecretory)
    Macroglobulinemia (IgM)
    Primary amyloidosis (usually Bence Jones protein)
    Heavy chain diseases (γ, α, μ, δ)
    Lichen myxedematosus (papular mucinosis) (IgG)
Clinically Occult (Asymptomatic or Presymptomatic) Forms
    Plasma-cell dyscrasias of unknown significance (PCDUS)
        With chronic infectious or inflammatory processes
        With nonreticular neoplasms
        With various other disorders
        In healthy persons (age-related incidence)
    Transient plasma-cell dyscrasias
        With infections
        With drug reactions
        With cardiac surgery

From Stone [11] with permission.

cell clone secretes only one class of H chain (γ, μ, α, δ, or ϵ) and one class of L chain (κ or λ) at any one time in its lifespan.

A disproportionate or unbalanced proliferation of one clone results in a corresponding increase in the serum level of its secreted molecular product (Fig. 3). This monoclonal Ig is usually detected by finding a tall symmetric "spike" with γ-, β-, or occasionally α_2-mobility on cellulose acetate electrophoresis of serum (SPE) or urine (UPE), but immunoelectrophoresis (IEP) is required to identify the H and L chain class of the protein. The magnitude of M-components is related to the number of cells in the body producing that component as well as to its catabolic characteristics; these proteins thus serve as valuable markers in diagnosis, staging, and management of patients.

Serum M-components are typically found in patients with symptomatic PCD (MM, Waldenström's macroglobulinemia [MW], primary systemic amyloidosis, or the various H chain diseases). Serum M-components without evidence of overtly neoplastic PCD are also found in association with a variety of other diseases and in a few healthy persons; in the latter circumstance, the incidence is age-related—1% of persons age 25 and 3% of those age 70. Although many asymptomatic cases remain unchanged for years and are therefore seemingly benign, a few represent incipient or "premyeloma" fortuitously discovered on routine SPE. It is impossible to predict the course in any individual patient, and clinically symptomatic MM may not evolve for as long as 20 years [25,26]. The designation "plasma-cell dyscrasia of unknown significance" (PCDUS) is therefore preferred for asymptomatic individuals with monoclonal serum components.

Patients with PCDUS usually have low levels of serum M-components that are stable with time and show only mild marrow plasmacytosis, normal levels of serum Igs, and no lytic bone lesions or Bence Jones (BJ) proteinuria (see Occult [Asymptomatic] Plasma-Cell Dyscrasias).

INTERPRETATION OF THE SERUM PROTEIN ELECTROPHORETIC (SPE) PATTERN

Normal human serum contains over 100 individual proteins, each having a specific function [27]. The normal concentrations of these proteins vary over a wide range ($\sim$ 6 logs) from a few micrograms to several grams per dL. In addition to Igs, serum proteins function as enzymes, proteinase inhibitors, complement components, kinin precursors, and transport substances for vitamins, hormones, lipids and metals. Only those proteins present in relatively high concentration in serum contribute to the electrophoretic contour [28]. Igs may migrate anywhere from the slow (cathodal) γ- to the α_2-globulin area (Fig. 4) [29].

Tips on Interpretation of the SPE Pattern

1) Normal values in most laboratories: albumin 3.8–5.0 g/dL; $\alpha_1 \sim 0.2$ g/dL; $\alpha_2 \sim 0.8$ g/dL; $\beta \sim 0.9$ g/dL; $\gamma \sim 1.2$ g/dL.

2) For recognition of M-proteins, *contour* of the pattern is more important than quantification of the various fractions.

3) Whenever possible, examine the stained membrane for presence of a discrete, homogeneous M-component rather than relying solely on the densitometric tracing (especially valuable for recognizing application artifacts).

4) M-components are best recognized by SPE; however, their H and L chain type must be established by immunologic methods (IEP).

5) Is hypogammaglobulinemia ($\gamma < 0.6$ g/dL) present? If so, this should be confirmed by IEP and quantification of serum Ig levels by radial immunodiffusion (RID). Careful examination of the urine for BJP should be performed; IEP is preferred.

6) Quantification of typical narrow, "church-spire" M-components is best done from the SPE pattern. Marked increases in Ig levels are notoriously

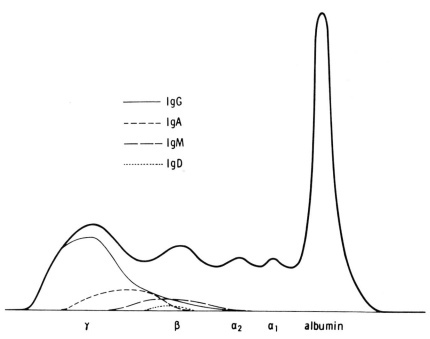

——— IgG
----- IgA
— —— IgM
············· IgD

γ　　　β　　α_2　α_1　albumin

Fig. 4.　Distribution of four human immunoglobulins on electrophoresis of serum. The IgE class has a similar mobility of IgD but cannot be represented quantitatively because of its low level in serum. (From Holborow [29].)

unreliable by RID (especially true for polymeric M-proteins—IgA and IgM of serum Ig).[3]

7) A decrease in albumin and increase in α_2-globulin are nonspecific findings and are present in many inflammatory processes and chronic diseases. Most α_2-"spikes" are not due to Ig M-components, but a few are—confirm with IEP.

8) IgA M-proteins often appear relatively heterogeneous (i.e., broadbased) due to polymer formation or differences in carbohydrate content; IgD M-proteins may have a similar appearance or may be present in such a low quantity that they are scarcely evident on the pattern. Whenever these are possibilities or when it is difficult to distinguish such situations from polyconal (diffuse) hypergammaglobulinemia, IEP with monospecific H and L chain antisera should be performed.

9) BJ proteinemia is rarely evident on SPE but can often be identified by serum IEP. The most likely cause of a "double spike" is retained BJP in a patient with renal failure who also has an intact monoclonal Ig molecule.

10) Causes of pseudo M-proteins:

   a) Gross hemolysis-large, often broad, α_2-peak (hemoglobin-haptoglobin complexes);
   b) chronic inflammatory or neoplastic disease or nephrotic syndrome—α_2-peak;
   c) hyperlipidemia—α_2- or β-peak;
   d) plasma—homogeneous component in slow-β region (fibrinogen);
   e) Marked Fe deficiency anemia—homogenous β-component ($\uparrow\uparrow$ transferrin) (very rare);
   f) bisalbuminemia (very rare).

MULTIPLE MYELOMA (PLASMA-CELL MYELOMA: MYELOMATOSIS)

Multiple myeloma (MM) is a progressive neoplastic disease characterized by marrow plasma-cell (or secretory B-cell) tumors and overproduction of intact monoclonal Igs (IgG, IgA, IgD, IgE) or BJP (free monoclonal κ- or λ-L chains), and often associated with numerous osteolytic lesions, hypercalcemia, anemia, renal damage, and increased susceptibility to bacterial infections. Persons over the age of 40 are most commonly affected. The criteria for diagnosis [30] are critically dependent on laboratory studies and are given in Table IV.

---

[3]Ed. note: See also [487].

MM is the prototype of "overt" or symptomatic PCD and, as has been noted, can be characterized according to the type of homogeneous Ig produced by the neoplastic clone of plasma cells (Table III) [11,23,28,31,32]. Myeloma accounts for approximately 1% of all malignancies and 10% of hematologic malignancies [33]. The annual incidence is 2–4 per 100,000 population [32]. Several studies suggest that myeloma is more common in black than white persons [34]; men and women are equally affected. The disorder has been reported in spouses [35–37], mother and daughter [38], and family and community "clusters" [39,40], but these are very rare. The usual patient is over 40 years of age (mean 62), although occasional reports of individuals in their teens or twenties have appeared [41–44,386]. Myeloma patients are said to have an increased incidence of other solid neoplasms, but this is questionable [45,46].

Symptoms and Signs

The usual mode of clinical presentation is in one of three ways: 1) The most common presentation relates to the presence of bone pain, especially in the spine, pelvis or ribs. 2) Less frequently, patients manifest renal failure of unknown etiology; this is particularly common in the "light chain disease" subgroup [30]. 3) Some patients may be seen because of the recent onset of recurrent bacterial infections—especially pneumococcal pneumonia [47]. Occasional patients present because of symptoms related to amyloid deposition [30] or with unusual central nervous system manifestations [48–53]. Aside from the inconstant presence of bone tenderness, physical examination usually is nonrevealing. Pallor may be noted if anemia is severe. Lymphadenopathy and hepatosplenomegaly [54] are notably absent unless the patient has amyloid. Neurological examination may disclose signs of spinal cord compression [30,52]. Joint findings are uncommon and usually due to amyloid arthritis; one patient with hemarthrosis as the presenting manifestation of myeloma has been reported [55].

TABLE IV. Multiple Myeloma: Criteria for Diagnosis

A: Demonstration of an M-protein in serum and/or urine
B1: Marrow plasma cells in sheets or clusters (i.e., marrow plasma cell tumors)
B2: Osteolytic lesions (unassociated with metastatic carcinoma or granulomatous disease)
B3: Bence Jones proteinuria in excess of 300 mg/day

Diagnosis of myeloma
    = A plus any one of the categories in B
    = B1 plus B2 (for "nonsecretory" cases; <1% of all myeloma)

Laboratory Findings

A mild to moderate normocytic-normochromic anemia usually is present, although hypochromic-microcytic red cell morphology may be seen if the patient has a coexisting iron reutilization defect ("anemia of chronic disease"), iron deficiency anemia, or sideroblastic state [56–58]. The direct Coombs' test is negative if the cells are thoroughly washed. Occasional plasma cells may be evident on careful examination of the blood smear but this finding is nonspecific [59–63]. True plasma-cell leukemia [64–73,387,388] is uncommon (see Case 1).

CASE 1. PLASMA-CELL LEUKEMIA

This 38-year-old housewife was seen in July 1976 with pneumonia and found to have leukocytosis with many plasma cells in the peripheral blood. She was hospitalized, at which time it was noted that her spleen was palpable 2 cm below the left costal margin. Physical examination was otherwise unremarkable except for signs of lung consolidation. She had no evidence of macroglossia or bone tenderness. The patient was not anemic, but peripheral blood smear revealed rouleau and leukocytosis (15,000/mm³) with 25% plasma cells. The bone marrow was hypercellular with clusters of plasma cells; it was estimated that these cells accounted for 30–35% of the nucleated marrow elements. SPE disclosed an M-spike (3.2 g/dL), which on IEP was found to be an IgG λ-Ig. The patient was also found to have λ-H chain BJ proteinuria (8.4 g/24 h). Calcium, creatinine, and uric acid determinations were normal and bone survey was negative.

The patient was treated with six courses of melphalan and prednisone from August of 1976 through February of 1977, with subsequent disappearance of peripheral blood plasma cells and a concomitant reduction in the serum M-spike from 3.2 to 1.3 g/dL on SPE. The λ-BJ proteinuria decreased markedly although it could still be detected by IEP. She maintained normal performance status and played tennis twice weekly. In May, 1977 it was found that the patient's serum M-spike had increased to 1.6 g/dL and the peripheral smear disclosed 20% plasma cells. Vincristine was added to the melphalan-prednisone regimen for the next 3 months. By September 1977, the serum M-spike had decreased to 1.0 g/dL. Hemoglobin was 12.8 g/dL with a hematocrit of 37%, and platelets were 102,000/mm³. However, her white count had decreased to 3,000/mm³. Bone marrow examination disclosed a hypercellular aspirate which contained 70–75% pleomorphic plasma cells in sheets and clusters. Repeat 24-hour urine showed 910 mg protein, which was essentially all λ-BJP. Bone films, uric acid, and calcium remained within normal limits, but her serum creatinine increased to 3.2 mg/dL. The patient was placed on VMCP (vincristine, melphalan, cyclophosphamide, prednisone) regimen for the next 3 months without major change in findings. She was then switched to vincristine, BCNU, adriamycin, and prednisone (VBAP) in June 1978. Severe leukopenia and thrombocytopenia developed from this treatment. However, after six courses of this chemotherapy regimen, BJ proteinuria decreased from 4.0 to 1.4 g/24 h.

SPE in October 1978 disclosed an M-spike of 1.4 g/dL with decreased background γ-globulin; the albumin was 4.9 g/dL and the total protein was 8.5 g/dL. The hematocrit was 36%, white count 9,500/mm³ with 66% polys, and platelets 152,500/mm³. No plasma cells were seen on peripheral smear. During the following year, the patient became refractory to further chemotherapy and numerous plasma cells again appeared in the peripheral blood. She expired 39 months after diagnosis.

Comment: Plasma cell leukemia is an unusual mode of presentation of myeloma. Most reports have emphasized the short survival of patients with this myeloma variant. This young woman illustrates that such is not always the case. She was treated for 3 years after presenting with plasma-cell leukemia and maintained near-normal functional status throughout most of her course, despite aggressive chemotherapy.

Plasma cells also may be found in the urine [74]. Except for the "light chain disease" (LCD) subgroup [30], rouleau on peripheral smear and an erythrocyte sedimentation rate (ESR) in excess of 100 mm/h are helpful early laboratory findings that frequently suggest the underlying disorder. Leukocyte and platelet counts are usually normal at the time of diagnosis [30,33,75,76]. Leukocyte alkaline phosphatase levels have been reported to be elevated in 60 of 62 patients with myeloma [77].

As noted above, the presence of a plasma-cell dyscrasia is most readily identified by the finding of a narrow band on cellulose acetate or agarose electrophoresis of serum or urine. It is important to note that *both* serum and urine must be analyzed by electrophoresis and IEP if a precise immunochemical diagnosis is to be made, since about 25% of myeloma patients have LCD, an entity in which only free homogeneous light chains (BJPs) are secreted by the abnormal monoclone [23,30]. Because BJPs are small molecules, they are usually filtered by the glomeruli and excreted in the urine but do not accumulate in serum unless renal failure supervenes. Thus, one cannot rely on the absence of an M-spike in serum to rule out MM (Fig. 5). Approximately 99% of myeloma patients have a demonstrable M-protein if both serum *and* urine are analyzed by electrophoretic and IEP techniques (Table V) [23,30,32,33,78]. Intracellular M-protein often can be demonstrated by immunofluorescence studies in the rare nonsecretory variant [79–87,389]. Sheets or clusters of marrow plasma cells and the presence of osteolytic lesions will identify such patients. In approximately half of patients with localized plasmacytoma, an M-component may not be present initially. In addition to bone [30,88], plasmacytomas have been described in the stomach, small and large intestine, nasopharynx, skin and subcutaneous tissues, breast, liver, spleen, lymph nodes, testis, thyroid, kidney, lung, pleura, heart, brain, and meninges [89–111,390–394]. The prognosis for patients with extramedullary plasmacytoma appears better than that for individuals presenting with "solitary" plasmacytoma of bone [91,110]. True plasmacytomas must be differentiated from reactive plasma cell infiltrates [112–114,395] and giant lymph node hyperplasia of the plasma cell type [115,116].

About half of myeloma patients will have monoclonal IgG serum proteins (Table V). In our experience, 26% of myeloma patients (18% of all patients

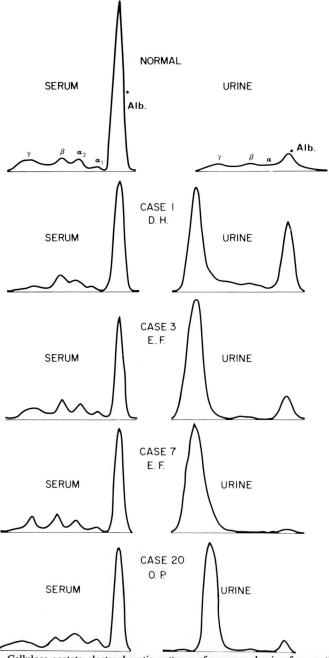

Fig. 5. Cellulose acetate electrophoretic patterns of serum and urine from patients with L chain myeloma. (From Stone [11].)

TABLE V. Categories of M-proteins in Myeloma

	Hobbs [78]	Osserman [23]	Kyle [33]	Dallas Series[a]
No. cases	212	351	537	217
IgG	53%	52%	59%	53%
IgA	25	22	23	19
IgD	1	1	1	1
BJ only (LCD)[b]	19	25	(17)	26
Biclonal	2	<1	—	—
No M-protein	—	—	<1	<1

[a]During the interval 1969–74, a total of 327 patients with plasma-cell dyscrasias were identified. Approximately 30% of those with IgG and 20% with IgA M-proteins did not have evidence of myeloma. Eleven percent of the total population had macroglobulinemia. None of these subgroups is included in the table above.
[b]LCD = light chain disease.

with PCD) produce only BJP and, therefore, have LCD [30]. This large subgroup of patients tends to be more difficult to diagnose, since such individuals usually have no evidence of an M-spike in serum (instead they generally display hypogammaglobulinemia) and tend not to have rouleau on peripheral smear. Identification and characterization of proteinuria thus becomes especially critical to the diagnosis of these myeloma patients (Fig. 5). LCD also is important to recognize because patients with this entity have a higher incidence of renal functional impairment and amyloidosis than other myeloma patients [30,78]. Approximately 20% of patients with myeloma have IgA proteins; these often appear relatively heterogeneous (i.e., broad-based) on SPE due to polymer formation or differences in carbohydrate content. L chain typing tends to be difficult in patients with monoclonal IgA proteins unless Bence Jones proteinuria is also present [31,117]. IgD accounts for only 1% of myeloma proteins; a typical M-spike may *not* be evident on SPE and λ-L chains are present in 80–90% of cases [118,119,396–399]. Only eleven cases of IgE myeloma have been reported [120,121,400].[4] Biclonal and even triclonal gammopathies occur rarely and have provided interesting models for the study of genetics and synthesis of H and L chains [122–126,401].

Approximately 70% of the entire group of myeloma patients has BJP identifiable in urine by sensitive electrophoretic and immunochemical tech-

[4]Ed. note: See also [488].

niques. BJP also may be demonstrable in serum in a small proportion of patients (Fig. 6) [30,31].

Detection of BJP

The clinician must bear in mind that not all proteinuria is albuminuria and that identification of abnormal proteinuria requires that the components be quantified and characterized by means of 24-hour urine protein excretion, cellulose acetate electrophoresis, and IEP. A variety of screening tests for identifying significant proteinuria are utilized in most laboratories. The commonly employed Dipstix method does not recognize most urine BJPs [30,31]. Thus, it has been frequent in our experience to obtain a negative protein by Dipstix in the face of 5 grams (or more) of BJ proteinuria per 24 hours. The classic heat precipitation test for BJP is obsolete, insensitive, and cumbersome to perform. As has been pointed out previously, the results of the heat test as carried out in most hospital laboratories often are actually misleading

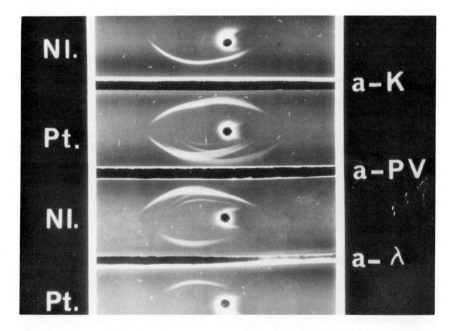

Fig. 6. Immunoelectrophoresis demonstrating κ-Bence Jones proteinemia. Anode on right. The polyvalent anti-immunoglobulin serum (a-PV) gives three arcs (IgG, IgA, and IgM) vs. normal serum (N1.). Note thickened, bowed arc of patient's serum developed with anti-κ) (a-κ) as well as extra major arc vs. the polyvalent reagent. (From Stone and Frenkel [30].)

[88]. For the past ten years, we have screened for urine protein, including BJ, by utilizing both the sulfosalicylic acid (SSA) and p-toluene sulfonic acid (TSA) methods [30]. SSA will precipitate BJ, as well as other urine proteins, if present in a concentration exceeding approximately 30 mg/dL. TSA is particularly useful in initial screening for BJP, since this reagent does not precipitate albumin when the latter is present in concentrations as high as 25 g/dL [127]. It should be pointed out that TSA is not specific for BJP or even for polyclonal Ig L chains; this reagent will precipitate other plasma proteins found in urine, especially transferrin [128]. However, combined use of the SSA and TSA tests provides a simple, quick, and inexpensive method of screening urine specimens for BJP. The diagnosis of LCD is particularly revealing in this regard. As noted, these myeloma patients ordinarily do not have serum M-spikes, rouleau, or markedly elevated ESRs. Because the Dipstix urine protein is frequently negative, the diagnosis of myeloma is often missed because appropriate screening tests for detection of BJP are not employed.

Quantitative determination of 24-hour urine protein excretion is important in any patient with BJ proteinuria because its presence may be an adverse prognostic factor in certain patients and because criteria for objective response to therapy rest, in part, on the demonstration of a 50% or greater decrease in serum or urine M-protein [129,130]. It may be necessary to concentrate the urine prior to performance of UPE or IEP analyses. This can be accomplished conveniently through the use of Minicon B15 concentrators after the appropriate concentrating factor is determined by initial screening with SSA and TSA. UPE will then disclose the proportion of albumin that is present, as well as documenting the presence of a tall narrow monoclonal spike in the β-, γ-, or α_2-region (Fig. 5). The components can then be typed for L chain class by the use of urine IEP (Fig. 7).

CASE 2. CHRONIC RENAL FAILURE OF UNKNOWN ETIOLOGY

This 64-year-old woman presented in 1970 with nausea and vomiting. She had a history of syphilitic heart disease, chronic alcoholism, and recurrent pneumonias (1953, 1960, and 1964). Her blood urea nitrogen had been normal in 1964 but was 66 mg/100 mL 15 months before her admission. Physical examination revealed only the murmurs of aortic regurgitation and stenosis. Her hemoglobin level was 7.9 g/dL, hematocrit value 22% with normal red cell morphology and no evidence of rouleau. The erythrocyte sedimentation rate was 32 mm/h. Plasma electrolytes were sodium 135 meq/L, potassium 5.4 meq/L, carbon dioxide 10 meq/L, and chloride 116 meq/L. The blood urea nitrogen was 78 mg/dL, serum creatinine 6.2 mg/dL, calcium 9.8 mg/dL, and uric acid 8.3 mg/dL. Urine protein was negative by Dipstix and the heat test for BJP was negative. SPE disclosed no evidence of a monoclonal spike. The urine was found to be 4+ by SSA and strongly positive by the TSA test, which led to the quantitative determination of 4.65 g/24 h urine protein excretion. UPE (Fig. 5) showed a tall symmetrical spike in the γ-

region; urine IEP (Fig. 7) demonstrated increased λ-L chains without evidence of type κ. λ-BJ proteinemia also was documented. Serum levels of IgG, IgA, and IgM were decreased; IgD and IgE were undetectable. Bone roentgenograms showed no lytic defects. Bone marrow aspiration revealed 77% mature plasma cells in sheets and clusters. Treatment with allopurinol and intermittent melphalan was instituted and the patient's urine protein excretion was 1.4 g/24 h after two years of therapy.

Comment: This patient presented with increasing renal failure, proteinuria, and anemia. The diagnosis was established when the proteinuria was quantified and defined. The discrepancy between the Dipstix and SSA methods is ascribable to the fact that the former does not detect most BJPs, whereas the latter does.

This case emphasized the unreliability of the heat precipitation test for BJP. This procedure was performed on urines from 18 patients in our LCD series [30], but only 6 were positive. The test requires strict control of pH and ionic strength, and a minimum protein concentration of 145 mg/dL. The TSA test is of much greater value as a screening procedure for BJ proteinuria. A positive result does not establish the presence of increased Ig L chains in

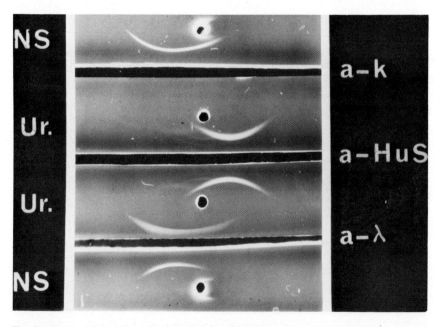

Fig. 7. Immunoelectrophoresis of unconcentrated urine from myeloma patient. Anode on right. Cellulose acetate electrophoretic patterns from this patient (Case 7) are shown in Figure 5. λ-Bence Jones protein is the major component demonstrable with only a small amount of albumin evident vs. the antihuman serum reagent (middle trough). NS = normal serum. (From Stone [11].)

the urine, since significant transferrinuria may cause a "false-positive" test; however, the latter is easily differentiated from BJP by IEP.

Normal urine protein excretion is less than 200 mg/24 h. Approximately 5–40 mg of this "normal" proteinuria consist of free Ig L chains, but these are *polyclonal* (i.e., heterogeneous) and present in the usual κ:λ ratio of 2:1. In the patient with nephrotic syndrome, the SSA test will be 4+ and the TSA test will usually be negative or only slightly positive, while UPE will disclose a pattern which appears similar to that of serum. IEP of urine from such a patient will disclose multiple-component proteinuria, predominately albumin; various other serum proteins will be present, and usually both κ- and λ-L chain determinants will be detected.

By contrast, in the patient with BJ proteinuria, both the SSA and TSA tests tend to be strongly positive. As noted previously, UPE and urine IEP confirm the presence of free monoclonal L chains. Except in the patient who has coexisting amyloidosis, significant albuminuria does not occur in patients with myeloma. The presence of marked albuminuria in addition to BJP should alert the physician to the probable presence of glomerular amyloid [30,131].

A few patients with BJ proteinuria but without other evidence of myeloma or primary amyloidosis have been reported [132–135], but the incidence of such nonmyelomatous BJ proteinuria is extremely low. *In general, the demonstration of significant (i.e., > 300 mg/24 h) Bence Jones proteinuria is a reliable, albeit not absolute, indication of malignancy in patients with plasma cell dyscrasias [30,136,402].*

Bone Marrow Findings

The average marrow aspirate from a patient with MM contains 30–35% plasma cells (normal < 5%) [33,137]. However, a normal marrow is also consistent with the diagnosis of myeloma. Occasionally, the aspirate may be hypocellular and simulate aplastic anemia [138], in such instances a core biopsy should be obtained. Marrow involvement tends to be patchy, especially in the early phases of the disease. Consequently, the specimen obtained may show no definite increase in plasma cells or, alternatively, only mild plasmacytosis [30,139]. Since allergic drug reactions (especially to sulfonamides) [403] and chronic diseases associated with ongoing immune responses are also associated with marrow plasmacytosis (e.g., rheumatoid arthritis, tuberculosis, ulcerative colitis) [140], we feel it is usually necessary to demonstrate sheets or multiple clusters (greater than ten per oil immersion field) of plasma cells (Fig. 8) in order to make the diagnosis of a malignant plasma-cell dyscrasia (Table IV) [30]. This approach to histologic diagnosis rests on the demonstration of marrow plasma cell tumors rather than on any attempt at cytologic differentiation between normal and malignant plasma cells [139,141]. Although there is no question that some myeloma patients have marrow plasma cells that are so anaplastic as to be clearly malignant, this is the exception. In most situations it is difficult to distinguish normal from malignant plasma cells, despite the claim of some investigators that nuclear-cytoplasmic dissociation as determined by electron or light microscopy is useful [142,143].

Similarly, it should be emphasized that one cannot reliably determine the Ig abnormality from plasma-cell morphology [30,139,141,144,404]. Identification of the type of associated M-protein production is an immunochemical diagnosis and not a histologic one.

Many different types of inclusions have been described in plasma cells from normal individuals and myeloma patients. Russell bodies are intracytoplasmic hyaline, acidophilic, PAS-positive spherules which are electron-dense and located within the cisternae of the endoplasmic reticulum [145–147,405]. They appear to be Igs, perhaps L chains [148]. Russell bodies also have been described in plasma cells from primary amyloid patients [141]. Plasma cells containing numerous cytoplasmic vacuoles have been termed "Mott cells," "grape cells," and "morula cells;" these appear to be aggregates of Russell bodies. Other inclusions including crystals [149,150] and Auer-

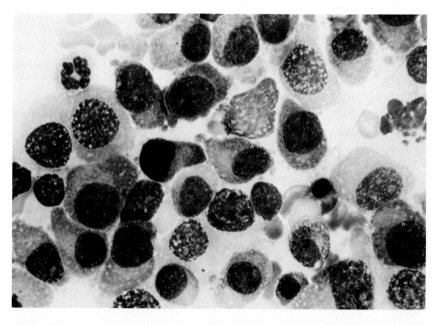

Fig. 8.   Bone marrow in myeloma. Pleomorphism of plasma cells is manifest by variation in cell size, nuclear-cytoplasmic ratio, and nuclear maturity. Many cells contain large nucleoli. (From Stone [11].)

like bodies [151,152] occur rarely. Unusual cases in which plasma cells appear to be phagocytic (containing red cells, polymorphonuclear leukocytes, platelets, and iron) have been reported [153–155,406]. Gaucher-like cells and acid phosphatase activity also have been described in myeloma [156,407].

Intracytoplasmic monoclonal Ig is demonstrable by the immunofluorescence [80,85–87] or immunoperoxidase [157,158] methods. Myeloma cells are usually negative for surface Ig [159]. The number of peripheral blood B lymphocytes has been found to be reduced in myeloma patients but may rise after treatment [160–163]. Some circulating B lymphocytes appear to bear the idiotypic determinants of the patient's myeloma protein [162–165]; this finding is of great potential significance. Involvement in the neoplastic monoclone may extend even to the pre-B cell stage [166]. Abnormalities in T-lymphocyte subpopulations also have been reported [408–410]. An *in vitro* assay that permits formation of colonies of human myeloma cells in soft agar has been developed [167] and may be useful in assessing susceptibility to various chemotherapeutic drugs.

An array of cytogenetic abnormalities in myeloma cells has been reported. Evidence indicates that genes on chromosome 14 may be involved in the regulation of lymphoid cell proliferation and lymphomas [168,411]. An abnormal chromosome 14 with extra bands at the end of the long arm (14q+) has been observed in myeloma as well as lymphomas [169–172]. This finding is not present in patients with myeloproliferative disorders and may represent a marker chromosome for lymphoid malignancy. A high incidence of aneuploidy has been detected in myeloma cells by the use of DNA flow cytometry [173,412].

Additional Studies

The recommended initial evaluation for a patient with known or suspected MM is listed in Table VI. Quantification of serum M-protein usually can be determined from the SPE pattern [31]. Reduction in the levels of normal serum Igs is generally present, reflecting the fact that these patients typically, but not always, manifest a poor antibody response following immunization [47,174–179,413]. In addition to the studies discussed previously, serum calcium, BUN and/or creatinine, uric acid, and electrolyte values should be obtained [30,180,181,414]. Some patients with myeloma and other gammopathies have a low anion "gap" [182–185,415,416]; if present, this may be a helpful diagnostic clue.[5] Determination of the creatinine clearance and renal biopsy should be considered if the patient has BJP, amyloid, or other renal disease [417–419]. Bone roentgenograms should be obtained to identify

[5]Ed. note: See also Chapter 3.

lytic lesions (Fig. 9). Osteosclerotic lesions are rare but do occur and may be associated with polyneuropathy [121,186,420–422]. Diffuse osteoporosis without lytic lesions is commonly seen; this finding is, of course, not diagnostic of myeloma [187–189]. Because of the predominantly lytic nature of bone destruction, bone scans are frequently negative in myeloma [423]. Occasional patients present with apparently "solitary" intraosseous lytic defects that are found to be plasmacytomas at biopsy (see Case 3). Although evidence of other marrow involvement may not be demonstrable initially, typical "multiple" myeloma develops within three years in most instances [30,88]. By contrast, extramedullary plasmacytomas may or may not be associated with identifiable M-proteins and progressive disease [89–111,390–394].

TABLE VI. Recommendations for the Diagnostic Evaluation of Patients with Plasma-Cell Dyscrasias

MANDATORY PROCEDURES

History
Physical examination
Laboratory tests
  CBC and platelet count
  Serum protein electrophoresis and immunoelectrophoresis
  Serum calcium, BUN/creatinine, uric acid, and electrolytes
  Urine protein screen (SSA/TSA)
  Quantitative 24-h urinary protein excretion
  Urine protein electrophoresis and immunoelectrophoresis
Radiographic examinations
  Chest
  Bone survey
Bone marrow aspirate/biopsy[a]

CONTINGENT PROCEDURES

ESR
Quantitative serum immunoglobulins
Creatinine clearance
Coagulation studies, bleeding time
Rectal biopsy for amyloid[b]
Serum viscosity determination
Serum cryoglobulin determination
Rheumatoid factor titer
Cold agglutinin titer
Other tissue biopsies: Lymph node, small bowel, etc.

[a]Whenever possible, both aspirate and biopsy should be obtained.
[b]Tissue should be examined by Congo red staining under polarized light and by electron microscopy.
From Stone [11].

CASE 3. "SOLITARY" INTRAMEDULLARY PLASMACYTOMA

This 38-year-old woman presented in 1970 because of the abrupt onset of pain in the left shoulder after minor trauma. Physical examination was within normal limits except for marked tenderness over the upper left arm without evidence of soft tissue swelling. Roentgenograms revealed a pathologic fracture in the proximal humerus through a solitary lytic defect which on biopsy was a plasmacytoma. CBC and routine blood chemistries were normal. SPE showed hypoalbuminemia and increased α_2-globulin but no monoclonal component. Urine protein excretion was 500 mg/24 h; the BJ heat test was negative, but the TSA test was positive. UPE (Fig. 5) showed a monoclonal component, identified by IEP as λ-BJP. The bone marrow contained 7% diffusely distributed plasma cells. A diagnosis of intramedullary plasmacytoma (? localized) was made and the patient received radiotherapy to the humeral lesion.

Two months later, the patient underwent an uneventful vaginal hysterectomy for cervical carcinoma *in situ*. She was lost to follow-up for 14 months when she returned with low back pain. Laboratory studies and bone marrow were unchanged from the previous findings, and bone survey revealed no new lesions. However, 24-hour urine protein excretion had risen to 1.6 g. IEP again confirmed marked λ-Bence Jones proteinuria. The patient was treated with intermittent courses of melphalan. During the next 2 years, her 24-hour urine protein excretion diminished to 420 mg/24 h and she remained well. She developed diffuse osteolytic lesions 2 years later and expired due to progressive myeloma in 1976.

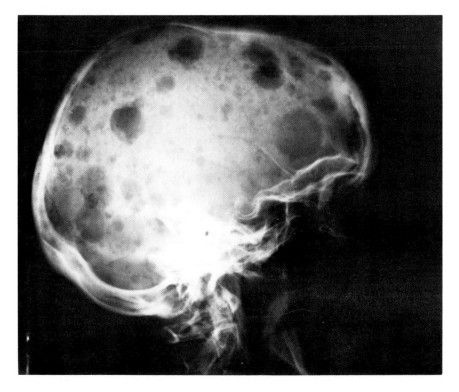

Fig. 9.   Multiple myeloma. Roentgenogram demonstrates numerous sharply defined, "punched-out" osteolytic lesions. (From Stone [11].)

Comment: This young woman initially appeared to have an isolated plasma cell tumor, but her subsequent course documented systemic involvement. Evidence for diffuse disease was supported by the quantitatively progressive λ-BJ proteinuria.

Typical diffuse myeloma eventually develops in most patients presenting with apparently "solitary" intraosseous plasmacytoma, although a decade or more may pass before this occurs. Eight patients in our LCD series presented with symptoms referable to "localized" plasmacytomas, and all but one demonstrated generalized involvement within 3 years of diagnosis [30].

Other studies listed in Table VI as "Contingent Procedures" should be obtained, if indicated.

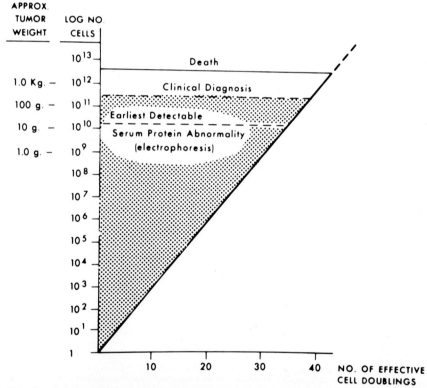

Fig. 10. Relation of tumor weight and cell number to the number of effective cell doublings from the initiation of a malignant monoclone. It should be emphasized that time is not shown on the abscissa of this graph, because the tumor-cell doubling time is not constant. The figure is designed to show the "iceberg" of preclinical doublings that go on prior to potential detection of an M-component on serum electrophoresis. Clinical diagnosis is generally about one or more logs above that point. (From Salmon [191].)

The dangers of intravenous pyelography (IVP) in myeloma patients with BJ proteinuria has been documented repeatedly [30,180,190]. This radiographic examination is most likely to be obtained in the patient with undiagnosed myeloma who presents with renal failure of "unknown" etiology (see Case 2). It is just this circumstance in which the identification and quantification of proteinuria becomes critical, since dehydration prior to IVP can lead to irreversible renal failure in patients with Bence Jones proteinuria. If an IVP is required in such a patient, he or she should not be dehydrated prior to the procedure.

On the basis of cell kinetic studies, Salmon [191,424] and others [425] have confirmed the fact that the amount of M-protein reflects the magnitude of the tumor-cell burden in myeloma patients (Figs. 10, 11). Thus, the serum

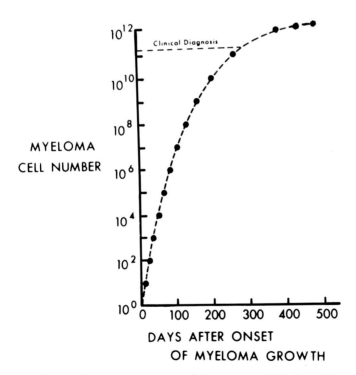

Fig. 11. Gompertzian curve of tumor growth for a patient with IgG multiple myeloma. The data points are computer-generated and placed at 1 log intervals, up to 10^{12} cells, and are based on back extrapolation from tumor-cell number determinations in the clinical phase of illness. In this patient, the preclinical phase appears to be less than 1 year in duration. (From Salmon [191].)

and/or urine M-components serve as markers that are useful not only in diagnosis but also in determination of the extent of disease. The initial staging criteria for myeloma patients which have been derived from such kinetic studies [129] are shown in Table VII. This staging system has been shown to provide helpful prognostic information [192,193,426].

Prognosis and Treatment

The disease is progressive, but optimal management improves both the quality and duration of life [30,32,122,129,130,191–197]. Life expectancy is related to the extent of disease at diagnosis, adequacy of supportive measures, and response to chemotherapy or other modalities [32,122,167,176,191–208,427–434]. The criterion for objective response to chemotherapy is usually taken as a 50% or greater decrement in the serum M-spike or urine BJP excretion. Serial determinations of M-protein quantity in serum and urine thus constitute an important aspect of management of myeloma patients. Death most often results from infection or renal failure [435]. Myeloma occasionally terminates in acute leukemia, a complication apparently related to prolonged treatment with alkylating agents [200,436,437].

TABLE VII. Myeloma Staging System

Stage I: Low cell mass (<0.6 × $10^{12}/M^2$ myeloma cells)[a]
All of the following
Hemoglobin > 10 g/100 mL
Serum calcium normal (≤ 12 mg/100 mL)
On roentgenogram, normal bone structure or solitary bone plasmacytoma only
Low M-component production rates
IgG < 5 g/100 mL
IgA < 3 g/100 mL
Bence Jones proteinuria < 4 g/24 h
Stage II: Intermediate cell mass (0.6 to 1.2 × $10^{12}/M^2$ myeloma cells)
Fitting neither Stage I nor Stage III
Stage III: High cell mass (>1.2 × $10^{12}/M^2$ myeloma cells)
One or more of the following
Hemoglobin < 8.5 g/100 mL
Serum calcium > 12 mg/100 mL
Advanced lytic bone lesions
High M-component production rates
IgG > 7 g/100 mL
IgA > 5 g/100 mL
Bence Jones proteinuria > 12 g/24 h
Subclassification
A = relatively normal renal function (serum creatinine < 2.0 mg/100 mL)
B = abnormal renal function (serum creatinine ≥ 2.0 mg/100 mL)

[a]10^{12} cells ~ 1 kg; M^2 = square meter of body surface area.
Modified from Durie and Salmon [129].

MACROGLOBULINEMIA

Macroglobulinemia of Waldenström (MW) is distinct from MM clinically as well as immunochemically. MW is a plasma-cell dyscrasia which involves cells that normally synthesize IgM Igs [23,122,209] (Table VIII). Approximately 12% of all patients with monoclonal gammopathies have MW [32,210]. This disorder resembles a lymphoma more than it does myeloma; modest generalized lymphadenopathy and hepatosplenomegaly are commonly noted in patients with MW [33,209,211,212]. "Plasmacytoid" lymphocytes are classically noted in the marrow of patients with MW, but as noted above, there is no reliable way by which the type of Ig abnormality can be predicted from marrow morphology in the plasma-cell dyscrasias [30,144]. Thus, we have seen patients with MW in whom many of the marrow elements appear as typical plasma cells indistinguishable from those seen in the usual myeloma patient; by contrast, other patients with MW have cells which resemble small lymphocytes like those noted in patients with chronic lymphocytic leukemia (CLL). Indeed, immunofluorescent studies have revealed that patients with MW have IgM surface Ig receptors demonstrable on peripheral blood lymphocytes as is found in 90–95% of patients with CLL [213]. However, unlike the latter, many lymphocytes from MW patients also display significant intracytoplasmic IgM synthesis and secretion. Although MW bears many similarities to CLL, it thus appears that a more differentiated or "intermediate" type of lymphoid cell is involved in the neoplastic process [214,215]. The cell type present in most patients with CLL resembles that of an antigen-reactive B lymphocyte, which has not differentiated to the point where significant intracytoplasmic synthesis and secretion of IgM has occurred. Substantial evidence indicates that the small B lymphocyte of CLL, the inter-

TABLE VIII. Waldenström's Macroglobulinemia

A plasma-cell dyscrasia specifically involving cells that normally synthesize IgM immunoglobulins
Clinically distinct from myeloma
    Resembles a lymphoma (lymphadenopathy and hepatosplenomegaly)
    Symptoms are 2° to the monoclonal protein (hyperviscosity syndrome)
    "Plasmacytoid" lymphocytes in marrow; B-cell leukemia similar to CLL[a]
    Lytic bone lesions rare (hypercalcemia rare)
    Significant Bence Jones proteinuria rare (renal failure rare)
Similar to myeloma
    Anemia common
    Increased susceptibility to bacterial infections
    Amyloidosis occurs

[a]CLL-chronic lymphocytic leukemia.
From Stone [11] with permission.

mediate or "plasmacytoid" lymphocyte of MW, and the typical plasma cell of MM (the latter lacking surface Ig receptors but having the fully developed apparatus for intracytoplasmic synthesis and secretion of Ig) form a spectrum of human B-cell neoplasia [216,217]. Preliminary studies have demonstrated that peripheral blood lymphocytes from patients with MW have increased adenosine deaminase (ADA) activity, a finding not seen in peripheral lymphocytes from patients with CLL or myeloma [218].

Several other features of MW distinguish it from a myeloma (Table VIII). First, lytic bone lesions are very rare in MW; thus, the bone pain and hypercalcemia are most uncommon. Although destructive bone lesions have been described rarely in "IgM myeloma," their presence should make one question the diagnosis of MW [53,219]. Second, heavy BJ proteinuria is infrequent in MW; thus, severe renal failure of the type so commonly encountered in myeloma patients tends to be uncommon [23,220].

The rarity of osteolytic lesions and heavy BJ proteinuria are two important features responsible for the relative benignity of MW as compared with myeloma. The third feature that distinguishes MW from most cases of myeloma involves the common occurrence of the hyperviscosity syndrome (vide infra) in the former.

MW also has features in common with myeloma (Table VIII). Thus, anemia and recurrent bacterial infections may be seen [174]. Amyloidosis occurs in MW, though it is less frequent than in myeloma. This lower frequency of tissue amyloid deposition may relate to the fact that marked imbalance in H-L chain synthesis is unusual in MW. In addition, 80% of monoclonal IgM proteins have κ-L chains; this type is less commonly associated with the presence of amyloid than λ-L chains [30,221].

In a significant proportion of patients, the monoclonal macroglobulins are antibodies directed to autologous IgG (rheumatoid factors) [20,222–225] or to the I red cell antigen (cold agglutinins) [226–229]. In such individuals, the presence of cryoglobulinemia or cold-antibody immunohemolytic anemia, respectively, may first draw attention to the presence of the underlying IgM plasma-cell dyscrasia. Rarely, a monoclonal macroglobulin may possess the properties of both a cold agglutinin and a cryoglobulin [230].

Hyperviscosity Syndrome[6]

Occasional patients with diffuse non-Hodgkin's lymphoma or chronic lymphocytic leukemia will be noted to have a serum IgM spike evident on SPE. In most instances these spikes are quantitatively small and reflect the fact that the involved clone of malignant B cells has some capacity to synthesize and secrete monoclonal IgM [231]. This circumstance has been re-

[6]Ed. note: See also Chapters 1 and 9 and [490].

ferred to as "macroglobulinemic lymphoma." By contrast, the quantitative values of serum M-spikes in patients with typical MW tend to be high; it is this group of patients which commonly manifest *"hyperviscosity syndrome"* (HVS).

IgM (mol wt 900,000 daltons) is an 18S pentamer of 4-chain subunits and has a high intrinsic viscosity; when present in serum at a concentration in excess of 4 g/dL, its relative viscosity rises almost exponentially [232]. MW accounts for approximately 90% of cases of HVS [233]. The differential diagnosis includes MM (where 5–10% of patients may develop HVS, especially those with IgG_3 and IgA proteins), rheumatoid arthritis, and polycythemia [233–242]. The two most important features of the HVS are that 1) it can be diagnosed by physical examination; and 2) most of the symptoms and findings are readily reversible by prompt removal of plasma (plasmapheresis or plasma exchange). The characteristic physical finding consists of enormous dilatation and tortuosity of the retinal veins ("sausaging") (Fig. 12). Patients with HVS tend to have a variety of other symptoms and findings,

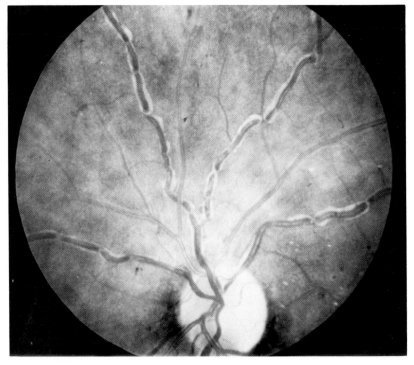

Fig. 12. Fundus in macroglobulinemia. Note retinal vein engorgement with "sausaging." (From Stone [11].)

particularly fatigue, skin and mucosal bleeding, and variable neurologic disorders. The determination of relative serum viscosity with an Ostwald viscosimeter is simple, rapid, and inexpensive. Moreover, viscosity measurements utilizing this method have been demonstrated to correlate closely with clinical findings in patients with macroglobulinemia [232]. Reduction of serum viscosity can be easily monitored during therapy with plasmapheresis [232,233,243] or cytotoxic drugs. Although the viscosity level at which signs and symptoms of HVS develop varies widely from patient to patient, it tends to be relatively constant in any one patient [232,438–440]. This has led to the concept of a "symptomatic threshold" and has made the serial determination of serum viscosity in patients with macroglobulinemia an important part of initial evaluation and subsequent management. It is not necessary to return the patient's relative serum viscosity to normal but only to keep it below his symptomatic threshold. Some patients with macroglobulinemia can be managed solely by plasmapheresis, although alkylating agents may also be employed to suppress IgM production [244].

Symptoms and Signs

The usual mode of presentation of MW is exemplified by the elderly patient who presents with manifestations of HVS: fatigue, generalized weakness, skin and mucosal bleeding, visual disturbances, headache, and a variety of other neurologic signs and symptoms [209,245]. A history or evidence of Sjögren's syndrome may be present. Cardiopulmonary abnormalities predominate in some patients and are associated with an increased plasma volume, which, together with the elevated serum viscosity, contribute to circulatory impairment [246,247]. The history of cold sensitivity or Raynaud's phenomenon is associated with the presence of a cryoglobulin or cold agglutinin. Recurrent bacterial infections constitute a major problem in some patients [174]. Physical examination frequently discloses purpura, modest generalized lymphadenopathy, and hepatosplenomegaly. As noted previously, diagnosis of HVS can be made by the finding of marked retinal venous engorgement and localized narrowing, which gives the sausage-like appearance.

Evidence of polyneuropathy is present in some patients [248,249,441]. Rarely, patients with the clinical features of MW are found to have serum monoclonal IgG or IgA Igs [250].

Laboratory Findings

Moderate anemia with profound rouleau and a very high ESR are characteristic. Leukopenia, relative lymphocytosis, and thrombocytopenia occasionally occur. The Sia test is usually positive but is nonspecific since it indicates only an increase in euglobulins.

Cryoglobulins, rheumatoid factor, or cold agglutinins may be present—in the latter instance, the direct Coombs' test may be positive and is of the "non-γ" variety.

Cryoglobulins are usually Igs that precipitate or gel at temperatures below 37°C and become soluble on rewarming [20,222–225,442]. Other non-Ig plasma proteins also may be present. Most commonly, such cryoglobulins are "mixed," i.e., they contain more than one Ig component, usually IgM and IgG. Almost all mixed IgM-IgG cryoglobulins possess high-titer rheumatoid factor activity [20,223]. In addition, such antigen-antibody complexes may be associated with hypocomplementemia. The finding of cryoglobulinemia suggests the presence of circulating immune complexes and/or a plasma-cell dyscrasia in any patient in whom it is identified. Care should be taken in collecting and processing the blood specimen when cryoglobulins (or cold agglutinins) are sought. This is particularly true with the mixed cryoproteins, many of which precipitate out at temperatures as high as 30–35°C. Whenever cryoglobulins are suspected, therefore, the blood should be allowed to clot and promptly centrifuged at 37°C. Cryoglobulins are found in a variety of disease states (Table IX) and may be associated with significant clinical

TABLE IX. Some Disorders Associated with Cryoglobulinemia

Myeloma and macroglobulinemia
Diffuse lymphoma and chronic lymphocytic leukemia
Connective tissue diseases
   Systemic lupus erythematosus
   Polyarteritis nodosa
   Sjögren's syndrome
   Rheumatoid arthritis
   Juvenile rheumatoid arthritis
   Ankylosing spondylitis
   Lyme arthritis
Renal disease (glomerulonephritis, nephrotic syndrome, renal tubular acidosis)
Cirrhosis and chronic active hepatitis
Sarcoidosis
Purpura-arthralgia syndrome
Infections
   Infectious mononucleosis
   Bacterial endocarditis
   Leprosy
   Cytomegalovirus
   Syphilis
   Hepatitis B
   Malaria
Status post-intestinal bypass surgery for obesity

From Stone [11] with permission.

findings (Table X). In patients with HVS *(vide supra),* the coexisting presence of a cryoglobulin may be responsible for marked temperature dependence of serum viscosity [223,439,440] (Fig. 13).

A melange of coagulation abnormalities and evidence of a platelet functional defect may be present (Table XI) [251,252]. A typical M-spike on SPE, which proves to be IgM by IEP, establishes the diagnosis. Variable amounts of low molecular weight (8S monomer) IgM may be present in

TABLE X. Manifestations of Cryoglobulinemia

Weakness
Purpura (dependent)
Arthralgias
Raynaud's phenomenon
Acrocyanosis (occ. peripheral gangrene)
Livedo reticularis
Cold urticaria
Cutaneous vasculitis with ulceration
Visual disturbances and retinal hemorrhages
Mucosal bleeding tendency
Cerebral thrombosis
Lymphadenopathy
Hepatosplenomegaly
Renal disease (proliferative glomerulonephritis, nephrotic syndrome, renal tubular acidosis)
None

From Stone [11] with permission.

TABLE XI. Hemostatic Abnormalities Associated with Macroglobulinemia and Other Monoclonal Gammopathies

Hemorrhagic abnormalities
  Abnormalities of platelets
    Thrombocytopenia
    Impaired function
  Abnormalities of plasma coagulation factors
    Inhibitors of coagulation
      Fibrin monomer aggregation
      Factor VIII
      Nonspecific—usually detected by thromboplastin generation test
      Other coagulation factors
      Factor X deficiency due to *in vivo* inactivation
    Depression of clotting factors
  Hyperviscosity syndrome
  Miscellaneous
Thrombotic abnormalities

From Lackner [251] with permission.

some patients. Immunoelectrophoretic study of concentrated urine frequently demonstrates a monoclonal L chain (κ in 80% of cases), but gross BJ proteinuria is uncommon. Bone x-rays may show osteoporosis but lytic lesions are very rarely present. The marrow shows a variable increase in plasma cells, lymphocytes, intermediate forms ("plasmacytoid" lymphocytes), and mast cells [253]. Periodic acid-Schiff (PAS)-positive intranuclear inclusions in the lymphoid cells are characteristic but nonspecific [254]. Lymph node biopsies are frequently interpreted as "pleomorphic lymphoma." Occasionally, the histologic appearance resembles that of histiocytic lymphoma, immunoblastic sarcoma, or hairy-cell leukemia [217,255,256]. It should be

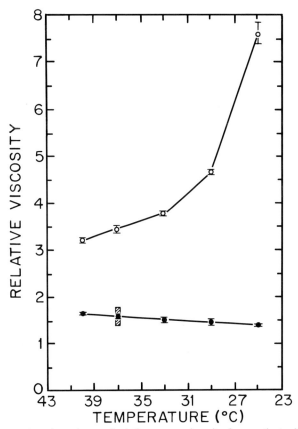

Fig. 13. Temperature dependence of relative serum viscosity from patient with macroglobulinemia and cryoglobulinemia. ○ = patient's serum. ● = normal serum. Brackets indicate range of duplicate determinations. Bar indicates normal range (1.4–1.8) at 37°C. (From Stone and Fedak J [223].)

emphasized that a definitive histopathologic diagnosis of MW cannot be made by light microscopy. Amyloidosis occurs in about 5% of patients. An association between nodular regenerative hyperplasia of the liver and macroglobulinemia has been recently reported [443].

Prognosis and Treatment

The course is variable but tends to be more benign than myeloma. If evidence of HVS is present, initial management consists of reducing serum viscosity by plasmapheresis or plasma exchange. Although only a temporary measure, plasmapheresis is the most effective and rapid means of reversing the bleeding and neurologic abnormalities caused by high circulating levels of IgM [232,233,243,244].

Chemotherapy with oral alkylating agents is effective on a long-term basis in the majority of patients. As is true in myeloma, serial quantification of the M-spike by SPE is critical in objective assessment of the response to treatment.

CASE 4. WALDENSTRÖM'S MACROGLOBULINEMIA (MW)

A 55-year-old white male machinist was well until August 1968, when he noted "cold feet" and hemorrhagic areas over the lower extremities. One month later, he developed severe generalized headaches, blurred vision, gingival bleeding, and epistaxis. At another hospital he was found to have modest generalized lymphadenopathy, hepatosplenomegaly, ataxia, purpura, marked engorgement of the retinal veins, and a mild anemia. Bone marrow aspiration disclosed 21% "lymphoid elements." SPE revealed a 6.5 g/dL monoclonal spike that consisted of IgM; IgG and IgA levels were reduced. The diagnosis of MW with hyperviscosity syndrome was made and the patient was treated with intermittent courses of chlorambucil over the ensuing 15 months. During this interval his hyperviscosity symptoms improved somewhat and the splenomegaly receded.

The patient was referred to this institution in January 1970. He still complained of headaches, visual disturbances, skin and mucosal bleeding, cold lower extremities and a "blotchy" color of the skin over the legs. He denied Raynaud's phenomenon and acrocyanosis. There was no history of arthralgias, arthritis or morning stiffness, dry eyes, xerostomia, paresthesias, bone pain, weight loss, or increased susceptibility to infections.

An attack of recurrent rheumatic fever led to a medical discharge from the military in 1943. The patient gave a history of long-standing allergic rhinitis but had never received hyposensitization therapy. He denied other allergies, asthma, and previous transfusions. The family history was noncontributory.

On physical examination the patient was obese with normal vital signs, petechiae over the left upper arm, and livido reticularis over the lower legs. There was no significant lymphadenopathy. Funduscopic examination disclosed severe venous engorgement with typical "sausaging" (Fig. 12). Marked sheathing of the retinal veins was evident; no hemorrhages were present and the optic discs were flat. Cardiac examination revealed an atrial gallop but no murmur. The liver edge was palpable 2 cm under the right costal margin, and the spleen was palpable 2 cm below the left costal margin. The joints were normal except for the presence of Heberden's nodes. Neurologic examination was unremarkable except for mild tandem-gait ataxia. The remainder of the physical examination was within normal limits.

Initial laboratory data included hemoglobin 13.2 g/dL, hematocrit 39%, white blood cell count 4,200/mm³ and platelets 150,000/mm³. Rouleau and occasional plasmacytoid lymphocytes were noted on peripheral smear. The ESR (Westergren) was 135 mm/h at 37°C and the Sia test was 4+. Relative serum viscosity was 6.5 at 37°C; large amounts of cryoglobulin were present, which caused a marked increase in viscosity below 30°C and opaque serum at 25°C. After 1 hour at 4°C, the serum solidified completely. SPE demonstrated a 3.8 g/dL homogeneous component in the γ-region. Urinary protein excretion was 360 mg/24 h and creatinine clearance was 117 mL/min. A concentrated urine specimen contained κ- but no evidence of λ-L chains by IEP. Bone marrow aspiration disclosed a hypercellular marrow with 10% plasma cells and focal clusters of lymphocytes. Intranuclear PAS positive inclusions were present in the latter. The patient's red cells were type A; his serum anti-B titer was 1:64. Direct Coombs' and cold agglutinin tests were negative. Clot retraction was decreased but other coagulation studies as well as routine chemistries, chest film, bone survey, and electrocardiogram were within normal limits. The patient underwent plasmapheresis with the removal of 3,300 mL of plasma over a 4-day period with reduction in relative serum viscosity to 3.5 and improvement in symptoms of hyperviscosity syndrome. Daily chlorambucil therapy was begun in the dosage of 2–4 mg/d, which produced modest granulocytopenia and maintained the relative serum viscosity between 3.0 and 3.5. The serum monoclonal component had decreased to 2.3 g/dL by September 1971. The patient remained asymptomatic although his cryoglobulinemia and retinopathy persisted. He expired from hepatitis in 1974.

Comment: This patient presented with typical MW and HVS. The hyperviscosity was enhanced by the presence of a cryoglobulin with high thermal sensitivity. His disease was controlled with plasmapheresis and alkylating agent therapy. Subsequent studies disclosed that this patient's cryoglobulin was an immune complex, the monoclonal IgM being an antibody to polyclonal IgG [20,223]. His serum gave a rheumatoid factor titer of 1:256,000 (bentonite flocculation method).

PRIMARY SYSTEMIC AMYLOIDOSIS[7]

It has been known for many years that 10–15% of patients with typical multiple myeloma have amyloid demonstrable in various organs at autopsy. More recently, it has become clear that most patients presenting with the manifestations of "primary" systemic amyloidosis of the non-hereditary type have an identifiable monoclonal Ig abnormality [30,221]. Amyloid deposition in these individuals tends to be distributed in the heart, tongue, gastrointestinal tract, skin, ligaments, and peripheral nerves [257]. However, involve-

[7]Ed. note: See also Chapter 11.

TABLE XII. Characterization of Human Amyloid Fibrils

Physical properties (common to all forms of amyloid)
  Polarized light: green birefringence with Congo red
  EM appearance: 70 to 100 Å nonbranching fibrils
  X-ray diffraction pattern: β-pleated sheet conformation
Chemical studies (two major types of amyloid proteins)
  Amyloid AL:Intact monoclonal immunoglobulin light chains and/or fragments from N-
    terminal (variable) region
    Patients with nonfamilial *primary* systemic or plasma cell dyscrasia-associated
      amyloidosis
    Approximately 15% of Bence Jones proteins apparently "amyloidogenic" ($\lambda > \kappa$)
  Amyloid AA: Not derived from L chains
    Patients with *secondary* amyloidosis (rheumatoid arthritis, bronchiectasis, tuberculosis,
      Hodgkin's and familial Mediterranean fever)
    Mol wt $\simeq$ 9,000 daltons
    No relationship to any known immunoglobulin fragment
    Origin obscure but appears related to minor component in normal serum (? acute-phase
      reactant)
  Additional types of amyloid proteins reported

Revised from Stone [11].

ment of liver, kidneys, spleen, and adrenals—a distribution more characteristic of "secondary" amyloidosis, may also occur. Because of this overlap
in distribution of amyloid, differentiation into "primary" and "secondary"
types on the basis of organ involvement is often difficult.

The principal reason for retaining the "primary" and "secondary" nomenclature rests on the demonstration of the chemically distinct nature of amyloid
fibrils found in patients in whom a recognizable, coexisting, chronic infectious or inflammatory disease is ("secondary") or is not ("primary") present.
Although amyloid fibrils from various sources share the same physical properties as delineated by Congo red staining under polarized light, electron
microscopy, and x-ray diffraction patterns, chemical studies have revealed
two major types of amyloid fibril proteins (Table XII).

In patients with nonfamilial "primary" systemic amyloidosis or PCD-
associated amyloidosis, the major constituent of the isolated amyloid fibril
protein usually consists of intact monoclonal Ig L chains and/or fragments
from their N-terminal (variable) region [258–260]. Therefore, the amyloid
in these patients (amyloid AL) appears to consist of extracellular deposits of
intact or fragmented BJP. In our experience, approximately 80% of patients
presenting with "primary" (i.e., without evidence of coexisting chronic infectious or inflammatory disease) systemic amyloidosis have identifiable M-

proteins in serum and/or urine. The most commonly observed M-protein abnormality consists of BJP exclusively [30,221]. Thus, accurate characterization of urinary proteins is critically important in this group of patients. Approximately 15% of BJP appear to be "amyloidogenic"; i.e., they have the property of precipitating as fibrillar material resembling amyloid following *in vitro* proteolytic digestion [444]. This amyloidogenic property is more commonly observed with λ- than with κ- monoclonal L chains [445].

Our previous study of 35 patients with L chain myeloma [30] included seven subjects who presented with primary systemic amyloidosis (see Case 5). The carpal-tunnel syndrome, macroglossia, congestive heart failure, arthralgias, peripheral neuropathy, and gastrointestinal bleeding were findings confined to the amyloid group. By contrast, patients without evidence of amyloid presented with the typical symptoms of myeloma (skeletal pain, renal failure, etc.).

The recent insights into the chemical nature of amyloid fibrils have clinical implications that are pertinent to our study. The amyloid patients presented with complaints directly relating to tissue deposition of amyloid, whereas the other LCD patients exhibited the usual symptoms and signs of myeloma. Yet the monoclonal L chain abnormality and degree of evident plasma-cell proliferation were similar in both groups [30]. These considerations emphasize that the distinction between "primary systemic amyloidosis" and "myeloma-associated amyloidosis" is vague, particularly when the M-protein disturbance involves overproduction of BJP. Both of these forms of amyloid have recently been designated "immunocyte-derived amyloid" by Glenner [444]. The experimental studies relating BJP and amyloid may explain the rather high incidence (20%) of amyloidosis in LCD. Amyloid has been identified only rarely in the remainder of our myeloma population, a finding similar to that of Hobbs [78].

The data are consistent with the hypothesis that LCD patients who synthesize and secrete BJPs possessing "amyloidogenic" properties tend to have an illness dominated by the features of primary amyloidosis instead of the usual manifestations noted in other myeloma patients. The resulting clinical picture would be, therefore, more dependent on the molecular structure of the individual BJP produced than on any intrinsic difference between primary amyloidosis and MM. Such a hypothesis does not dictate that every patient producing "amyloidogenic" L chains need necessarily develop clinical amyloidosis; some clearly do not [258,260,444], suggesting that additional factors play a role in the tissue deposition of amyloid fibrils [261].

In contrast to primary amyloidosis, patients with amyloidosis "secondary" to rheumatoid arthritis, bronchiectasis, tuberculosis, Hodgkin's disease, and familial Mediterranean fever (FMF), have as the major constituent in their amyloid fibrils a protein (called Protein AA) which is not derived from Ig L chains (Table XII) [262,263]. Its origin is obscure, but it appears to be related to some minor component present in normal serum [264,446]. Amyloid AA has been found in fibroblasts [265], plasma cells and Kupffer cells [266], and polymorphonuclear leukocytes [267]. Amyloid AA has been isolated from an occasional patient with "primary" or "idiopathic" amyloidosis [268].

Additional chemical types of amyloid have been described, particularly those noted in association with tumors of endocrine glands (e.g., medullary thyroid carcinoma and islet-cell tumors of the pancreas) [269,270]. Another chemically distinct type of amyloid (protein A_{SCA}) has been described recently in individuals with senile cardiac amyloidosis [271]. Prealbumin is the major protein in fibrils from patients with hereditary amyloid other than FMF [447–450]. Thus "amyloid" appears to be a generic term applying to fragments of many different proteins which can be deposited in tissues as fibrils (Table XIII).

Symptoms and Signs

Presenting manifestations are variable and depend on the organ or system which is predominantly involved. Thus, intractable low-output cardiac failure

TABLE XIII. Classification of Amyloidosis According to Major Protein Constituent of Fibrils

Type	Protein component
Primary systemic amyloid (nonhereditary)	AL (BJP)
Amyloid associated with plasma-cell dyscrasias	AL (BJP)
Secondary systemic amyloid	AA
Hereditary amyloid (FMF)	AA
Hereditary amyloid (except FMF)	Prealbumin
Senile amyloid (cardiac)	A_{SCA}
Amyloid associated with endocrine tumors (MTC)	Peptide hormone (precalcitonin)
Localized amyloid	?

AL = amyloid related to monoclonal immunoglobulin L chains; BJP = Bence Jones protein; AA = amyloid A (nonimmunoglobulin derived); FMF = familial Mediterranean fever; SCA = senile cardiac amyloid; MTC = medullary thyroid carcinoma.

with or without conduction defects and arrhythmias, macroglossia, gastrointestinal bleeding or diarrhea, carpal-tunnel syndrome, arthralgias associated with periarticular thickening, autonomic or peripheral neuropathy, skin plaques and purpura, hepatosplenomegaly, or massive proteinuria may be seen [272–275,451–454].

Diagnosis

Amyloidosis can be diagnosed only by biopsy [276]. The finding of fibrillar material in urinary sediments is nonspecific, and this method should not be employed to establish the diagnosis [277]. Tissue should be stained with Congo red and examined under polarized light for presence of the characteristic yellow-green birefringence [276,455]. The typical fibrillar structure is well demonstrated by electron microscopy. Biopsy of rectal mucosa is the safest and most convenient screening procedure [272]. In any patient found to have "primary" amyloid, a careful search should be made for the presence of a homogeneous Ig or L chain in both serum and concentrated urine [30]. Bence Jones proteinuria without an accompanying serum M-spike is the abnormality most frequently encountered. Coagulation studies may be prolonged in a rare amyloid patient due to a deficiency of factor X [278,456].

The bone marrow should be examined for evidence of plasmacytosis as well as amyloid. Evidence of "functional" hyposplenism (consisting of the triad of findings of abnormal red cell forms with Howell-Jolly bodies on peripheral blood smear, reduced or absent splenic uptake following injection of ^{99m}Tc-sulfur colloid, and splenomegaly) has been documented in approximately 20% of our amyloid patients [30,279]. Circulating immune complexes and immunofluorescence findings on renal biopsies have been reported but are not characteristic for one particular type of amyloid [457,458]. Amyloid-related BJP binds dinitrophenyl lysine, and this property may prove to be useful as a diagnostic test [459]. Primary amyloidosis can be distinguished from the secondary form by the permanganate reaction [460].

Treatment of amyloidosis is unsatisfactory [444,445,461]. A recent report suggests that about 50% of patients with primary systemic amyloidosis treated with alkylating agents improve but that survival is not prolonged when compared to untreated controls [280]. Colchicine may be of benefit in certain patients [281,282].

CASE 5. PRIMARY SYSTEMIC AMYLOIDOSIS

In this 59-year-old man, bilateral carpal-tunnel syndrome (surgically relieved), hoarseness, a thick tongue, and bilateral submandibular swelling developed during the year prior to admission.

On physical examination the patient's tongue was indurated and enlarged as were the submandibular glands. The jugular veins were distended, and cardiomegaly was present. Scrotal and pretibial edema also was noted. The hemoglobin level was 14.2 g/dL, hematocrit value was 42%, white blood cell count 8,200/mm³, platelets 265,000/mm³, and ESR 15 mm/h. Rouleau was absent on the peripheral blood smear. Blood chemistry studies were within normal limits. SPE showed hypoalbuminemia and hypogammaglobulinemia. Serum levels of IgG, IgA, and IgM were low; IgD and IgE were undetectable. Urine protein was negative by Dipstix but 4+ by SSA; quantitative urine protein excretion was 4.5 g/24 h. BJP was present by both the heat and TSA tests. UPE demonstrated a typical M-spike in the fast γ-region, which accounted for more than 90% of the protein present; IEP showed a marked increase in λ-L chains, a small amount of albumin and no evidence of κ-determinants. Serum IEP revealed λ-BJ proteinemia. Voltage was normal on the electrocardiogram, and a bone survey revealed no abnormalities.

Needle biopsy of the tongue showed marked infiltration with amyloid. A bone marrow aspirate demonstrated 75% pleomorphic plasma cells in sheets and clusters.

Intermittent melphalan therapy was started. The 24-hour urine protein excretion was reduced to 650 mg 10 months later and 260 mg 16 months after institution of therapy, although λ-BJP remained the major urine protein component. The macroglossia did not change. However, claudication of thigh muscles developed, and the patient died from refractory congestive heart failure 18 months after diagnosis.

Postmortem examination disclosed a 690-g heart with extensive amyloidosis. Amyloid also was present in the tongue, esophagus, liver, spleen, kidneys, and small arterioles of the muscles. Only occasional renal glomeruli were involved with amyloid, and there was no evidence of myeloma kidney.

Comment: This patient presented with the classic features of primary systemic amyloidosis: bilateral carpal-tunnel syndrome, macroglossia, and congestive heart failure in the absence of a coexisting chronic disease. His persistent muscle pain on exertion was ischemic in origin due to amyloid infiltration of arterioles with subsequent limited capacity for vasodilation during exercise.

The association between amyloid, BJP, and marrow plasmacytosis has been stressed by many investigators. Strong support for the role of Ig components in the pathogenesis of amyloidosis has come from the studies of Glenner et al., who established the identity of fragments of monoclonal Ig L chains (BJPs) and certain amyloid fibril proteins [444,445].

This case is an excellent example of the close relationship between nonhereditary primary systemic amyloidosis and multiple myeloma. As is true in most patients with this type of amyloid, the initial clinical manifestations and subsequent course were dominated by the sequelae of amyloid deposition. It is noteworthy that this patient did not have anemia, lytic bone lesions, or evidence of severe renal functional impairment despite diffuse infiltration of his marrow by plasma cells and profound BJ proteinuria.

HEAVY CHAIN DISEASES

As noted previously, most monoclonal proteins are structurally similar to normal antibody molecules. By contrast, the heavy chain diseases (HCDs) are disorders in which incomplete monoclonal Igs ("true paraproteins") occur [462]. These unusual plasma-cell dyscrasias are characterized by the over-production of homogeneous gamma (γ), alpha (α), mu (μ), or delta (δ) Ig H chains. Abnormal lymphocytes or plasma cells secrete the various H chain components. The cliinical picture tends to be more similar to a lymphoma than to MM. Most of the H chain proteins are fragments of their normal H chain counterparts with internal deletions of variable length; these deletions appear to result from structural mutations [283]. Epsilon (ε) HCD is yet to be described.

IgG Heavy Chain (γ-Chain) Disease (γ-HCD)

More than 60 cases have been reported, primarily in elderly men [117,283]. However, the disease has occasionally been seen in childhood. Associated chronic disorders include rheumatoid arthritis, Sjögren's syndrome, systemic lupus erythematosus, tuberculosis, myasthenia gravis, hypereosinophilic syndrome, autoimmune hemolytic anemia, and thyroiditis. The clinical picture resembles that of a malignant lymphoma with lymphadenopathy and hepatosplenomegaly as usual findings. Anemia, leukopenia, thrombocytopenia, eosinophilia, and circulating atypical lymphocytes or plasma cells are common findings. Fever, recurrent infections, and reduction in normal Ig levels are also seen. Palatal edema is present in approximately one fourth of patients. The bone marrow and lymph node histopathology is variable. Lytic lesions are absent on bone x-rays in most patients. Amyloid deposits have rarely been found at autopsy.

The diagnosis is based on electrophoretic and IEP demonstration of free homogeneous H chain fragments of IgG in serum and urine. Evidence of associated monoclonal L chain production is usually absent [463]. Fifty percent of patients have monoclonal serum components (often appearing broad and heterogeneous) in excess of 1 g/dL and 50% have proteinuria greater than 1 g/24 h. Heavy chain proteins belonging to each of the four IgG subclasses have been reported, but the G3 subclass is especially common [462]. The course is variable—from a few months to more than 5 years. Death usually results from bacterial infection or progressive malignancy. Chemotherapy with alkylating agents or corticosteroids, and radiotherapy, sometimes yield transient remissions.

IgA Heavy Chain (α-Chain) Disease (α-HCD)

This is the most common of the HCD and tends to appear in young persons, most being between the ages of 10 and 30 years [284,285,462]. It is geographically limited almost entirely to the Middle East and bears a close relationship to "Mediterranean lymphoma" [286]. The disorder has been described in the United States [287]. The clinical picture is strikingly uniform, almost all patients presenting with the diffuse abdominal lymphoma and malabsorption syndrome. Histopathologic examination discloses massive infiltration of the intestine and mesenteric nodes with lymphocytes, plasma cells, and/or immunoblasts. The cellular infiltrate may be pleomorphic and not overtly malignant by histopathologic criteria. Peripheral nodes, marrow, liver, and spleen usually are not involved. No osteolytic lesions are seen on bone x-rays. A discrete M-spike may not be observed on routine SPE, but free α-chains are demonstrable by conventional IEP in 80% of cases; special immunochemical techniques are required to make the diagnosis in the remainder [288].

The abnormal protein is usually present in intestinal secretions and may be found in concentrated urine. As in γ-HCD, there is usually no evidence of BJP [463]. Several well-documented instances of prolonged remission have been reported following corticosteroid, cytotoxic drug, and broadspectrum antibiotic therapy. In view of the responses to antibiotics alone, and the peculiar geographic incidence of the disorder, α-HCD might, in fact, represent an aberrant immune response to a parasite or other microorganism which is not, in all cases, neoplastic [285]. A respiratory-tract form of the disease has rarely been described [289].

IgM Heavy Chain (μ-Chain) Disease (μ-HCD)

This variant represents the least common of the HCDs [117,283,290,291]. The clinical picture usually has been that of long-standing chronic lymphocytic leukemia or other lymphoproliferative disorder. Affected patients have primarily visceral organ involvement (spleen, liver, abdominal lymph nodes) with little peripheral lymphadenopathy. Vacuolated plasma cells are present in the bone marrow in two thirds of patients, but these vacuoles do not contain the abnormal protein [464]. BJ proteinuria (type κ), pathologic fractures, and amyloidosis may occur. Routine SPE usually is normal or shows hypo-γ-globulinemia. The diagnosis is made by the finding of a rapidly migrating serum component which reacts with antiserum to μ-chains but not with antisera to L chains. Free μ-chains are only rarely found in the urine. However, as noted, κ-BJ proteinuria may be present (10 of 15 patients) [291]. In those patients with associated BJP, the monoclonal κ-L chains are not structurally linked to the μ-chains even though they appear to be synthesized by the same cells that produce the μ-HCD proteins [464]; the reason for this failure of assembly is unclear.

IgD Heavy Chain (δ-Chain) Disease (δ-HCD)

A single case has been reported recently [465]. The patient was an elderly man with a clinical picture similar to multiple myeloma. Marked marrow plasmacytosis and osteolytic lesions in the skull were present. A small M-component was evident on SPE that reacted with a monospecific anti-IgD antiserum but not with other antisera of H or L chain specificity. Proteinuria was absent. Death occurred due to renal failure. The principal histopathologic finding in the kidney was a thickening of the glomerular basement membrane, presumably resulting from deposition of the abnormal protein.

The principal features of the H chain diseases are summarized in Table XIV.

LICHEN MYXEDEMATOSUS (PAPULAR MUCINOSIS)

This rare skin disease, also known as scleromyxedema, is characteristically associated with dermal deposits of mucin and a slow-migrating (cathodal) IgG monoclonal Ig in serum [122,292,293]. Most of these homogeneous IgG proteins bear λ-L chains. Other evidence of myeloma usually is absent, although myeloma-type therapy with alkylating agents has resulted in remission of the skin disorder in some patients. Certain IgG, λ-proteins from patients with lichen myxedematosus have an internal deletion of the Fd portion of the γ-H chain. These paraproteins do not share idiotypic specificity, suggesting that they are not antibodies to the same antigenic determinant [466].

OCCULT (ASYMPTOMATIC) PLASMA-CELL DYSCRASIAS

Plasma-Cell Dyscrasias of Unknown Significance (PCDUS)

As noted previously, the advent of SPE as a routine diagnostic test during the past 15 years has led to the relatively common finding of a homogeneous Ig in serum of patients with a wide variety of "nonmyelomatous" disorders [22,23,30,33,122,294–296,467]. These fortuitously discovered M-proteins have been documented in patients with chronic infectious and inflammatory diseases, nonreticular neoplasms, storage diseases, and many other disorders. Most of these individuals do not have additional evidence of multiple myeloma or other "overt" plasma-cell dyscrasias at the time these serum M-

TABLE XIV. Heavy Chain Diseases

	γ	α	μ	δ
First described	1964	1968	1970	1980
Approx. no. cases	>60	>150	15	1
Geographic incidence	North America, Europe	Mediterranean region and Middle East	North America, Europe	Europe
Age	Av ~50 yr (9–76)	Most 10–30 yr	Adults: Middle age–elderly	70 yr
Clinical picture	Lymphadenopathy, hepato-splenomegaly, swelling of uvula, bacterial infections, anemia	Malabsorption syndrome, diffuse abdominal lymphoma	Lymphoproliferative disorder, often CLL[a]; visceral lymphadenopathy	Renal failure
Histology	Variable-pleomorphic lymphoid infiltrates of lymph nodes and marrow	Variable-pleomorphic lymphoid infiltrates of small intestine and mesenteric nodes	Vacuolated plasma cells in marrow (10/15)	Plasma cells in marrow

	γ-chain	α-chain	μ-chain	δ-chain
SPE	Small M-peak (heterogeneous)	M-peak may or may not be evident	Normal or hypogamma-globulinemia	M-peak present
Serum IEP	Free γ-chains	Free α-chains in 80%; others require special studies	Free μ-chains	Free δ-chains
BJP	No[b]	No[b]	Yes: 10/15—all K	No
Osteolytic lesions	Rare	No	Yes: 5/15	Yes
Prognosis	Unfavorable: Death from bacterial infection or progressive malignancy in few months > 5 yr	Favorable: May be reversible with antibiotics; patients with progressive disease often respond to cytotoxic chemotherapy	Fair with CLL-type Rx	Death from renal failure

[a]CLL = chronic lymphocytic leukemia.
[b]See text.

spikes are found. However, it appears that 5–10% of such instances occur in patients with "presymptomatic" myeloma, in which the serum M-protein abnormality is discovered because an SPE was obtained (see Case 6). Unfortunately, no reliable method is presently available to distinguish this small group of "premyeloma" individuals from those with stable, nonprogressive plasma-cell dyscrasias [25,26,297,467]. Moreover, evolution to *full-blown myeloma* may take as long as 20 years to occur.

CASE 6. EVOLUTION OF PCDUS INTO MYELOMA

This 74-year-old black woman had been followed since 1962 for multiple complaints, mainly related to musculoskeletal pain. Initial evaluation showed evidence of degenerative joint disease (DJD), obesity, and mild hypertension. In 1971, she was found to have a small monoclonal serum spike on routine SPE. She was referred to the Hematology Clinic and was first seen in March 1973, at which time SPE confirmed the presence of a γ-spike of 2.3 g/dL with normal albumin and otherwise normal serum protein pattern. IEP disclosed that the spike consisted of a monoclonal IgG, κ-Ig. IgA was normal and there was a mild decrease in IgM; IgD and IgE were undetectable. IEP of concentrated urine showed no evidence of significant proteinuria or BJP. A 24-hour quantitative urine protein determination showed <200 mg. The metastatic bone survey was negative, and a bone marrow performed in March 1973 was normal (3% plasma cells). The patient's CBC, platelet count, and routine blood chemistries also were within normal limits. A rectal biopsy was negative for amyloid. She was felt to have a plasma-cell dyscrasia of unknown significance. She was followed in the clinic without evident change in status; serial SPE demonstrated a stable M-spike in the range of 2.3 to 2.5 g/dL. Except for ongoing lower extremity joint pain related to her DJD, she did well until October 1978, when a follow-up SPE demonstrated that the γ-M-spike had increased to 4.1 g/dL during the past year. The patient had also developed a mild normocytic, normochromic anemia (hemoglobin 9.4 g/dL, hematocrit 30%); white cell and platelet counts, as well as calcium, uric acid, BUN, and creatinine were within normal limits. A bone survey demonstrated DJD and diffuse osteoporosis but no lytic lesions. Because of the marked increase in a previously stable spike, a bone marrow was performed which revealed a hypercellular marrow with 50% plasma cells in sheets and clusters. She was started on chemotherapy with melphalan and prednisone.

Comment: Although most patients with PCDUS do not progress to overt myeloma, a few do. This patient was observed for 7 years before myeloma could be diagnosed; periodic reexamination is the only means presently available to identify the change in status in such patients.

With the recognition that some (? most) monoclonal Igs in humans and experimental animals appear to be true antibodies (see Monoclonal Igs as Antibodies), it seems likely that many M-proteins in patients with PCDUS may, in fact, represent monoclonal antibody responses. This conclusion is also supported by the finding of serum M-proteins in healthy individuals; in this case, the incidence is age-related. Thus, 1% of normal persons age 25 and 3% of individuals age 70 have such monoclonal Igs detectable in their serum. In the majority of cases of PCDUS, the Ig abnormality present is IgG. That this is a common finding is illustrated by the fact that approximately 30% of patients having serum monoclonal IgG components identified in our laboratory have been those in whom PCDUS was present (Table V). IgA and IgM M-components may be found in this group of patients but are less common.

It is important to evaluate the patient having a fortuitiously discovered serum M-spike for other evidence of myeloma. The criteria for the diagnosis of myeloma (Table IV) must be borne in mind in this regard. Features which we have found helpful in differentiating patients with myeloma from those with PCDUS are shown in Table XV.

By definition, patients with an apparently nonprogressive or stable plasma-cell dyscrasia (PCDUS) do not have sheets or clusters of marrow plasma cells, significant Bence Jones proteinuria, or lytic bone lesions. Similarly, such individuals would not be expected to have amyloidosis or unexplained renal failure. Some persons with asymptomatic monoclonal gammopathy have a subnormal antibody response following primary immunization [298]. Since the quantity of the M-component bears a direct relationship to the tumor-cell burden, patients with nonprogressive plasma cell dyscrasias generally tend to have lower serum M-spikes than those seen in myeloma patients. In this regard, it may be helpful to note that the average patient with IgG myeloma has a 4.3 g/dL serum M-spike, while the average serum M-component in patients with IgA myeloma is approximately 2.8 g/dL [78]. The most characteristic feature of patients with these apparently "benign" plasma cell tumors is the absence of a rise in the serum M-component on serial SPE analyses. We generally repeat the SPE at 4–6 month intervals. Only in the

TABLE XV. Findings Useful in Distinguishing Overt From Occult Plasma-Cell Dyscrasias (PCD)

Favor Overt PCD
    Marrow plasma cells in sheets or clusters
    Bence Jones proteinuria (> 300 mg/24 h)
    Lytic bone lesions
    Systemic amyloidosis
    Rising serum M-spike
    Progressive unexplained renal failure
    Recurrent bacterial infections
    Reduced levels of normal serum immunoglobulins
Favor Occult PCD
    Minor marrow plasmacytosis (no sheets or clusters)
    Absence of Bence Jones proteinuria
    Absence of osteolytic lesions
    Absence of systemic amyloidosis
    Stable, small serum M-spike (< 2.5 g/dL), especially if IgG
    Normal levels of serum immunoglobulins
    Age > 70 yr (3% incidence)

From Stone [11] with permission.

event of a significant increase in the quantity of serum M-protein (greater than 0.5 g/dL) do we repeat the diagnostic evaluation for meyloma (Table VI).

Patients with PCDUS should be distinguished from the myeloma population, since the former should not receive cytotoxic chemotherapy, while most patients with overt disease require such treatment. Occasional patients with findings that meet the diagnostic criteria for myeloma have an indolent or "smoldering" course and should not be treated [468]. Even in those few PCDUS patients with premyeloma, the evolution to clinically significant disease may require many years to occur, as has been noted. Because of the uncommon but well-documented development of acute granulocytic and monocytic leukemias in treated myeloma patients who have responded to therapy with alkylating agents [200,299–301,436,437], patients with PCDUS should not be treated until they demonstrate unequivocal evidence of malignancy.

MONOCLONAL Igs AS ANTIBODIES

In humans and animals, the usual antibody response to injected antigen is heterogeneous. This heterogeneity is reflected at various levels (class, subclass, L chain type, electrophoretic mobility, affinity constant, etc). During the past decade, however, evidence has accumulated that antibodies to certain antigens may be much less heterogeneous than previously thought. Indeed it appears that monoclonal antibodies may arise during the course of a normal immune response [5,20,302]. Krause, Haber, and their co-workers have demonstrated that high concentrations of monoclonal antibodies appear in the sera of some rabbits immunized with streptococcal and pneumococcal polysaccharides (Fig. 14). Such antibodies are observed to be homogeneous by a variety of physicochemical criteria. There is no other evidence of a plasma-cell dyscrasia in these animals, but the serum antibody levels to the immunizing antigen may rise to concentrations of 30–60 mg/mL. Moreover, they decrease with time unless the rabbits are further challenged with antigen (Fig. 14).

Monoclonal antibodies (or antibodies with restricted heterogeneity) also have been documented in humans without evidence of plasma-cell dyscrasias. Thus, most antibodies to Factor VIII (found in hemophiliacs, postpartum women and elderly patients) are of the IgG_4 subclass; many antibodies to polysaccharide antigens belong to the IgG_2 subclass; and the IgM components of mixed cryoglobulins are often monoclonal antibodies to autologous IgG [222,224,225,469].

Transient plasma-cell dyscrasias (Table III) have been encountered in humans [122,303,304,467] and, as noted previously, stable nonprogressive plasma-cell dyscrasias are frequently seen in patients with a variety of other disorders. Although defined antigenic specificities have only rarely been documented in these populations, some may represent monoclonal antibody responses to unrecognized antigens.

Antibody activity associated with human and murine myeloma proteins was first demonstrated unequivocally in 1967 [305–308]. Since then, a number of other examples have been demonstrated in patients with monoclonal gammopathies [5,20,309–317,441,470–473] (Table XVI) and in mice with induced plasma-cell tumors [5,318,319,474].

Although the possibility that myeloma proteins might represent the products of a directed immune response has been raised on clinical grounds alone [23,320–327], the number of patients with documented antigen-binding M-proteins in whom the antigen appeared meaningful has been sparse. Two examples are noteworthy: one patient with a history of recurrent episodes of rheumatic fever who developed myeloma with an IgG M-protein having

TABLE XVI. Antigens Reactive With Human Monoclonal Immunoglobulins From Patients with Monoclonal Gammopathies

Antigen	Ig class
Blood group antigens	
I, i	IgM, IgA
Sp_1	IgM
A_1	IgM
P	IgM
Streptolysin O	IgG
Staphylolysin	IgG
Klebsiella	IgM
Brucella	IgG
Rubella	IgG
IgG	IgM, IgG, IgA
Immune complexes	IgM
Fibrin monomer	IgG
Lipoproteins	IgA, IgG
Transferrin	IgG
Albumin	IgM, IgG
α_2-macroglobulin	IgG
Dnp	IgM, IgG, IgA
Cardiolipids	IgM
Phosphorylcholine	IgM
Riboflavin	IgG
Myelin	IgM
Phospholipid	IgM

Antigens included are those for which evidence of specificity is strongest.
Revised from Nisonoff et al. [5].

antistreptolysin activity [310]; and another patient who had received two injections of unpurified horse serum 6 years apart and who, years later, developed myeloma with an IgG M-component having specificity for horse α_2-macroglobulin [314].

We have discussed the data relating to the structural similarity between M-proteins and typical antibody Ig molecules. Antigen-binding activity of myeloma and macroglobulinemia proteins is chemically indistinguishable

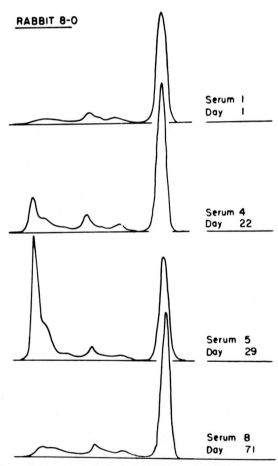

Fig. 14. Tracings of the densitometric scan of the zone electrophoretic patterns for sera collected before, during, and after immunization of a rabbit with streptococcal vaccine. (From Osterland [485].)

from that observed with conventionally induced antibodies and has been found in all three major classes of Igs (IgG, IgM, and IgA). The determinants thus far identified include representatives from each of the classical types of antigen molecules: proteins, polysaccharides, and haptens. Protein and polysaccharide antigens may represent meaningful responses since they are constituents of autoantigens or exogenous antigens with which a host is likely to come in contact. Such findings suggest that an expanded clone of cells is more likely to undergo neoplastic transformation. While normal clones are antigen-regulated and pathologic ones presumably are not, antigen can nonetheless be involved in the developmental history of the abnormal clone up to the time at which the neoplastic event occurs. The virtual inability to induce myeloma in the murine system when germ-free mice are employed supports the role of an expanded clone as a necessary prerequisite to the development of a malignant plasma-cell dyscrasia [216]. Genetic factors also may play an important role in pathogenesis of human monoclonal gammopathies. A high frequency of the α_1-antitrypsin PiMZ phenotype has been reported among patients with myeloma or lymphoma who have serum and/ or urine M-components [328].

The significance of demonstrated binding activity for haptens, some of which do not occur naturally, is less clear. Although the history of immunochemistry abounds with studies that demonstrate that combination of antibody with antigen is specific and generally restricted to the inducing antigen or structurally related similar compounds (cross-reactivity), some investigators have recently raised the possibility that antibody combining sites might be multispecific (polyfunctional) [329–331]. This point remains highly controversial. The number of monoclonal proteins examined for antibody activity is limited by available assays for a rather small number of antigens. In addition, detection of binding activity is frequently more difficult for homogeneous Igs than for usual heterogeneous antibodies.

Thus, some (? most) monoclonal proteins are antibodies, but the biologic significance of this interesting finding in the pathogenesis of monoclonal gammopathies awaits further investigation.

UNUSUAL PATHOPHYSIOLOGIC MANIFESTATIONS OF MONOCLONAL GAMMOPATHIES

An array of intriguing syndromes and laboratory findings are occasionally found in patients with monoclonal gammopathies. Some occur rather frequently (e.g., myeloma renal failure and hypercalcemia) but most are unusual. The majority are related to physicochemical (including antibody) properties of the M-component (Table XVII).

TABLE XVII. Pathophysiologic Manifestations of Monoclonal Gammopathies

Clinical or laboratory finding	Probable mechanism	References
I. Related to physiocochemical (including antibody) properties of M-components		
Mixed cryoglobulinemia	Usually monoclonal IgM with anti-IgG activity; occasionally IgM anti-IgA, IgG anti-IgG, or IgA anti-IgG; high-titer "rheumatoid factor" activity present	20,222–225, 305,307,309, 335,442,469
Chronic cold agglutinin disease	Usually IgM antibody directed to I antigen on red cell membrane, some anti-i. Rarely IgA antibody	226–230, 336,472,473
Hemorrhagic syndromes associated with circulating anticoagulants and/or platelet function defects	Complex (? immune) of M-protein with various coagulation factors or platelets	251,252,337–340, 470,471
Polyneuropathy	Deposition of IgM or IgG on nerve sheath, probably immune complex; motor neuropathy with λ-light chain disease	248,249,341, 420–422,441, 475–477
Hyperlipidemia	Antilipoprotein antibody, IgA or IgG	342–347
Xanthoderma	Antiflavin antibody, IgG	316
Sudden death after x-ray contrast agent injected	Intravascular precipitation of IgM by drug; ? immune	348
Hyperviscosity syndrome	IgM M-components with high intrinsic viscosity; IgA or IgG M-components which spontaneously aggregate at high concentrations	20,223,232–247, 438–440
Renal Failure	Free monoclonal light chain (Bence Jones) monomers or dimers in large excess which are filtered by kidney and result in renal damage (tubular atrophy); other factors, esp. dehydration and hypercalcemia, may contribute	30,180,181,190, 199,202,203, 349–359,402, 417–419,424, 435,484
Renal tubular acidosis ± Fanconi syndrome	Proximal tubule damage associated with certain Bence Jones proteins with tendency to form intracellular crystals	30,149, 360–365

Primary systemic amyloidosis	Proteolytic cleavage of certain Bence Jones proteins having variable fragment with propensity to deposit in blood vessels and other tissues (Bence Jones dimer a primitive antibody?)	30,131,221, 257–262,270, 272–275,278–280, 444,445,451–453, 456–461,478–480
Cryoglobulinemia	M-component which precipitates or gels below 37°C	222,224,225,230, 310,336,366,481, 482
Biclonal or triclonal gammopathy	Multiple M-components produced by a single clone of secretory B cells; also seen with renal failure and consequent retention of excess free L chains in serum in a patient with intact M-component, usually IgG or IgA	123–126,351,401
Multiple organ dysfunction	Systemic light chain deposition (not amyloid)	367,483
Systemic capillary leak	IgG, mechanism unknown	368
Low anion gap	Cationic M-protein binds anions; may occur in patients with asymptomatic serum spikes as well as in those with myeloma	182–185,415,416
Hypercalcemia (asymptomatic)	M-component binds calcium, IgG	369,370
Hyponatremia (asymptomatic)	M-component binds sodium, IgG; spurious hyponatremia with increased serum viscosity (IgM, IgA, or IgG)	183,371
Decreased chemotaxis	IgA; ? steric hindrance of cell receptors	372
Low serum levels of normal IgG	Hypercatabolism of all IgG due to high concentration IgG M-component	12
II. Related to products other than M-component which may be released from B cell monoclones or mononuclear phagocytes		
Hypercalcemia	Release of osteoclast activating factor (OAF) by plasma cells with consequent mobilization of calcium from bone	204,373,374
Antibody-deficiency syndrome	Secretion of specific mitotic inhibitor (chalone) that blocks proliferation of normal (background) B-cell clones; may involve monocyte-macrophage suppressor cells	375–380

Revised and expanded from Salmon [332].

CONCLUDING STATEMENT

Major advances in the understanding of myeloma, macroglobulinemia, and related disorders have occurred during the past two decades. These advances have taken place simultaneously with an explosive increase in knowledge of the immune system. Many significant questions remain to be answered at both the clinical and basic science levels. It seems likely that the study of monoclonal gammopathies will continue to provide important insights to the clinician, the cellular immunologist, and the immunochemist [491].

ACKNOWLEDGMENTS

This work was supported in part by the following grants: NIH 1 P01 CA 17065-03, CA 18132 (NCI-DHEW), USPHS CA 09082, American Cancer Society ET-62, the Damon Runyon Memorial Fund, and the Tri Delta Cancer Research Fund.

REFERENCES

1. Jones HB: On a new substance occurring in the urine of a patient with mollities ossium. Philos Trans R Soc Lond [Biol] 138:55, 1848.
2. Porter RR: The hydrolysis of rabbit γ-globulin and antibodies with crystalline papain. Biochem J 73:119, 1959.
3. Edelman GM: Dissociation of γ-globulin. J Am Chem Soc 81:3155, 1959.
4. Spiegelberg HL: Biological activities of immunoglobulins of different classes and subclasses. Adv Immunol 19:259, 1974.
5. Nisonoff A, Hopper JE, Spring SB: "The Antibody Molecule." New York: Academic Press, 1975.
6. Putnam FW: Immunoglobulins. In Putnam FW (ed): "The Plasma Proteins." Ed 2, vol 3. New York: Academic Press, 1977, chs 1–3.
7. Capra JD, Edmundson AB: The antibody combining site. Sci Am 236:50, 1977.
8. Poljak RJ: Studies on the three-dimensional structure of immunoglobulins. In Litman GW, Good RA (eds): "Immunoglobulins. Comprehensive Immunology." Vol 5. New York: Plenum, 1978, ch 1.
9. Cunningham-Rundles C: The secretory component and the J chain. In Litman GW, Good RA (eds): "Immunoglobulins. Comprehensive Immunology." Vol 5. New York: Plenum, 1978, ch 5.
10. Bach JF: "Immunology." New York: Wiley, 1978, p 178.
11. Stone MJ: Multiple myeloma, macroglobulinemia, and related plasma cell dyscrasias. In Race GJ (ed): "Laboratory Medicine." Vol 4. Hagerstown: Harper & Row, 1979, ch 24.
12. Waldmann TA, Strober W: Metabolism of immunoglobulins. Clin Immunobiol 3:71, 1976.
13. Plaut AG: Microbial IgA proteases. N Engl J Med 298:1459, 1978.
14. Siegal FP: Cytoidentity of the Lymphoreticular Neoplasms. In Twomey JJ, Good RA (eds): "The Immunopathology of Lymphoreticular Neoplasms. Comprehensive Immunology." Vol 4. New York: Plenum, 1978, ch 10.
15. Gupta S, Good RA: Markers of human lymphocyte subpopulations in primary immunodeficiency and lymphoproliferative disorders. Semin Hematol 17:1, 1980.

16. Ishizaka K, Ishizaka T: Immunoglobulin E: Biosythesis and immunological mechanisms of IgE-mediated hypersensitivity. In Gupta S, Good RA (eds): "Cellular, Molecular, and Clinical Aspects of Allergic Disorders. Comprehensive Immunology." Vol 6. New York: Plenum, 1979, ch 5.
17. Edelman GM, Gally JA: The nature of Bence Jones proteins. Chemical similarities to polypeptide chains of myeloma globulins and normal γ-globulins. J Exp Med 116:207, 1962.
18. Solomon A: Bence-Jones proteins and light chains of immunoglobulins. New Engl J Med 294:17, 91, 1976.
19. Fudenberg HH, Pink JRL, Wang A-C, Douglas SD: "Basic Immunogenetics." Ed 2. New York: Oxford, 1978.
20. Stone MJ: Studies on monoclonal antibodies. I. The specificity and binding properties of a Waldenström macroglobulin with anti-γG activity. J Lab Clin Med 81:393, 1973.
21. Osserman EF, Fahey JL: Plasma cell dyscrasias. Current clinical and biochemical concepts. Am J Med 44:256, 1968.
22. Bergsagel DE: Plasma cell neoplasms—general considerations. In Williams WJ, Beutler E, Erslev AJ, Rundles RW, (eds): "Hematology." Ed 2. New York: McGraw-Hill, 1977, ch 121.
23. Osserman EF: Multiple myeloma and related plasma cell dyscrasias. In Samter M (ed): "Immunological Diseases." Ed 3. Boston: Little, Brown, 1978, ch 25.
24. Kagan E, Jacobson RJ, Yeung KY, Haidak DH, Nachnani GH: Asbestos-associated neoplasms of B cell lineage. Am J Med 67:325, 1979.
25. Kyle RA, Bayrd ED: "Benign" monoclonal gammopathy: A potentially malignant condition? Am J Med 40:426, 1966.
26. Kyle RA: Monoclonal gammopathy of undetermined significance. Natural history in 241 cases. Am J Med 64:814, 1978.
27. Alper CA: Plasma protein measurements as a diagnostic aid. N Engl J Med 291:287, 1974.
28. Kyle RA, Greipp PR: The laboratory investigation of monoclonal gammopathies. Mayo Clin Proc 53:719, 1978.
29. Holborow EJ, Reeves WG: "Immunology in Medicine." London: Academic Press, 1977, p 84.
30. Stone MJ, Frenkel EP: The clinical spectrum of light chain myeloma. A study of thirty-five patients with special reference to the occurrence of amyloidosis. Am J Med 58:601, 1975.
31. Franklin EC: Electrophoresis and immunoelectrophoresis in the evaluation of homogeneous immunoglobulin components. Clin Immunobiol 3:21, 1976.
32. Bergsagel DE: Plasma cell myeloma. In Williams WJ, Beutler E, Erslev AJ, Rundles RW (eds): "Hematology." Ed 2. New York: McGraw-Hill, 1977, ch 122.
33. Kyle RA, Bayrd ED: "The Monoclonal Gammopathies. Multiple Myeloma and Related Plasma-Cell Disorders." Springfield: Charles C. Thomas, 1976.
34. McPhedran P, Heath CW Jr, Garcia J: Multiple myeloma incidence in metropolitan Atlanta, Georgia: Racial and seasonal variations. Blood 39:866, 1972.
35. Kyle RA, Heath CW Jr, Carbone P: Multiple myeloma in spouses. Arch Intern Med 127:944, 1971.
36. Pietruszka M, Rabin BS, Srodes C: Multiple myeloma in husband and wife. Lancet 1:314, 1976.
37. Kardinal CG: Multiple myeloma in a husband and wife. JAMA 239:22, 1978.
38. Goldstone AH, Wood JK, Cook MK: Myeloma in mother and daughter. Acta Haematol 49:176, 1973.
39. Maldonado JE, Kyle RA: Familial myeloma. Report of eight families and a study of serum proteins in their relatives. Am J Med 57:875, 1974.

40. Kyle RA, Herber L, Evatt BL, Heath CW Jr: Multiple myeloma. A community cluster. JAMA 213:1339, 1970.
41. Hewell GM, Alexanian R: Multiple myeloma in young persons. Ann Intern Med 84:441, 1976.
42. Kaplan J: Multiple myeloma in young persons. Ann Intern Med 85:133, 1976.
43. Hyun BH: Multiple myeloma in the young. Ann Intern Med 85:260, 1976.
44. Clough V, Delamore IW, Whittaker JA: Multiple myeloma in a young woman. Ann Intern Med 86:117, 1977.
45. Migliore PJ, Alexanian R: Monoclonal gammopathy in human neoplasia. Cancer 21:1127, 1968.
46. Stegman R, and Alexanian R: Solid tumors in multiple myeloma. Ann Intern Med 90:780, 1979.
47. Zinneman HH, Hall WH: Recurrent pneumonia in multiple myeloma and some observations on immunologic response. Ann Intern Med 41:1152, 1954.
48. Gavrilescu K, Papakrivopoulos A: IgG myeloma in cerebrospinal fluid with a total protein of 32 mg/100 ml. Br Med J 4:156, 1967.
49. Maldonado JE, Kyle RA, Ludwig J, Okazaki H: Meningeal myeloma. Arch Intern Med 126:660, 1970.
50. Spiers ASD, Halpern R, Ross SC, Neiman RS, Harawi S, Zipoli TE: Meningeal myelomatosis. Arch Intern Med 140:256, 1980.
51. Poon MC, Prchal JT, Murad TM, Galbraith JG: Multiple myeloma masquerading as chromophobe adenoma. Cancer 43:1513, 1979.
52. Benson WJ, Scarffe JH, Todd IDH, Palmer M, Crowther D: Spinal-cord compression in myeloma. Br Med J 1:1541, 1979.
53. Fudenberg HH, Virella G: Multiple myeloma and Waldenström macroglobulinemia: Unusual presentations. Semin Hematol 17:63, 1980.
54. Thomas FB, Clausen KP, Greenberger NJ: Liver disease in multiple myeloma. Arch Intern Med 132:195, 1973.
55. Mintz G, Robles-Saavedra EJ, Enriquez RD, Jimenez FJ, Juan L: Hemarthrosis as the presenting manifestation of true myeloma joint disease. Arthritis Rheum 21:148, 1978.
56. Cline MJ, Berlin NI: Studies of the anemia of multiple myeloma. Am J Med 33:510, 1962.
57. Hoffbrand AV, Hobbs JR, Kremenckuzky S, Mollin DL: Incidence and pathogenesis of megaloblastic erythropoiesis in multiple myeloma. J Clin Pathol 20:699, 1967.
58. MacSween JM, Langley GR: Light chain disease (hypogammaglobulinemia and Bence Jones proteinuria) and sideroblastic anemia-preleukemic chronic granulocytic leukemia. Can Med Assoc J 106:995, 1972.
59. Ginsberg DM: Circulating plasma cells in multiple myeloma. A method for detection and review of the problem. Ann Intern Med 57:843, 1962.
60. Barnett EV, Stone G, Swisher SN, Vaughan JH: Serum sickness and plasmacytosis. A clinical, immunologic and hematologic analysis. Am J Med 35:113, 1963.
61. Schmidt JJ, Robinson HJ, Pennypacker CS: Peripheral plasmacytosis in serum sickness. Ann Intern Med 59:542, 1963.
62. Han T, Chawla PL, Sokal JE: Sulfapyridine-induced serum-sickness-like syndrome associated with plasmacytosis, lymphocytosis and multiclonal gamma-globulinopathy. N Engl J Med 280:547, 1969.
63. Moake JL, Landry PR, Oren ME, Sayer BL, Heffner LT: Transient peripheral plasmacytosis. Am J Clin Pathol 62:8, 1974.
64. Anderson J, Osgood EE: Acute plasmacytic leukemia responsive to cyclophosphamide. JAMA 193:188, 1965.
65. Mullinax F, Mullinax GL, Himrod B: RNA metabolism and protein synthesis in plasma cell leukemia. Am J Med 42:302, 1967.

66. Pruzanski W, Platts ME, Ogryzlo MA: Leukemic form of immunocytic dyscrasia (plasma cell leukemia). A study of ten cases and a review of the literature. Am J Med 47:60, 1969.

67. Polliack A, Rachmilewitz D, Zlotnick A: Plasma cell leukemia. Unassembled light and heavy chains in the urine. Arch Intern Med 134:131, 1974.

68. Kyle RA, Maldonado JE, Bayrd ED: Plasma cell leukemia. Report on 17 cases. Arch Intern Med 133:813, 1974.

69. Shaw MT, Twele TW, Nordquist RE: Plasma cell leukemia: Detailed studies and response to therapy. Cancer 33:619, 1974.

70. Bernier GM, Berman JH, Fanger MW: Plasma cell leukemia with excretion of half-molecules of immunoglobulin A ($\alpha_1 \lambda_1$). Ann Intern Med 86:572, 1977.

71. Zawadzki ZA, Kapadia S, Barnes AE: Leukemic myelomatosis (plasma cell leukemia). Am J Clin Pathol 70:605, 1978.

72. Woodruff RK, Malpas JS, Paxton AM, Lister TA: Plasma cell leukemia (PCL): A report on 15 patients. Blood 52:839, 1978.

73. Isobe T, Ikeda Y, Ohta H: Comparison of sizes and shapes of tumor cells in plasma cell leukemia and plasma cell myeloma. Blood 53:1028, 1979.

74. Riggs SA, Minuth AN, Nottebohm GA, Rossen RD, Suki WN: Plasma cells in urine. Occurrence in multiple myeloma. Arch Intern Med 135:1245, 1975.

75. Zimelman AP: Thrombocytosis in multiple myeloma. Ann Intern Med 78:970, 1973.

76. Chikkappa G, Chanana AD, Chandra P, Cronkite EP, Thompson KH: Cyclic oscillation of blood neutrophils in a patient with multiple myeloma. Blood 55:61, 1980.

77. Brook J, Dreisbach PB: Leukocyte alkaline phosphatase levels in multiple myeloma. J Lab Clin Med 90:114, 1977.

78. Hobbs JR: Immunochemical classes of myelomatosis. Br J Haematol 16:599, 1969.

79. Coltman CA: Multiple myeloma without a paraprotein. Report of a case with observations on chromosomal composition. Arch Intern Med 120:687, 1967.

80. Hurez D, Preud'homme JL, Seligmann M: Intracellular "monoclonal" immunoglobulin in non-secretory human myeloma. J Immunol 104:263, 1970.

81. Guillan RA, Ranjini R, Zelman S, Hocker EV, Smalley RL: Multiple myeloma with hypogammaglobulinemia. Electron microscopic and chromosome studies. Cancer 25:1187, 1970.

82. Gach J, Simar L, Salmon J: Multiple myeloma without M-type proteinemia. Report of a case with immunologic and ultrastructure studies. Am J Med 50:835, 1971.

83. Azar HA, Zaino EC, Pham TD, Yannopoulos K: "Nonsecretory" plasma cell myeloma: observations on seven cases with electron microscopic studies. Am J Clin Pathol 58:618, 1972.

84. River GL, Tewksbury DA, Fudenberg HH: "Nonsecretory" multiple myeloma. Blood 40:204, 1972.

85. Arend WP, Adamson JW: Nonsecretory myeloma. Immunofluorescent demonstration of paraprotein within bone marrow plasma cells. Cancer 33:721, 1974.

86. Mancilla R, Davis GL: Nonsecretory multiple myeloma. Immunohistologic and ultra-structural observations on two patients. Am J Med 63:1015, 1977.

87. Joyner MV, Cassuto JP, Dujardin P, Schneider M, Ziegler G, Euller L, Masseyeff R: Non-excretory multiple myeloma. Br J Haematol 43:559, 1979.

88. Snapper I, Kahn A: "Myelomatosis." Baltimore: University Park Press, 1971.

89. Edwards GA, Zawadzki ZA: Extraosseous lesions in plasma cell myeloma. Am J Med 43:194, 1967.

90. Ghosh ML, Sayeed A: Unusual cases of myelomatosis. Scand J Haematol 12:147, 1974.

91. Wiltshaw E: The natural history of extramedullary plasmacytoma and its relation to solitary myeloma of bone and myelomatosis. Medicine 55:217, 1976.

92. Remigio PA, Klaum A: Extramedullary plasmacytoma of stomach. Cancer 27:562, 1971.

93. Godard JE, Fox JE, Lerrinson MJ: Primary gastric plasmacytoma. Am J Digest Dis 18:508, 1973.
94. Goeggel-Lamping C, Kahn SB: Gastrointestinal polyposis in multiple myeloma. JAMA 239:1786, 1978.
95. Douglass HO Jr, Sika JV, LeVeen HH: Plasmacytoma: A not so rare tumor of the small intestine. Cancer 28:456, 1971.
96. Nielsen SM, Schenken JR, Cawley LP: Primary colonic plasmacytoma. Cancer 30:261, 1972.
97. Robinson KP: Plasmacytoma and plasma cell polyposis of the colon. Proc R Soc Med 62:46, 1969.
98. Chan KP, Tam CS: Plasmacytoma. Report of a case. Cancer 23:694, 1969.
99. Kotner LM, Wang CC: Plasmacytoma of the upper air and food passages. Cancer 30:414, 1972.
100. Johnson WH, Taylor BG: Solitary extramedullary plasmacytoma of the skin. Cancer 26:65, 1970.
101. Rodriquez JM, Lam S, Silber R: Multiple myeloma with cutaneous involvement. JAMA 237:2625, 1977.
102. Rosenberg B, Attie JN, Mandelbaum HL: Breast tumor as the presenting sign of multiple myeloma. N Engl J Med 269:359, 1963.
103. Stavem P, Hjort PF, Elgjo K, Sommerschild H: Solitary plasmocytoma of the spleen with marked polyclonal increase of gamma G, normalized after splenectomy. Acta Med Scand. 188:115, 1970.
104. Suissa L, Losa J, Linn B: Plasmacytoma of lymph nodes. A case report. JAMA 197:136, 1966.
105. Levin HS, Mostofi FK: Symptomatic plasmacytoma of the testis. Cancer 25:1193, 1970.
106. Shimaoka K, Gailani S, Tsukada Y, Barcos M: Plasma cell neoplasm involving the thyroid. Cancer 41:1140, 1978.
107. Gardner-Thorpe C. Presumed plasmacytoma of clivus producing isolated hypoglossal nerve palsy. Br Med J 2:405, 1970.
108. CPC-MGH, Case 3–1973. N Engl J Med 288:150, 1973.
109. Hughes JC, Votaw ML: Pleural effusion in multiple myeloma. Cancer 44:1150, 1979.
110. Corwin J, Lindberg RD: Solitary plasmacytoma of bone vs. extramedullary plasmacytoma and their relationship to multiple myeloma. Cancer 43:1007, 1979.
111. Soumerai S, Gleason EA: Asynchronous plasmacytoma of the stomach and testis. Cancer 45:396, 1980.
112. Soga J, Saito K, Suzuki N, Sakai T: Plasma cell granuloma of the stomach. A report of a case and review of the literature. Cancer 25:618, 1970.
113. Bahadori M, Liebow AA: Plasma cell granulomas of the lung. Cancer 31:191, 1973.
114. Eimoto T, Yanaka M, Kurosawa M, Ikeya F: Plasma cell granuloma (inflammatory pseudotumor) of the spinal cord meninges. Cancer 41:1929, 1978.
115. Yu GSM, Carson JW: Giant lymph-node hyperplasia, plasma-cell type, of the mediastinum, with peripheral neuropathy. Am J Clin Pathol 66:46, 1976.
116. Weisenberger DD, DeGowin RL, Gibson DP, Armitage JO: Remission of giant lymph node hyperplasia with anemia after radiotherapy. Cancer 44:457, 1979.
117. Franklin EC, Buxbaum J: Immunoglobulin structure, synthesis, secretion, and relation to neoplasms of B cells. Clin Haematol. 6:503, 1977.
118. Jancelwicz Z, Takatsuki K, Sugai S, Pruzanski W: IgD myeloma: Review of 133 cases. Arch Intern Med 135:87, 1975.
119. Valenzuela R, Govindarajan S, Tubbs R, Deodhar S, Bukowski R: IgD myeloma. Report of a case with unusual clinical and immunologic features. Am J Clin Pathol 72:246, 1979.

120. Ogawa M, Kochwa S, Smith C, Ishizaka K, McIntyre OR: Clinical aspects of IgE myeloma. N Engl J Med 281:1217, 1969.
121. Rogers JS, Spahr J, Judge DM, Varano LA, Eyster ME: IgE Myeloma with osteoblastic lesions. Blood 49:295, 1977.
122. Farhangi M, Osserman EF: Biology, clinical patterns, and treatment of multiple myeloma and related plasma-cell dyscrasias. In Twomey JJ, Good RA (eds): "The Immunopathology of Lymphoreticular Neoplasms. Comprehensive Immunology." Vol 4. New York: Plenum 1978, ch 22.
123. Rudders RA, Yakulis V, Heller P: Double myeloma. Production of both IgG type lambda and IgA type lambda myeloma proteins by a single plasma cell line. Am J Med 55:215, 1973.
124. Dalal FR, Winsten S: Double light-chain disease: A case report. Clin Chem 25:190, 1979.
125. Hopper JE, Haren JM, Kmiecik TE: Evidence for shared idiotypy expressed by the IgM, IgG and IgA serum proteins of a patient with a complex multiple paraprotein disorder. J Immunol 122:2000, 1979.
126. Hopper JE, Noyes C, Hsu R, Heinrickson R, Gallagher W: Shared N-terminal sequences in monoclonal IgM$_\kappa$ and IgG$_\kappa$ proteins from a patient with a complex multiple paraprotein disorder. J Immunol 122:2007, 1979.
127. Cartwright GE: "Diagnostic Laboratory Hematology." Ed 4. New York: Grune & Stratton, 1968, p 411.
128. Guest WG, Stone MJ: Urine transferrin masquerading as Bence Jones protein in the nephrotic syndrome of primary amyloidosis. Clin Res 22:529A, 1974.
129. Durie BGM, Salmon SE: A clinical staging system for multiple myeloma. Cancer 36:842, 1975.
130. Kyle RA, Elveback LR: Management and prognosis of multiple myeloma. Mayo Clin Proc 51:751, 1976.
131. Ooi BS, Pesce AJ, Pollak VE, Mandalenakis N: Multiple myeloma with massive proteinuria and terminal renal failure. Am J Med 52:538, 1972.
132. Dammacco F, Waldenström J: Bence Jones proteinuria in benign monoclonal gammapathies. Acta Med Scand 184:403, 1968.
133. Kyle RA, Maldonado JE, Bayrd ED: Idiopathic Bence Jones proteinuria—a distinct entity? Am J Med 55:222, 1973.
134. Cronstedt J, Carling L, Ostberg H: Idiopathic light chain dyscrasia—a new distinct entity? Acta Med Scand 196:445, 1974.
135. Mallick NP, Dosa S, Acheson EJ, Delamore IW, McFarlane H, Seneviratre CJ, Williams G: Detection, significance, and treatment of paraprotein in patients presenting with "idiopathic" proteinuria without myeloma. Q J Med (New Series) 47:145, 1978.
136. Perry MC, Kyle RA: The clinical significance of Bence Jones proteinuria. Mayo Clin Proc 50:234, 1975.
137. Kyle RA: Multiple myeloma. Review of 869 cases. Mayo Clin Proc 50:29, 1975.
138. James TN, Monto RW: Multiple myeloma simulating aplastic anemia. Am J Med 17:50, 1954.
139. Azar HA: The myeloma cell. Azar HA, Potter M (eds): In "Multiple Myeloma and Related Disorders." Vol 1. Hagerstown: Harper & Row, 1973, ch 2.
140. Bernstein JS, Nixon DD: Ulcerative colitis disguised as multiple myeloma. Am J Digest Dis 9:625, 1964.
141. Block MH: "Text-Atlas of Hematology." Philadelphia: Lea & Febiger, 1976, pp 544–563.
142. Graham RC Jr, Bernier GM: The bone marrow in multiple myeloma: Correlation of plasma cell ultrastructure and clinical state. Medicine 54:225, 1975.

143. Bernier GM, Graham RC Jr: Plasma cell asynchrony in myeloma: Correlation of light and electron microscopy. Semin Hematol 13:239, 1976.
144. Brecher G, Tanaka Y, Malmgren RA, Fahey JL: Morphology and protein synthesis in multiple myeloma and macroglobulinemia. Ann NY Acad Sci 113:642, 1964.
145. Ashley DJB: "Evans' Histopathological Appearances of Tumors." Ed 3, Vol 1. Edinburgh: Churchill Livingstone, 1978, p 210.
146. Welsh RA: Electron microscopic localization of Russell bodies in the human plasma cell. Blood 16:1307, 1960.
147. Brunning RD, Parkin J: Intranuclear inclusions in plasma cells and lymphocytes from patients with monoclonal gammopathies. Am J Clin Pathol 66:10, 1976.
148. Blom J, Mansa B, Wiik A: A study of Russell bodies in human monoclonal plasma cells by means of immunofluorescence and electron microscopy. Acta Pathol Microbiol Scand 84:335, 1976.
149. Costanza DJ, Smoller M: Multiple myeloma with the Fanconi Syndrome. Am J Med 34:125, 1963.
150. Kalderon AE, Boggars HA, Diamond I, Cummings FJ, Kaplan SR, Calabresi P: Ultrastructure of myeloma cells in a case with crystalcryoglobulinemia. Cancer 39:1475, 1977.
151. Dameshek W, Gunz F: "Leukemia." Ed 2. New York: Grune & Stratton, 1964, p 256.
152. Stone MJ, Reese MH: Unpublished observations.
153. Abramson N, von Kapff C, Ginsberg AD: The phagocytic plasma cells. N Engl J Med 283:248, 1970.
154. Lerner RG, Parker JW: Dysglobulinemia and iron in plasma cells. Ferrokinetics and electron microscopy. Arch Intern Med 121:284, 1968.
155. Fitchen JH, Lee S: Phagocytic myeloma cells. Am J Clin Pathol 71:722, 1979.
156. Scullin DC, Shelburne JD, Cohen HJ: Pseudo-Gaucher cells in multiple myeloma. Am J Med 67:347, 1979.
157. Pinkus GS, Said JW: Specific identification of intracellular immunoglobulin in paraffin sections of multiple myeloma and macroglobulinemia using an immunoperoxidase technique. Am J Pathol 87:47, 1977.
158. Taylor CR, Russell R, Chandor S: An immunohistologic study of multiple myeloma and related conditions, using an immunoperoxidase method. Am J Clin Pathol 70:612, 1978.
159. Burns GF, Worman CP, Roberts BE, Raper CGL, Barker CR, Cawley JC: Terminal B cell development as seen in different human myelomas and related disorders. Clin Exp Immunol 35:180, 1979.
160. Lindstrom FD, Hardy WR, Eberle BJ, Williams RC Jr: Multiple myeloma and benign monoclonal gammopathy: differentiation by immunofluorescence of lymphocytes. Ann Intern Med 78:837, 1973.
161. Abdou NL, Abdou NI: Immunoglobulin receptors on human leukocytes. IV. Differences between bone marrow and blood cells in multiple myeloma and chronic lymphocytic leukemia: Effects of therapy. J Lab Clin Med 82:611, 1973.
162. Abdou NI, Abdou NL: The monoclonal nature of lymphocytes in multiple myeloma. Effects of therapy. Ann Intern Med 83:42, 1975.
163. Chen Y, Bhoopalm N, Yakulis V, Heller P: Changes in lymphocyte surface immunoglobulins and the effect of an RNA-containing plasma factor. Ann Intern Med 83:625, 1975.
164. Warner TFCS, Krueger RE: Circulating lymphocytes and the spread of myeloma. Lancet 1:1174, 1978.
165. Biberfeld P, Mellstedt H, Petterson D: Immunocytochemical studies of human myeloma cells by light and electron microscopy. Isr J Med Sci 15:687, 1979.
166. Kubagawa H, Vogler LB, Capra JD, Conrad ME, Lawton AR, Cooper MD: Studies on the clonal origin of multiple myeloma. J Exp Med 150:792, 1979.

167. Hamburger A, Salmon SE: Primary bioassay of human myeloma stem cells. J Clin Invest 60:846, 1977.
168. McCaw BK, Hecht F, Harnden DG, Teplitz RL: Somatic rearrangement of chromosome 14 in human lymphocytes. Proc Natl Acad Sci USA 72:2071, 1975.
169. Lawler SD: Chromosomes in haematology. Br J Haematol 36:455, 1977.
170. Liang W, Rowley JD: 14q+ marker chromosomes in multiple myeloma and plasma-cell leukemia. Lancet 1:96, 1978.
171. Fukuhara S, Rowley JD, Variakojis D, Sweet DL: Banding studies on chromosomes in diffuse "histiocytic" lymphomas: Correlation of 14q+ marker chromosome with cytology. Blood 52:989, 1978.
172. Liang W, Hopper JE, Rowley JD: Karyotypic abnormalities and clinical aspects of patients with multiple myeloma and related paraproteinemic disorders. Cancer 44:630, 1979.
173. Latreille J, Barlogie B, Dosik G, Johnston DA, Drewinko B, Alexanian R: Cellular DNA content as a marker of human multiple myeloma. Blood 55:403, 1980.
174. Fahey JL, Scoggins R, Utz JP, Szwed DF: Infection, antibody response and gamma globulin components in multiple myeloma and macroglobulinemia. Am J Med 35:698, 1963.
175. Cone L, Uhr JW: Immunological deficiency disorders associated with chronic lymphocytic leukemia and multiple myeloma. J Clin Invest 43:2241, 1964.
176. Alexanian R, Migliore PJ: Normal immunoglobulins in multiple myeloma: Effect of melphalan chemotherapy. J Lab Clin Med 75:225, 1970.
177. Myers BR, Hirschman SZ, Axelrod JA: Current patterns of infection in multiple myeloma. Am J Med 52:87, 1972.
178. Twomey JJ: Infections complicating multiple myeloma and chronic lymphocytic leukemia. Arch Intern Med 132:562, 1973.
179. Nolan CM, Baxley PJ, Frasch CE: Antibody response to infection in multiple myeloma. Implications for vaccination. Am J Med 67:331, 1979.
180. DeFronzo, RA, Humphrey LR, Wright JR, Cooke CR: Acute renal failure in multiple myeloma. Medicine 54:209, 1975.
181. DeFronzo RA, Cooke CR, Wright JR, Humphrey RL: Renal function in patients with multiple myeloma. Medicine 57:151, 1978.
182. Murray T, Long W, Narins RG: Multiple myeloma and the anion gap. N Engl J Med 292:574, 1975.
183. Emmett, M, Narins RG: Clinical use of the anion gap. Medicine 56:38, 1977.
184. DeTroyer AD, Stolarczyk A, de Beyl DZ, Stryckmans P: Value of anion-gap determination in multiple myeloma. N Engl J Med 296:858, 1977.
185. Schnur MJ, Appel GB, Karp G, Osserman EF: The anion gap in asymptomatic plasma cell dyscrasias. Ann Intern Med 86:304, 1977.
186. Mangalik A, Veliath AJ: Osteosclerotic myeloma and peripheral neuropathy. A case report. Cancer 28:1040, 1971.
187. Buonocore E, Solomon A, Kerley HE: Pseudomyeloma. Radiology 95:41, 1970.
188. Maldonado JE, Riggs BL, Bayrd ED: Pseudomyeloma. Is association of severe osteoporosis with serum monoclonal gammopathy an entity or a coincidence? Arch Intern Med 135:267, 1975.
189. Law IP: Pseudomyeloma: a separate entity or a coincidence? Arch Intern Med 136:118, 1976.
190. Byrd L, Sherman RL: Radiocontrast-induced acute renal failure: A clinical and pathophysiologic review. Medicine 58:270, 1979.
191. Salmon SE: Immunoglobulin synthesis and tumor kinetics of multiple myeloma. Semin Hematol 10:135, 1973.

192. Woodruff RK, Wadsworth J, Malpas JS, Tobias JS: Clinical staging in multiple myeloma. Br J Haematol 42:199, 1979.
193. Durie BGM, Salmon SE, Moon TE: Pretreatment tumor mass, cell kinetics, and prognosis in multiple myeloma. Blood 55:364, 1980.
194. McIntyre OR: Multiple myeloma. N Engl J Med 301:193, 1979.
195. Alexanian R: Plasma cell neoplasms. Curr Probl Cancer 3(5):1, 1978.
196. Bergsagel DE: Treatment of plasma cell myeloma. Ann Rev Med 30:431, 1979.
197. Colls BM, Darlow BA: Multiple myeloma—prognosis, treatment and survival in an eight year study. Aust NZ J Med 9:262, 1979.
198. Alexanian R, Gehan E, Haut A, Saiki J, Weick J: Unmaintained remissions in multiple myeloma. Blood 51:1005, 1978.
199. Solomon A: Bence Jones proteins and light chains of immunoglobulins. XV. Effect of corticosteroids on synthesis and excretion of Bence Jones protein. J Clin Invest 61:97, 1978.
200. Bergsagel DE, Bailey AJ, Langley GR, MacDonald RN, White DF, Miller AB: The chemotherapy of plasma-cell myeloma and the incidence of acute leukemia. N Engl J Med 301:743, 1979.
201. Cornell DJ, McIntyre OR, Kochwa S, Weksler BB, Pajok TF: Response to therapy in IgG myeloma patients excreting lambda or kappa light chains: CALGB experience. Blood 54:23, 1979.
202. Misiani R, Remuzzi G, Bertani T, Licini R, Levoni P, Crippa A, Mecca G: Plasmaphoresis in the treatment of acute renal failure in multiple myeloma. Am J Med 66:684, 1979.
203. Johnson WJ, Kyle RA, Dahlberg PJ: Dialysis in the treatment of multiple myeloma. Mayo Clin Proc 55:65, 1980.
204. Siris ES, Sherman WH, Baquiran DC, Schlatterer JP, Osserman EF, Canfield RE: Effects of dichloromethylene diphosphonate on skeletal mobilization of calcium in multiple myeloma. N Engl J Med 302:310, 1980.
205. Mellstedt H, Ahre A, Bjorkholm M, Holm G, Johansson B, Strander H: Interferon therapy in myelomatosis. Lancet 1:245, 1979.
206. Austrian R: Pneumococcal vaccine: Development and progress. Am J Med 67:547, 1979.
207. Shildt RA, Rubin RN, Schiffman G: Pneumococcal immunization of patients with plasma cell dyscrasias and lymphoma. Proc 22nd Ann Meeting Am Soc Hematol Blood 54 (suppl):209a, 1979.
208. Salmon SE, Hamburger AW, Soehlen B, Durie BGM, Alberts DS, Moon TE: Quantitation of differential sensitivity of human-tumor stem cells to anticancer drugs. N Engl J Med 298:1321, 1978.
209. Bergsagel DE: Macroglobulinemia. In: Williams WJ, Beutler E, Erslev AJ, Rundles RW (eds): "Hematology." Ed 2. New York: McGraw-Hill, 1977, ch 123.
210. Pick AI, Schoenfeld Y, Frohlichmann R, Weiss H, Vana D, Schreibman S: Plasma cell dyscrasia. Analysis of 423 patients. JAMA 241:2275, 1979.
211. MacKenzie MR, Fudenberg HH: Macroglobulinemia. An analysis of forty patients. Blood 39:874, 1972.
212. Krajny M, Pruzanski W: Waldenström's macroglobulinemia. Review of 45 cases. Can Med Assoc J 114:899, 1976.
213. Preud'Homme JL, Seligmann M: Immunoglobulins on the surface of lymphoid cells in Waldenström's macroglobulinemia. J Clin Invest 51:701, 1972.
214. Pangalis GA, Nathwani BN, Rappaport H: Malignant lymphoma, well-differentiated lymphocytic. Its relationship with chronic lymphocytic leukemia and macroglobulinemia of Waldenström. Cancer 39:999, 1977.

215. Smith JL, Gordon J, Newell DG, Whisson M: The biosynthesis and characterization of unreleased IgM in a case of CLL. Br J Haematol 37:217, 1977.
216. Salmon SE, Seligmann M: B-cell neoplasia in man. Lancet 2:1230, 1974.
217. Lukes RJ, Parker JW, Taylor CR, Tindle BH, Cramer AD, Lincoln TL: Immunologic approach to non-Hodgkin's lymphomas and related leukemias. Analysis of the results of multiparameter studies of 425 cases. Semin Hematol 15:322, 1978.
218. Sidi Y, Boer P, Pick I, Pinkhas J, Sperling O: Increased adenosine deaminase activity in peripheral lymphocytes in Waldenström's macroglobulinemia. Lancet 1:500, 1979.
219. Leb L, Grimes ET, Balogh K, Merritt JA: Monoclonal macroglobulinemia with osteolytic lesions. Cancer 39:227, 1977.
220. Morel-Maroger L, Basch A, Danon F, Verroust P, Richet G: Pathology of the kidney in Waldenström's macroglobulinemia. N Engl J Med 283:123, 1970.
221. Isobe T, Osserman EF: Patterns of amyloidosis and their association with plasma-cell dyscrasia, monoclonal immunoglobulins and Bence-Jones proteins. N Engl J Med 290:473, 1974.
222. Grey HM, Kohler PF: Cryoimmunoglobulins. Semin Hematol 10:87, 1973.
223. Stone MJ, Fedak JE: Studies on monoclonal antibodies. II. Immune complex (IgM-IgG) cryoglobulinemia: The mechanism of cryoprecipitation. J Immunol 113:1377, 1974.
224. Brouet JC, Clauvel JP, Danon F, Klein M, Seligmann M: Biologic and clinical significance of cryoglobulins: A report of 86 cases. Am J Med 57:775, 1974.
225. Zinneman HH: Cryoglobulins and pyroglobulins. In Litman GW, Good RA (eds): "Immunoglobulins. Comprehensive Immunology." Vol 5. New York: Plenum, 1978, ch 14.
226. Ritzmann SE, Levin WC: Cold agglutinin disease: A type of primary macroglobulinemia: A new concept. Tex Rep Biol Med 20:236, 1962.
227. Frank MM, Atkinson JP, Gadek J: Cold agglutinins and cold-agglutinin disease. Ann Rev Med 28:291, 1977.
228. Pruzanski W, Shumak KH: Biologic activity of cold-reacting autoantibodies. N Engl J Med 297:538, 583, 1977.
229. Isbister JP, Cooper DA, Blake HM, Biggs JC, Dixon RA, Penny R: Lymphoproliferative disease with IgM lambda monoclonal protein and autoimmune hemolytic anemia. Am J Med 64:434, 1978.
230. Tsai C-M, Zopf DA, Yu RK, Wistar R, Ginsberg V: A Waldenström macroglobulin that is both a cold agglutinin and a cryoglobulin because it binds N-acetylneurominosyl residues. Proc Natl Acad Sci USA 74:4591, 1977.
231. Alexanian R: Monoclonal gammopathy in lymphoma. Arch Intern Med 135:62, 1975.
232. Fahey JL, Barth WF, Solomon A: Serum hyperviscosity syndrome. JAMA 192:464, 1965.
233. Bloch KJ, Maki DG: Hyperviscosity syndromes associated with immunoglobulin abnormalities. Semin Hematol 10:113, 1973.
234. Capra JD, Kunkel HG: Aggregation of γG3 proteins: relevance to the hyperviscosity syndrome. J Clin Invest 49:610, 1970.
235. MacKenzie MR, Fudenberg HH, O'Reilly RA: The hyperviscosity syndrome. I. In IgG Myeloma. The role of protein concentration and molecular shape. J Clin Invest 49:15, 1970.
236. Pruzanski W, Watt JG: Serum viscosity and hyperviscosity syndrome in IgG multiple myeloma. Report on 10 patients and a review of the literature. Ann Intern Med 77:853, 1972.
237. Lindsley H, Teller D, Noonan B, Peterson M, Mannik M: Hyperviscosity syndrome in multiple myeloma. A reversible concentration-dependent aggregation of the myeloma protein. Am J Med 54:682, 1973.

238. Anderson IS, Yeung K-Y, Hillman D, Lessin LS: Multiple myeloma in a patient with sickle cell anemia. Interacting effects on blood viscosity. Am J Med 59:568, 1975.
239. McGrath MA, Penny R: Paraproteinemia. Blood hyperviscosity and clinical manifestations. J Clin Invest 58:1155, 1976.
240. Phillips MJ, Harkness J: Plasma and whole blood viscosity. Br J Haematol 34:347, 1976.
241. McCann SR, Zinneman HH, Oken MM, Leary MC, Swaim WR, Moore M: IgM pyroglobulinemia with erythrocytosis presenting as hyperviscosity syndrome. I. Clinical features and viscometric studies. Am J Med 61:316, 1976.
242. Preston FE, Cooke KB, Foster ME, Winfield DA, Lee D: Myelomatosis and the hyperviscosity syndrome. Br J Haematol. 38:517, 1978.
243. Solomon A, Fahey J: Plasmapheresis therapy in macroglobulinemia. Ann Intern Med 58:789, 1963.
244. Editorial: Plasmapheresis in macroglobulinemia. Lancet 2:807, 1977.
245. McCallister BD, Bayrd ED, Harrison EG, McGuckin WF: Primary macroglobulinemia. Am J Med 43:394, 1967.
246. MacKenzie M, Brown E, Fudenberg H, Goodenday L: Waldenström's macroglobulinemia: Correlation between expanded plasma volume and increased serum viscosity. Blood 35:394, 1970.
247. Alexanian R: Blood volume in monoclonal gammopathy. Blood 49:301, 1977.
248. Propp RP, Means E, Deibel R, Sherer G, Barron K: Waldenström's macroglobulinemia and neuropathy. Deposition of M-component on myelin sheaths. Neurology 25:980, 1975.
249. Dellagi K, Brouet J-C, Danon F: Cross-idiotypic antigens among monoclonal immunoglobulin M from patients with Waldenström's macroglobulinemia and polyneuropathy. J Clin Invest 64:1530, 1979.
250. Tursz T, Brouet J-C, Flandrin G, Danon F, Clauvel J-P, Seligmann M: Clinical and pathologic features of Waldenström's macroglobulinemia in seven patients with serum monoclonal IgG or IgA. Am J Med 63:499, 1977.
251. Lackner H: Hemostatic abnormalities associated with dysproteinemia. Semin Hematol 10:125, 1973.
252. Brody JI, Haidar ME, Rossman RE: A hemorrhagic syndrome in Waldenström's macroglobulinemia secondary to immunoadsorption of factor VIII. Recovery after splenectomy. N Engl J Med 300:408, 1979.
253. Yoo D, Lessin LS, Jensen WN: Bone-marrow mast cells in lymphoproliferative disorders. Ann Intern Med 88:753, 1978.
254. Dutcher TF, Fahey JL: The histopathology of the macroglobulinemia of Waldenström. J Natl Cancer Inst 22:887, 1959.
255. Choi YJ, Yeh G, Reiner L, Spielvogel A: Immunoblastic sarcoma following Waldenström's macroglobulinemia. Am J Clin Pathol 71:121, 1979.
256. Golde DW, Saxon A, Stevens RH: Macroglobulinemia and hairy-cell leukemia. N Engl J Med 296:92, 1977.
257. Franklin EC: Amyloidosis. In Williams WJ, Beutler E, Erslev AJ, Rundles RW (eds): "Hematology." Ed 2. New York: McGraw-Hill, 1977, ch 125.
258. Glenner GG, Ein D, Eanes ED, Bladen HA, Terry W, Page DL: Creation of "amyloid" fibrils from Bence Jones proteins in vitro. Science 174:712, 1971.
259. Terry WD, Page DL, Kimura S, Isobe T, Osserman EF, Glenner GG: Structural identity of Bence Jones and amyloid fibril proteins in a patient with plasma cell dyscrasia and amyloidosis. J Clin Invest 52:1276, 1973.
260. Glenner GG, Terry WD, Isersky C: Amyloidosis: Its nature and pathogenesis. Semin Hematol 10:65, 1973.
261. Glenner GG, Ein D, Terry WD: The immunoglobulin nature of amyloid. Am J Med 52:141, 1972.

262. Rosenthal CJ, Franklin EC: Amyloidosis and amyloid proteins. Recent Adv Clin Immunol 1:41, 1977.
263. Meyerhoff J: Familial Mediterranean fever: Report of a large family, review of the literature, and discussion of the frequency of amyloidosis. Medicine 59:66, 1980.
264. Husby G, Natvig JB: A serum component related to nonimmunoglobulin protein AS, a possible precursor of the fibrils. J Clin Invest 53:1054, 1974.
265. Linder E, Anders RF, Natvig JB: Connective tissue origin of the amyloid-related protein SAA. J Exp Med 144:1336, 1976.
266. Wantanabe S, Jaffe E, Pollock S, Sipe J, Glenner GG: Amyloid AA protein. Cellular distribution and appearance. Am J Clin Pathol 67:540, 1977.
267. Rosenthal CJ, Sullivan L: Serum amyloid A. Evidence for its origin in polymorphonuclear leukocytes. J Clin Invest 62:1181, 1978.
268. Pras M, Zaretzky J, Frangione B, Franklin EC: AA protein in a case of "Primary" or "Idiopathic" amyloidosis. Am J Med 68:291, 1980.
269. Sletten K, Westermark P, Natvig JB: Characterization of amyloid fibril proteins from medullary carcinoma of the thyroid. J Exp Med 143:993, 1976.
270. Franklin EC: Some unsolved problems in the amyloid diseases. Am J Med 66:365, 1979.
271. Westermark P, Natvig JB, Johansson B: Characterization of an amyloid fibril protein from senile cardiac amyloid. J Exp Med 146:631, 1977.
272. Kyle RA, Bayrd ED: Amyloidosis: Review of 236 cases. Medicine 54:271, 1975.
273. Ridolfi RL, Bulkley BH, Hutchins PM: The conduction system in cardiac amyloidosis. Clinical and pathologic features of 23 patients. Am J Med 62:677, 1977.
274. Kelly JJ, Kyle RA, O'Brien PC, Dyck PJ: The natural history of peripheral neuropathy in primary systemic amyloidosis. Ann Neurol 6:1, 1979.
275. Battle WM, Rubin MR, Cohen S, Snape WJ: Gastrointestinal-motility dysfunction in amyloidosis. N Engl J Med 301:24, 1979.
276. Cohen AS: The diagnosis of amyloidosis. In Cohen AS, (ed): "Laboratory Diagnostic Procedures in the Rheumatic Diseases" Ed 2. Boston: Little, Brown, 1975, ch 12.
277. Shirahama T, Skinner M, Cohen AS, Benson MD: Uncertain value of urinary sediments in the diagnosis of amyloidosis. N Engl J Med 297:821, 1977.
278. Greipp PR, Kyle RA, Bowie EJW: Factor X deficiency in primary amyloidosis. Resolution after splenectomy. N Engl J Med 301:1050, 1979.
279. Stone MJ, Hirsch VJ, Shapiro G, Sheehan R, Streilein JW, Frenkel EP: Functional hyposplenism in amyloidosis: A diagnostic clue (in preparation).
280. Kyle RA, Greipp PR: Primary systemic amyloidosis: Comparison of melphalan and prednisone versus placebo. Blood 52:818, 1978.
281. Shirahama T, Cohen AS: Blockage of amyloid induction by colchicine in an animal model. J Exp Med 140:1102, 1974.
282. Ravid M, Robson M, Kedar I: Prolonged colchicine treatment in four patients with amyloidosis. Ann Intern Med 87:568, 1977.
283. Frangione B, Franklin EC: Heavy chain diseases: Clinical features and molecular significance of the disordered immunoglobulin structure. Semin Hematol 10:53, 1973.
284. Seligmann M, Mihaesco E, Hurez D, Mihaesco C, Preud'homme JL, Rambaud JC: Immunochemical studies in four cases of alpha chain disease. J Clin Invest 48:2374, 1969.
285. Seligmann M, Rambaud JC: α-Chain disease: A possible model for the pathogenesis of human lymphomas. In Twomey JJ, Good RA (eds): "The Immunopathology of Lymphoreticular Neoplasms. Comprehensive Immunology" Vol 4. New York: Plenum, 1978, ch 14.
286. Doe WF: Alpha chain disease. Clinicopathological features and relationship to so-called Mediterranean lymphoma. Br J Cancer 31 (suppl II):350, 1975.

287. Cohen HJ, Gonzalvo A, Krook J, Thompson TT, Kremer WB: New presentation of alpha heavy chain disease: North American polypoid gastrointestinal lymphoma. Cancer 41:1161, 1978.
288. Doe WF, Danon F, Seligmann M: Immunodiagnosis of alpha chain disease. Clin Exp Immunol 36:189, 1979.
289. Florin-Christensen A, Doniach D, Newcomb PB: Alpha-chain disease with pulmonary manifestations. Br Med J 2:413, 1974.
290. Franklin EC: μ-Chain disease. Arch Intern Med 135:71, 1975.
291. Brouet J-C, Seligmann M, Danon F, Belpomme D, Fine J-M: μ-Chain disease. Report of two new cases. Arch Intern Med 139:672, 1979.
292. Feldman P, Shapiro L, Pick AI, Slatkin MH: Scleromyxedema: A dramatic response to melphalan. Arch Dermatol 99:51, 1969.
293. Danby FW, Danby CWE, Pruzanski W: Papular mucinosis with IgG (κ) M component. Can Med Assoc J 114:920, 1976.
294. Zawadzki ZA, Edwards GA: Nonmyelomatous monoclonal immunoglobulinemia. Prog Clin Immunol 1:105, 1972.
295. Isobe T, Osserman EF: Pathological conditions associated with plasma cell dyscrasias. A study of 806 cases. Ann NY Acad Sci 190:507, 1971.
296. Solomon A: Homogeneous (monoclonal) immunoglobulins in cancer. Am J Med 63:169, 1977.
297. Lindstrom FD, Dahlstrom U: Multiple myeloma or benign monoclonal gammopathy? A study of differential diagnostic criteria in 44 cases. Clin Immunol Immunopathol 10:168, 1978.
298. Weits J, De Gast GC, The TH, Esselink MT, Van Der Giessen M, Mandema E: Class- and subclass-specific antibody response to hemocyanin in nonmalignant paraproteinemia. J Lab Clin Med 94:458, 1979.
299. Kyle RA, Pierre RV, Bayrd ED: Multiple myeloma and acute myelomonocytic leukemia: Report of four cases possibly related to melphalan. N Engl J Med 283:1121, 1970.
300. Kyle RA, Pierre RV, Bayrd ED: Multiple myeloma and acute leukemia associated with alkylating agents. Arch Intern Med 135:185, 1975.
301. Rosner F: Multiple myeloma and acute leukemia: Review of 104 cases. Proc Am Soc Hematol Blood (suppl) 52:597, 1978.
302. Krause RM, Kindt TJ: Antibodies with molecular uniformity. In Putnam FW (ed): "The Plasma Proteins." Ed 2, vol 3. New York: Academic Press, 1977, ch 4.
303. Clubb JS, Posen S, Neale FC: Disappearance of a serum paraprotein after parathyroid-ectomy. Arch Intern Med 114:616, 1964.
304. Del Carpio J, Espinoza LR, Lanter S, Osterland CK: Transient monoclonal proteins in drug hypersensitivity reactions. Am J Med 66:1051, 1979.
305. Metzger H: Characterization of a human macroglobulin. V. A Waldenström macroglobulin with antibody activity. Proc Natl Acad Sci USA 57:1490, 1967.
306. Eisen HN, Little JR, Osterland CK, Simms ES: A myeloma protein with antibody activity. Cold Spring Harbor Symp Quant Biol 32:75, 1967.
307. Stone MJ, Metzger H: The valence of a Waldenström macroglobulin antibody and further thoughts on the significance of paraprotein antibodies. Cold Spring Harbor Symp Quant Biol 32:83, 1967.
308. Cohn M: Natural history of the myeloma. Cold Spring Harbor Symp Quant Biol 32:211, 1967.
309. Grey HM, Kohler PF, Terry WD, Franklin EC: Human monoclonal γG-cryoglobulins with anti-γ-globulin activity. J Clin Invest 47:1875, 1968.
310. Seligmann M, Danon F, Basch A, Bernard J: IgG myeloma cryoglobulin with anti-streptolysin activity. Nature 220:711, 1968.

311. Potter M: Myeloma proteins (M-components) with antibody-like activity. N Engl J Med 284:831, 1971.
312. Seligmann M, Brouet JC: Antibody activity of human myeloma globulins. Semin Hematol 10:163, 1973.
313. Potter M: Antigen binding M-components in man and mouse. In Azar HA, Potter M (eds): "Multiple Myeloma and Related Disorders." Vol 1. Hagerstown: Harper & Row, 1973, ch 4.
314. Seligmann M, Sassy C, Chevalier A: A human IgG myeloma protein with anti-α_2 macroglobulin antibody activity. J Immunol 110:85, 1973.
315. Hauptman S, Tomasi TB: A monoclonal IgM protein with antibody-like activity for human albumin. J Clin Invest 53:932, 1974.
316. Farhangi M, Osserman EF: Myeloma with xanthoderma due to an IgG monoclonal antiflavin antibody. N Engl J Med 294:177, 1976.
317. Freedman M, Merrett R, Pruzanski W: Human monoclonal immunoglobulins with antibody-like activity. Immunochemistry 13:193, 1976.
318. Dixon JA, Sugai S, Talal N: An unusual mouse myeloma protein binding native DNA. Clin Exp Immunol 19:347, 1975.
319. Potter M: Antigen-binding myeloma proteins of mice. Adv Immunol 25:141, 1977.
320. Osserman EF, Takatsuki K: Considerations regarding the pathogenesis of the plasmacytic dyscrasias. Series Haematol (Suppl Scand J Haematol) 4:28, 1965.
321. Baitz T, Kyle RA: Solitary myeloma in chronic osteomyelitis. Arch Intern Med 113:872, 1964.
322. Joseph RR, Tourtellotte CD, Barry WE, Smalley RV, Durant JR: Prolonged immunological disorder terminating in hematological malignancy: a human analogue of animal disease? Ann Intern Med 72:699, 1970.
323. Penny R, Hughes S: Repeated stimulation of the reticuloendothelial system and the development of plasma-cell dyscrasias. Lancet 1:77, 1970.
324. Wohlenberg H: Osteomyelitis and plasmacytoma. N Engl J Med 283:822, 1970.
325. Woodroffe AJ: Multiple myeloma associated with long history of hyposensitisation with allergen vaccines. Lancet 1:99, 1972.
326. Editorial: Antigenic stimulation and myeloma. Lancet 1:252, 1978.
327. Schafer AI, Miller JB: Association of IgA multiple myeloma with pre-existing disease. Br J Haematol 41:19, 1979.
328. Ananthakrishnan R, Biegler B, Dennis PM: Alpha$_1$-antitrypsin phenotypes in paraproteinaemias. Lancet 1:561, 1979.
329. Richards FF, Konigsberg WH: Speculation—how specific are antibodies? Immunochemistry 10:545, 1973.
330. Richards FF, Konigsberg WH, Rosenstein RW, Varga JM: On the specificity of antibodies. Science 187:130, 1975.
331. Richards FF, Rosenstein RW, Varga JM, Konigsberg WH: Antibody combining regions. In Litman GW, Good RA (eds): "Immunoglobulins. Comprehensive Immunology." Vol 5. New York: Plenum, 1978, ch 4.
332. Salmon SE: "Paraneoplastic" syndromes associated with monoclonal lymphocyte and plasma cell proliferations. Ann NY Acad Sci 230:228, 1974.
333. Osterland CK: Biological properties of myeloma proteins. Arch Intern Med 135:32, 1975.
334. Waldenström JG: "Paraneoplasia. Biological Signals in the Diagnosis of Cancer." New York: Wiley, 1978.
335. Theofilopoulos AN, Dixon FJ: The biology and detection of immune complexes. Adv Immunol 28:89, 1979.
336. Kuenn JW, Weber R, Teague PO, Keitt AS: Cryopathic gangrene with an IgM lambda cryoprecipitating cold agglutinin. Cancer 42:1826, 1978.

337. Glueck HI, Hong R, Forristal J, Wittkenstein E, Miller MA, Brinker B: A circulating anticoagulant in γ_1A-multiple myeloma: Its modification by penicillin. J Clin Invest 44:1866, 1965.
338. Cohen I, Amir J, Ben-shaul Y, Pick A, DeVries A: Plasma cell myeloma associated with an unusual myeloma protein causing impairment of fibrin aggregation and platelet function in a patient with multiple malignancy. Am J Med 48:766, 1970.
339. Galanakis DK, Ginzler EM, Fikrig SM: Monoclonal IgG anticoagulants delaying fibrin aggregation in two patients with systemic lupus erythematosus (SLE). Blood 52:1037, 1978.
340. Hurtubise PE, Coots MC, Jacob DJ, Muhleman AF, Glueck HI: A monoclonal IgG$_4$ (λ) with factor V inhibitory activity. J Immunol 122:2119, 1979.
341. CPC-MGH, Case 31-1977. N Engl J Med 297:266, 1977.
342. Levin WC, Aboumrad MH, Ritzmann SE, Brantly C: γ-Type I myeloma and xanthomatosis. Arch Intern Med 114:688, 1964.
343. Cohen L, Blaisdell RK, Djordjevich J, Ormiste V, Dobrilovic L: Familial xanthomatosis and hyperlipidemia, and myelomatosis. Am J Med 40:299, 1966.
344. James W, Harlan WR: Plasma cell disease and xanthomatosis. Trans Am Clin Climatol Assoc 79:115, 1967.
345. Ozer FL, Telatar H, Telatar F, Muftuoglu E: Monoclonal gammopathy with hyperlipidemia. Am J Med 49:841, 1970.
346. Lewis LA, deWolfe VG, Butkus A, Page IH: Autoimmune hyperlipidemia in a patient. Atherosclerotic course and changing immunoglobulin pattern during 21 years of study. Am J Med 59:208, 1975.
347. Wilson DE, Flowers CM, Hershgold EJ, Eaton RP: Multiple myeloma, cryoglobulinemia and xanthomatosis. Distinct clinical and biochemical syndromes in two patients. Am J Med 59:721, 1975.
348. Harboe M, Folling I, Haugen OA, Bauer K: Sudden death caused by interaction between a macroglobulin and a divalent drug. Lancet 2:285, 1976.
349. Levi DF, Williams RC, Lindstrom FD: Immunofluorescent studies of the myeloma kidney with special reference to light chain disease. Am J Med 44:922, 1968.
350. Heptinstall RH: Amyloidosis, multiple myeloma, Waldenström's macroglobulinemia, mixed IgG-IgM cryoglobulinemia, and benign monoclonal gammopathy. In "Pathology of the Kidney." Ed 2. Boston: Little, Brown, 1974, ch 20.
351. Zinneman HH, Seal US: Double spike in myeloma serum due to retention of light chains. Arch Intern Med 124:77, 1969.
352. Jensen K: Metabolism of Bence Jones proteins in non-myeloma patients with normal renal function. Scand J Clin Lab Invest 25:281, 1970.
353. Rudders RA, Bloch KJ: Myeloma renal disease: Evaluation of the role of muramidase (lysozyme). Am J Med Sci 262:79, 1971.
354. Mogielnicki RP, Waldmann TA, Strober W: Renal handling of low molecular weight proteins. I. L-chain metabolism in experimental renal disease. J Clin Invest 50:901, 1971.
355. Waldmann, TA, Strober W, Mogielnicki RP: The renal handling of low molecular weight proteins. II. Disorders of serum protein catabolism in patients with tubular proteinuria, the nephrotic syndrome, or uremia. J Clin Invest 51:2162, 1972.
356. Clyne DH, Pesce AJ, Thompson RE, Pollak VE: Nephrotoxicity of Bence Jones protein in the rat: Importance of isoelectric point. Clin Res 25:628A, 1977.
357. McGeoch J, Smith JF, Ledingham J, Ross B: Inhibition of active transport sodium-potassium—A.T.P.ase by myeloma protein. Lancet 2:17, 1978.
358. Tan M, Epstein W: Polymer formation during the degradation of human light chain and Bence-Jones proteins by an extract of the lysosomal fraction of human kidney. Immunochemistry 9:9, 1972.

359. Pascal RR: Renal manifestations of extrarenal neoplasms. Human Pathol 11:7, 1980.
360. Engle RL, Wallis LA: Multiple myeloma and the adult Fanconi syndrome. Am J Med 22:5, 1957.
361. Headley RN, King JS Jr, Cooper MR, Felts JH: Multiple myeloma presenting as adult Fanconi syndrome. Clin Chem 18:293, 1972.
362. Maldonado JE, Velosa JA, Kyle RA, Wagoner RD, Holley KE, Salassa RM: Fanconi syndrome in adults. A manifestation of a latent form of myeloma. Am J Med 58:354, 1975.
363. Smithline N, Kassirer JP, Cohen JJ: Light-chain nephropathy. N Engl J Med 294:71, 1976.
364. Gennari FJ, Cohen JJ: Renal tubular acidosis. Ann Rev Med 29:521, 1978.
365. Seldin DW, Wilson JD: Renal tubular acidosis. In Stanbury JB, Wyngaarden JB, Fredrickson DS (eds): "The Metabolic Basis of Inherited Disease." Ed 4. New York: McGraw-Hill, 1978, ch 70.
366. Wintrobe MM, Buell MV: Hyperproteinemia associated with multiple myeloma. With report of a case in which an extraordinary hyperproteinemia was associated with thrombosis of the retinal veins and symptoms suggesting Raynaud's disease. Bull Johns Hopkins Hosp 52:156, 1933.
367. Randall RE, Williamson WC, Mullinax F, Tung MY, Still WJS: Manifestations of systemic light chain deposition. Am J Med 60:293, 1976.
368. Atkinson JP, Waldmann TA, Stein SF, Gelfand JA, MacDonald WJ, Heck LW, Cohen EL, Kaplan AP, Frank MM: Systemic capillary leak syndrome and monoclonal IgG gammopathy. Medicine 56:225, 1977.
369. Lindgarde F, Zettervall O: Hypercalcemia and normal ionized serum calcium in a case of myelomatosis. Ann Intern Med 78:396, 1973.
370. Jaffe JP, Mosher DF: Calcium binding by a myeloma protein. Am J Med 67:343, 1979.
371. Bloth B, Christensson T, Mellstedt H: Extreme hyponatremia in patients with myelomatosis. An effect of cationic paraproteins. Acta Med Scand 203:273, 1978.
372. Van Epps DE, Williams RC: Suppression of leukocyte chemotaxis by human IgA myeloma components. J Exp Med 144:1227, 1976.
373. Mundy GR, Raisz LG, Cooper RA, Schechter G, Salmon SE: Evidence for the secretion of an osteoclast stimulating factor in myeloma. N Engl J Med 291:1041, 1974.
374. Yoneda T, Mundy GR: Monocytes regulate osteoclast-activating factor production by releasing prostaglandins. J Exp Med 150:338, 1979.
375. Tanapatchaiyapong P, Zolla S: Humoral immunosuppressive substance in mice bearing plasmacytomas. Science 186:748, 1974.
376. Broder S, Humphrey R, Durm M, Blackman M, Meade B, Goldman C, Strober W, Waldmann T: Impaired synthesis of polyclonal (nonparaprotein) immunoglobulins by circulating lymphocytes from patients with multiple myeloma. Role of suppressor cells. N Engl J Med 293:887, 1975.
377. Kolb JP, Arrian S, Zolla-Pazner S: Suppression of the humoral immune response by plasmacytomas: Mediation by adherent mononuclear cells. J Immunol 118:702, 1977.
378. Paglieroni T, MacKenzie MR: Studies on the pathogenesis of an immune defect in multiple myeloma. J Clin Invest 59:1120, 1977.
379. Waldmann TA, Blaese RM, Broder S, Krakauer RS: Disorders of suppressor immunoregulatory cells in the pathogenesis of immunodeficiency and autoimmunity. Ann Intern Med 88:226, 1978.
380. Broder S, Waldmann TA: The suppressor-cell network in cancer. N Engl J Med 299:1281,1335, 1978.
381. Yasuda N, Kanoh T, Uchino H: J chain synthesis in human myeloma cells: Light and electron microscopic studies. Clin Exp Immunol 40:573, 1980.

382. Kutteh WH, Prince SJ, Mestecky J: Tissue origins of human polymeric and monomeric IgA. J Immunol 128:990, 1982.
383. Eisen HN: "Immunology." Ed 2. Hagerstown: Harper & Row, p 366, 1980.
384. Cuzick J: Radiation-induced myelomatosis. N Engl J Med 304:204, 1981.
385. Schafer AI, Miller JB: Association of IgA multiple myeloma with pre-existing disease. Br J Haematol 41:19, 1979.
386. Lazarus HM, Kellermeyer RW, Aikawa M, Herzig RH: Multiple myeloma in young men. Cancer 46:1397, 1980.
387. Rogers JS, Shah S: Spontaneous splenic rupture in plasma cell leukemia. Cancer 46:212, 1980.
388. Preud'homme JL, Labaume S, Praloran V: Synthesis of abnormal heavy chains in Bence-Jones plasma cell leukemia with intracellular IgG. Blood 56:1136, 1980.
389. Bartoloni C, Flamini G, Logroscino C, Guidi L, Scuderi F, Gambassi G, Terranova T: IgD (Kappa) "nonsecretory" multiple myeloma: Report of a case. Blood 56:898, 1980.
390. Peison B, Benisch B, Williams MC, Newman R: Primary extramedullary plasmacytoma of the omentum associated with recurrent adenocarcinoma of the colon: First case report. Human Pathol 11:399, 1980.
391. Preud'homme JL, Galian A, Danon F, Marti R, Rambaud JC: Extramedullary plasmacytoma with gastric and lymph node involvement: An immunological study. Cancer 46:1753, 1980.
392. Medini E, Rao Y, Levitt SH: Solitary extramedullary plasmacytoma of the upper respiratory and digestive tracts. Cancer 45:2893, 1980.
393. Buss DH, Marshall RB, Holleman IL, Myers RT: Malignant lymphoma of the thyroid gland with plasma cell differentiation (plasmacytoma). Cancer 46:2671, 1980.
394. Addis BJ, Isaacson P, Billings JA: Plasmacytoma of lymph nodes. Cancer 46:340, 1980.
395. West SG, Pittman DL, Coggin JT: Intracranial plasma cell granuloma. Cancer 46:330, 1980.
396. Ford HC, Casey BR, Walker S, Mason A: Multiple Myeloma with an IgD kappa monoclonal protein. Am J Clin Pathol 74:105, 1980.
397. Schulman P, Sun T, Sharer L, Hyman P, Vinciguerra V, Feinstein M, Blanck R, Susin M, Degnan TJ: Meningeal involvement in IgD myeloma with cerebrospinal fluid paraprotein analysis. Cancer 46:152, 1980.
398. Jennette JC, Wilkman AS, Benson JD: IgD myeloma with intracytoplasmic crystalline inclusions. Am J Clin Pathol 75:231, 1981.
399. Johnston JB, Weinerman B, Cooney T, Bowman DM, Pettigrew NM, Orr K: IgD kappa plasma cell dyscrasias. Extraosseous manifestations including isolated leptomeningitis. Am J Clin Pathol 77:60, 1982.
400. Endo T, Okumura H, Kikuchi K, Munakata J, Otake M, Nomura T, Asakawa H: Immunoglobulin E (IgE) multiple myeloma. A case report and review of the literature. Am J Med 70:1127, 1981.
401. Bouvet JP, Liacopoulos P, Pillot J, Banda R, Tung E, Wang AC: Three M-components IgA λ + IgG κn + IgG κh in one patient (DA): Lack of shared idiotypic determinants between IgA and IgG, and the presence of an unusual κh chain of 30,000 M.W. J Immunol 125:213, 1980.
402. Kyle RA, Greipp PR: "Idiopathic" Bence Jones proteinuria. Long-term follow-up in seven patients. N Engl J Med 306:564, 1982.
403. Wheelan KR, Cooper B, Stone MJ: Multiple hematologic abnormalities associated with sulfasalazine (Azulfidine). Ann Intern Med (in press).
404. Reed M, McKenna RW, Bridges R, Parkin J, Frizzera G, Brunning RD: Morphologic manifestations of monoclonal gammopathies. Am J Clin Pathol 76:8, 1981.

405. Hsu SM, Hsu PL, McMillan PN, Fanger H: Russell Bodies. A light and electron microscopic immunoperoxidase study. Am J Clin Pathol 77:26, 1982.
406. Ludwig H, Pavelka M: Phagocytic plasma cells in a patient with multiple myeloma. Blood 56:173, 1980.
407. Bataille R, Durie BGM, Sany J, Salmon SE: Myeloma bone marrow acid phosphatase staining: A correlative study of 38 patients. Blood 55:802, 1980.
408. Hoover RG, Hickman S, Gebel HM, Rebbe N, Lynch RG: Expansion of Fc receptor-bearing T lymphocytes in patients with immunoglobulin G and immunoglobulin A myeloma. J Clin Invest 67:308, 1981.
409. Ozer H, Han T, Henderson ES, Nussbaum A, Sheedy D: Immunoregulatory T cell function in multiple myeloma. J Clin Invest 67:779, 1981.
410. Oken MM, Kay NE: T-cell subpopulations in multiple myeloma: Correlation with clinical disease status. Br J Haematol 49:629, 1981.
411. Sandberg AA: Chromosome changes in the lymphomas. Human Pathol 12:531, 1981.
412. Latreille J, Barlogie B, Johnston D, Drewinko B, Alexanian R: Ploidy and proliferative characteristics in monoclonal gammopathies. Blood 59:43, 1982.
413. Savage DG, Lindenbaum J, Garrett TJ: Biphasic pattern of bacterial infection in multiple myeloma. Ann Intern Med 96:47, 1982.
414. Stone MJ, Lieberman ZH, Chakmakjian ZH, Matthews JL: Coexistent multiple myeloma and primary hyperparathyroidism. JAMA 247:823, 1982.
415. Keshgegian AA: Anion Gap and immunoglobulin concentration. Am J Clin Pathol 74:282, 1980.
416. Nanji AA, Campbell DJ, Pudek MR: Decreased anion gap associated with hypoalbuminemia and polyclonal gammopathy. JAMA 246:859, 1981.
417. Talreja D, Slater LM, Dara P, Branson H, Armentrout SA: Multiple myeloma complicated by myelomatous obstructive uropathy. Cancer 46:1893, 1980.
418. Border WA, Cohen AH: Renal biopsy diagnosis of clinically silent multiple myeloma. Ann Intern Med 93:43, 1980.
419. Tubbs RR, Gephardt GN, McMahon JT, Hall PM, Valenzuela R, Vidt DG: Light chain nephropathy. Am J Med 71:263, 1981.
420. Driedger H, Pruzanski W: Plasma cell neoplasia with osteosclerotic lesions. A study of five cases and a review of the literature. Arch Intern Med 139:892, 1979.
421. Driedger H, Pruzanski W: Plasma cell neoplasia with peripheral polyneuropathy. A study of five cases and a review of the literature. Medicine 59:301, 1980.
422. Bardwick PA, Zvaifler NJ, Gill GN, Newman D, Greenway GD, Resnick DL: Plasma cell dyscrasia with polyneuropathy, organomegaly, endocrinopathy, M protein, and skin changes: The POEMS Syndrome. Medicine 59:311, 1980.
423. Wahner HW, Kyle RA, Beabout JW: Scintigraphic evaluation of the skeleton in multiple myeloma. Mayo Clin Proc 55:739, 1980.
424. Durie BGM, Cole PW, Chen HS, Himmelstein KJ, Salmon SE: Synthesis and metabolism of Bence Jones protein and calculation of tumour burden in patients with Bence Jones myeloma. Br J Haematol 47:7, 1981.
425. Drewinko B, Alexanian R, Boyer H, Barlogie B, Rubinow SI: The growth fraction of human myeloma cells. Blood 57:333, 1981.
426. Merlini G, Waldenström, JG, Jayakar SD: A new improved clinical staging system for multiple myeloma based on analysis of 123 treated patients. Blood 55:1011, 1980.
427. Mill WB, Griffith R: The role of radiation therapy in the management of plasma cell tumors. Cancer 45:647, 1980.

428. Gutterman JU, Blumenschein GR, Alexanian R, Yap HY, Buzdar AU, Cabanillas F, Hortobagyi GN, Hersh EM, Rasmussen SL, Harmon M, Kramer M, Pestka S: Leukocyte interferon-induced tumor regression in human metastatic breast cancer, multiple myeloma, and malignant lymphoma. Ann Intern Med 93:399, 1980.
429. Houwen B, Ockhuizen T, Marrink J, Nieweg HO: Vindesine therapy in melphalan-resistant multiple myeloma. Eur J Cancer 17:227, 1981.
430. Karp JE, Humphrey RL, Burke PJ: Timed sequential chemotherapy of Cytoxan-refractory multiple myeloma with Cytoxan and adriamycin based on induced tumor proliferation. Blood 57:468, 1981.
431. Alexanian R, Salmon S, Gutterman J, Dixon D, Bonnet J, Haut, A: Chemoimmunotherapy for multiple myeloma. Cancer 47:1923, 1981.
432. Woodruff R: Treatment of multiple myeloma. Cancer Treat Rev 8:225, 1981.
433. Broun GO, Petruska PJ, Hiramoto RN, Cohen HJ: Cisplatin, BCNU, cyclophosphamide, and prednisone in multiple myeloma. Cancer Treatm Rep 66:237, 1982.
434. Hoogstraten B: Multiple myeloma. A therapeutic enigma. Am J Clin Oncol 5:13, 1982.
435. Kapadia SB: Multiple myeloma: A clinicopathologic study of 62 consecutively autopsied cases. Medicine 59:380, 1980.
436. Gonzalez F, Trujillo JM, Alexanian R: Acute leukemia in multiple myeloma. Ann Intern Med 86:440, 1977.
437. Casciato DA, Scott JL: Acute leukemia following prolonged cytotoxic agent therapy. Medicine 58:32, 1979.
438. Mannik M: Blood viscosity in Waldenström's macroglobulinemia. Blood 44:87, 1974.
439. MacKenzie MR, Babcock J: Studies of the hyperviscosity syndrome. II. Macroglobulinemia. J Lab Clin Med 85:227, 1975.
440. MacKenzie MR, Lee TK: Blood viscosity in Waldenström macroglobulinemia. Blood 49:507, 1977.
441. Latov N, Sherman WH, Nemni R, Galassi G, Shyong JS, Penn AS, Chess L, Olarte MR, Rowland LP, Osserman EF: Plasma-cell dyscrasia and peripheral neuropathy with a monoclonal antibody to peripheral-nerve myelin. N Engl J Med 303:618, 1980.
442. Levo Y: Nature of cryoglobulinaemia. Lancet 1:285, 1980.
443. Wanless IR, Solt LC, Kortan P, Deck JHN, Gardiner GW, Prokipchuk EJ: Nodular regenerative hyperplasia of the liver associated with macroglobulinemia. Am J Med 70:1203, 1981.
444. Glenner GG: Amyloid deposits and amyloidosis. The β-fibrilloses. N Engl J Med 302:1283, 1333, 1980.
445. Gorevic PD, Franklin EC: Amyloidosis. Ann Rev Med 32:261, 1981.
446. Bausserman LL, Herbert PN, McAdam KPWJ: Heterogeneity of human serum amyloid A proteins. J Exp Med 152:641, 1980.
447. Benson MD: Partial amino acid sequence homology between an heredofamilial amyloid protein and human plasma prealbumin. J Clin Invest 67:1035, 1981.
448. Pras M, Franklin EC, Prelli F, Frangione B: A variant of prealbumin from amyloid fibrils in familial polyneuropathy of Jewish origin. J Exp Med 154:989, 1981.
449. Tawara S, Araki S, Toshimori K, Nakagawa H, Ohtaki S: Amyloid fibril protein in type 1 familial amyloidotic polyneuropathy in Japanese. J Lab Clin Med 98:811, 1981.
450. Glenner GG: Amyloidosis: The hereditary disorders, including Alzheimer's disease. J Lab Clin Med 98:807, 1981.
451. Kelly JJ, Kyle RA, O'Brien PC, Dyck PJ: The natural history of peripheral neuropathy in primary systemic amyloidosis. Ann Neurol 6:1, 1979.
452. Dikman SH, Churg J, Kahn T: Morphologic and clinical correlates in renal amyloidosis. Human Pathol 12:160, 1981.

453. Finkelstein SD, Fornasier VL, Pruzanski W: Intrahepatic cholestasis with predominant pericentral deposition in systemic amyloidosis. Human Pathol 12:470, 1981.
454. Dorman SA, Gamelli RL, Benziger JR, Trainer TD, Foster RS: Systemic amyloidosis involving two renal transplants. Human Pathol 12:735, 1981.
455. Carson FL, Kingsley WB: Nonamyloid green birefringence following Congo red staining. Arch Pathol Lab Med 104:333, 1980.
456. Furie B, Voo LA, McAdam KPWJ, Furie BC: Mechanism of factor X deficiency in systemic amyloidosis. N Engl J Med 304:827, 1981.
457. Akoglu E, Akoglu T, Gurcay A, Turgan C, Anil H: Circulating immune complexes in systemic amyloidosis. Clin Immunol Immunopathol 20:321, 1981.
458. Jerath RS, Valenzuela R, Guerrero I, Deodhar SD, Vidt DB: Immunofluorescence findings in human renal amyloidosis. Am J Clin Pathol 74:630, 1980.
459. Bertram J, Gualtieri RJ, Osserman EF: Amyloid-related Bence Jones proteins bind dinitrophenyl L-lysine (DNP). In Glenner GG, Pinlo e Costa P, de Freitas F (eds): "Amyloid and Amyloidosis." Amsterdam: Excerpta Medica, 1980, p 351.
460. Wright JR, Calkins E: Clinical-pathologic differentiation of common amyloid syndromes. Medicine 60:429, 1981.
461. Osserman EF, Sherman WH, Kyle RA: Further studies of therapy of amyloidosis with Dimethylsulfoxide (DMSO). In Glenner GG, Pinlo e Costa P, de Freitas F (eds): "Amyloid and Amyloidosis." Amsterdam: Excerpta Medica, 1980, p 563.
462. Seligmann M et al: Heavy chain diseases: Current findings and concepts. Immunol Rev 48:145, 1979.
463. Preud'homme JL, et al: Cellular immunoglobulins in human γ and α heavy chain diseases. Clin Exp Immunol 37:282, 1979.
464. Zucker-Franklin D, Franklin EC: Ultrastructural and immunofluorescence studies of the cells associated with μ chain disease. Blood 37:257, 1971.
465. Vilpo JA, Irjala K, Viljanen MK, Klemi P, Kouvonen I, Ronnemaa T: δ-Heavy chain disease. A study of a case. Clin Immunol Immunopathol 17:584, 1980.
466. Wells JV, Fudenberg HH, Epstein WL: Idiotypic determinants on the monoclonal immunoglobulins associated with papular mucinosis. J Immunol 108:977, 1972.
467. Carter A, Tatarsky I: The physiopathological significance of benign monoclonal gammopathy: A study of 64 cases. Br J Haematol 46:565, 1980.
468. Kyle RA, Greipp PR: Smoldering multiple myeloma. N Engl J Med 302:1347, 1980.
469. Ginder PA, Middendorf DF, Abdou NI: Pancytopenia with mixed cryoglobulinemia: Evidence for anti-precursor cell activity of cryoglobulin—Effects of plasmapheresis. J Clin Immunol 2:55, 1982.
470. Thiagarajan P, Shapiro SS, De Marco L: Monoclonal immunoglobulin Mλ coagulation inhibitor with phospholipid specificity: Mechanism of a lupus anticoagulant. J Clin Invest 66:397, 1980.
471. Veenhoven WA, Van Der Schans GST, Nieweg HO: Monoclonal immunoglobulins with affinity for platelets and their relationship to malignant lymphoma. Cancer 49:40, 1982.
472. Von Dem Borne AEGK, Moi JJ, Joustra-Maas N, Pegels JG, Langenhuijsen MMAC, Engelfriet CP: Autoimmune haemolytic anaemia with monoclonal IgM (κ) anti-P cold autohaemolysins. Br J Haematol 50:345, 1982.
473. Kabat EA, Liao J, Shyong J, Osserman EF: A monoclonal IgMλ macroglobulin with specificity for lacto-N-tetraose in a patient with bronchogenic carcinoma. J Immunol 128:540, 1982.
474. Rudikoff S, Potter M: Immunoglobulin heavy chains from anti-inulin myeloma proteins: Evidence for a new heavy chain joining segment. J Immunol 127:191, 1981.

475. Dalakas MC, Engel WK: Polyneuropathy with monoclonal gammopathy: Studies of 11 patients. Ann Neurol 10:45, 1981.
476. Besinger UA, Toyka KV, Anzil AP, Fateh-Moghadam A, Neumeier D, Rauscher R, Heininger K: Myeloma neuropathy: Passive transfer from man to mouse. Science 213:1027, 1981.
477. Delauche MC, Clauvel JP, Seligmann M: Peripheral neuropathy and plasma cell neoplasias: A report of 10 cases. Br J Haematol 48:383, 1981.
478. Trump DL, Allen H, Olson J, Wright J, Humphrey RL: Epidermolysis Bullosa Acquisita. Association with amyloidosis and multiple myeloma. JAMA 243:1461, 1980.
479. CPC-MGH. Case 27–1981. N Engl J Med 305:33, 1981.
480. Isobe T, Takatsuki K, Tishendorf FW, Birken S, Osserman EF: Plasma Cell myeloma, hyperviscosity and amyloidosis associated with a serum $IgG_3\lambda$ and urinary excretion of two fragments related to the variable portion of λ light chains. Clin Immunol Immunopathol 19:55, 1981.
481. Langlands DR, Dawkins RL, Matz LR, Cobain TJ, Goatcher P, Papadimitriou JM, Cohen ML: Arthritis associated with a crystallizing cryoprecipitable IgG paraprotein. Am J Med 68:461, 1980.
482. Vallat JM, Desproges-Gotteron R, Leboutet MJ, Loubet A, Gualde N, and Treves R: Cryoglobulinemic neuropathy: A pathological study. Ann Neurol 8:179, 1980.
483. Preud'homme JL, Morel-Maroger L, Brouet JC, Cerf M, Mignon F, Guglielmi P, Seligmann M: Synthesis of abnormal immunoglobulins in lymphoplasmacytic disorders with visceral light chain deposition. Am J Med 69:703, 1980.
484. Fer MF, McKinney TD, Richardson RL, Hande KR, Oldham RK, Greco FA: Cancer and the kidney: Renal complications of neoplasms. Am J Med 71:704, 1981.
485. Osterland CK, Miller EJ, Karakawa WW, Krause RM: Characteristics of streptococcal antibody isolated from hyperimmune rabbits. J Exp Med 123:599, 1966.
486. Hahn GS: Antibody structure, function, and active sites. In Ritzmann SE (ed.) "Physiology of Immunoglobulins: Diagnostic and Clinical Aspects." New York: Alan R. Liss, 1982, pp 193–304.
487. Ritzmann SE: Quantitation of normal and abnormal serum IgG, A, and M by radial immunodiffusion, nephelometry, and turbidimetry. In Ritzmann SE (ed): "Physiology of Immunoglobulins: Diagnostic and Clinical Aspects." New York: Alan R. Liss, 1982, pp 139–156.
488. Wicher KJ: IgE: Diagnostic and clinical manifestations. In Ritzmann SE (ed): "Physiology of Immunoglobulins: Diagnostic and Clinical Manifestations." New York: Alan R. Liss, 1982, pp 305–351.
489. Leder P: The genetics of antibody diversity. Scientific American, May 1982, pp 102–115.
490. Wolf RE, Levin WC, Ritzmann SE: Thermoproteins. In Ritzmann SE, Daniels JC (eds): "Serum Protein Abnormalities: Diagnostic and Clinical Aspects," 2nd printing. New York: Alan R. Liss, Inc., 1982, pp 487–512.
491. Salmon SE (ed): Myeloma and related disorders. Clin Haematol 11:1–238, 1982.

Pathology of Immunoglobulins: Diagnostic and
Clinical Aspects, pages 237–259
© 1982 Alan R. Liss, Inc., 150 Fifth Avenue, New York, NY 10011

9

Disorders of Hyperviscosity

Jeffrey Crawford, MD, and Harvey Jay Cohen, MD

The symptoms and clinical syndrome of hyperviscosity[1] may be the result of numerous factors and their interactions. Chapter 1 described the definition of viscosity and its measurement *in vitro*. In order to fully understand the diseases associated with increased viscosity and the clinical manifestations created, one must first consider the contribution of other determinants of blood flow *in vivo*.

The science of rheology, or the study of fluid deformation and flow, has yielded great insight into the properties of blood [88]. However, in a clinical setting, any rheologic data must be considered in terms of hemodynamics, or the flow of blood in the circulatory system. Blood flow can be expressed as the ratio of the pressure differential divided by the resistance of a system. While blood viscosity is one parameter of resistance, the vascular system also provides resistance to flow. In arteries, the intrinsic elasticity of the smooth muscle layer appears to be a major factor governing flow and determining critical closing pressure, or that pressure required to maintain flow. Other hemodynamic factors such as pulsatile flow, cardiac output, and turbulent flow due to high flow rates or anatomic alterations are of obvious importance and have been reviewed [1].

Under physiologic conditions, the major factor determining flow is the vessel diameter. By Poisueille's law (Chapter 1) flow is directly proportional to the fourth power of the radius of the vessel. Because of its non-Newtonian behavior, blood would be expected to increase in viscosity as the vessel radius and shear rate decrease. However, the reverse is true since viscosity actually falls with a decrease in vessel diameter below 200 μm, the size of a small artery. This is known as the Fähraeus effect [2]. It results from alterations of the cellular elements of blood during flow through the circulation. Axial streaming, or the higher concentration of red cells in the center of flow compared to that along the wall layer, becomes more prominent as vessel diameter decreases. At branch vessels, plasma skimming occurs so

[1]Ed. note: See also [98].

that the branch vessel has a lower hematocrit and, therefore, lower viscosity than the parent vessel (Fig. 1). As vessel diameter continues to decrease, the viscosity of whole blood approaches that of plasma.

The Fåhraeus effect seems to be valid in capillaries with diameters as small as 5–10 μm (average capillary—6μm). Below that size there is an inversion phenomenon described by Dintenfass wherein blood viscosity dramatically increases [3]. This probably relates to the attainment of a critical relationship between red cell size and vessel size. At this point a certain pressure or yield stress must be applied to deform the cells so that they will pass through the vessel. Since the red cells may traverse the capillaries as a "plug" rather than as a fluid suspension, some investigators feel that this phenomenon should not be expressed as viscosity but as "resistance to flow" [4]. Despite disagreement as to the proper mathematical model for capillary flow, Dintenfass's observation remains a clinically important concept. It is easy to visualize how altered cell number or deformability could affect capillary transit. In addition, a major effect of increased plasma viscosity would be increased protein and protein-red cell interaction within the capillary.

Finally, it must be remembered that measurements of viscosity *in vitro* are performed in a steady state. Within the circulation, however, viscosity changes occur, even within the capillary, as transmural fluid shifts occur [5]. While the physiology of microcirculatory hemodynamics is still being defined, a spectrum of disorders associated with major alterations of the blood elements has led to insight into pathologic flow states clinically known as the hyperviscosity syndromes (Table I).

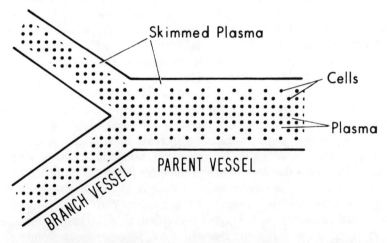

Fig. 1.   As blood flows through a branching vessel, the cell number decreases to a greater extent than the plasma volume. Therefore, cell concentration is lower than in the parent vessel.

TABLE I. Alteration of Blood Elements Associated With Increased Blood Viscosity

Cellular elements
    Hematocrit—polycythemia, neonatal hyperviscosity syndrome
    Altered red cell shape/viscosity—e.g., sickle cell anemia
    Massive white count elevation with leukemia
    Thrombocytosis
Plasma elements
    Lipid—hyperlipoproteinemia
    Fibrinogen—hyperfibrinogenemia, cryofibrinogenemia
    Globulins—macroglobulinemia, myeloma, polyclonal hyperviscosity syndrome

VISCOSITY AND HEMATOCRIT

In his classic paper, Wells carefully pointed out that although the hyperviscosity syndrome has clinically come to be synonymous with serum protein disorders, in fact, polycythemia is a more common cause of blood hyperviscosity [6]. The relationship between hematocrit and relative viscosity can be seen in Figure 2A [7]. Using an Ostwald viscometer, one can also determine the *in vitro* relationship of hematocrit and viscosity to blood flow rate, expressed as hemoglobin transport (Fig. 2B). At low levels of viscosity, hemoglobin transport increases as the hematocrit increases to an optimum around 45%. However, further increases in hematocrit actually decrease hemoglobin transport due to the increased blood viscosity and decreased flow rate. Multiple hemodynamic factors such as increased cardiac output and decreased peripheral vascular resistance may help maintain adequate hemoglobin transport in anemic states. However, in polycythemic states, the physiologic adjustments that can maintain adequate oxygenation are more limited.

As previously discussed, the potential for a hyperviscous state secondary to an increased hematocrit is attenuated by the Fåhraeus effect. However, patients with polycythemia often have hematocrit values greater than 60% and may present with symptoms of retarded blood flow and decreased oxygenation of tissue [89]. As in serum hyperviscosity states (to be discussed later) polycythemia patients frequently present with cerebral symptoms of lethargy and obtundation along with retinal changes of dilated tortuous vessels. However, bleeding disorders are less frequent, while thrombotic and cardiovascular events appear to be more common than in serum hyperviscosity syndromes. Clinically, phlebotomy to lower the hematocrit is quite effective in reversing symptoms.

As a correlate to the adult situation, polycythemia in newborns may present with characteristic findings known as the *neonatal hyperviscosity syndrome.* Manifestations may include plethora, cyanosis, respiratory distress, cardio-

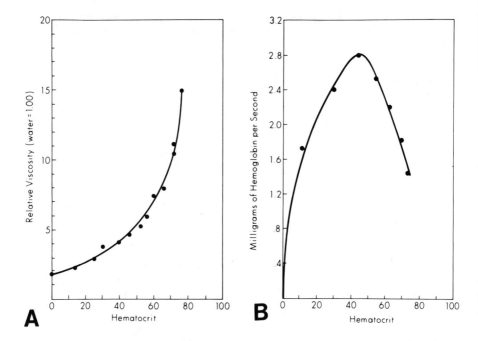

Fig. 2. (A) The relationship between hematocrit and relative viscosity. (B) The relationship of hematocrit to blood flow rate, as expressed by mg hemoglobin/sec. (Adapted from the data of Stone [7].)

megaly, edema, seizures, and lethargy. A favorable response to phlebotomy is also seen in these patients [8].

More controversial is the question of the impact of an elevated hematocrit in the high normal range with or without a decrease in plasma volume. One report suggested that such individuals have a decrease in cerebral blood flow of more than 25%, which can be returned to the normal range when the hematocrit is lowered from between 47% and 53% to 43% (with a concomitant return of whole blood viscosity to normal)[9]. This study has been criticized for oversimplifying the relationship of cerebral blood flow to hematocrit [10]. More recently, two other studies have shown clinical improvement in cerebral symptoms [90] or psychometric testing [91] which correlated with improved cerebral blood flow after phlebotomy in patients with secondary polycythemia. However, total cerebral oxygen carriage did not change [90].

VISCOSITY AND RED CELL SHAPE

A major factor in microcirculatory blood flow is the elasticity of the red blood cell. If one studies red cells in a saline solution to eliminate protein-induced red cell aggregation, little rise in viscosity occurs until very low shear rates are achieved. However, if one transforms these cells into spindle-shaped cells, the viscosity of the red cell-saline suspension dramatically increases at low shear rates [11]. Such cells retain the same volume as normal cells and are equally deformable at high shear rates. The major distinction appears to be that this shape change creates increased cell-cell interaction at lower shear rates. In contrast, in the situation of volume loss from the red cell, as in incubating normal cells in hypertonic media, increased viscosity occurs at all shear rates. This relates directly to the degree of increase in mean corpuscular hemoglobin concentration and a resultant decrease in cellular deformability. The clinical correlation of these two observations can be seen in pyruvate kinase deficiency and hereditary spherocytosis, respectively.

The manifestations of red cell hyperviscosity are often limited to a shortened red cell survival and the consequences of hemolysis. However, the clinical consequences of an alteration in red cell shape can be quite devastating, as in sickle cell anemia. While evidence exists for reduced red cell deformability secondary to membrane loss and altered intrinsic membrane flexibility during sickling and unsickling, a major determinant is the irreversibly sickled cell, in which the most striking abnormality is the high hemoglobin concentration and internal viscosity secondary to polymerized deoxyhemoglobin S [12]. The rheological difficulties these nondeformable cells undergo have been directly related to the vaso-occlusive phenomena that occur within the microvasculature of the spleen, kidney, retina, and bone [92].

VISCOSITY AND OTHER BLOOD CELL ELEMENTS

Leukocytes have a higher intrinsic viscosity than red cells, but their contribution to whole blood viscosity is generally insignificant due to their relatively small total volume. However, in patients with leukemia and marked white count elevation, leukocyte thrombi can occur in pulmonary and cerebral vessels [13]. In one report, leukemia patients are described with symptoms of hyperviscosity including auditory and visual disturbances, gait abnormalities, and altered sensorium [14]. Whole blood viscosity measurement showed a 50% or greater increase over normal. Response in clinical symptomatology occurred with leukapheresis and return of the white count and viscosity to more normal levels. This syndrome has been described in chronic lymphocytic leukemia, acute leukemia, and chronic granulocytic leukemia. In chronic lymphocytic leukemia the white count is usually greater than 500,000/mm^3 before any symptoms are seen, whereas in the acute disorders, it is often in the range of 200,000/mm^3. The difference probably relates to the difference in cell size, but other factors such as membrane deformability require further investigation.

With respect to thrombocytosis, the evidence for hyperviscosity is more circumstantial. Even massive platelet count elevations (greater than 1 million/mm^3), produce a platelet layer of only a few millimeters in a Wintrobe tube relative to the normal 40-mm red cell layer. Therefore, a dramatic effect on whole blood viscosity is not usually seen. However, Dintenfass has shown that platelet aggregates dramatically increase the capillary radius at which the inversion phenomenon occurs and resistance to flow increases [15]. Additionally, studies of thrombocytosis in myeloproliferative disorders have shown the presence of spontaneous circulating platelet aggregates [16]. Symptoms in these patients have included transient cerebral ischemic attacks, amaurosis, digital ischemia, venous thrombosis, and confusion which reverse with platelet antiaggregating agents. However, the distinction between microcirculatory hyperviscosity from thrombocytosis and microthrombi from platelet aggregates becomes a difficult differential point. Similar symptoms may arise from leukocyte aggregates activated in the setting of pancreatitis and other inflammatory disorders [93].

PLASMA ELEMENTS AND VISCOSITY

Little consideration has been given to the contribution of lipids to plasma viscosity [94]. One study in patients with primary hyperlipoproteinemia showed a linear correlation between increasing total lipids and plasma viscosity [17]. This concentration-dependent rise in viscosity appears to be true for both very low-density lipoprotein and low-density liproprotein fractions. However, the change in plasma viscosity even in severe derangements of lipids such as type IIb hyperlipoproteinemia is generally less than 20% above normal. In addition to plasma viscosity, whole blood viscosity and erythrocyte flexibility are altered by hyperlipoproteinemia and can be reversed with clofibrate [18]. Whether this degree of hyperviscosity relates to the abdominal pain seen in some patients with severe hypertriglyceridemia remains a question [19].

An elevated plasma viscosity in hospitalized patients is frequently secondary to an elevated fibrinogen level [20,21]. Fibrinogen has the highest intrinsic viscosity among the plasma proteins. This relates partially to its molecular weight, but predominantly to its shape as a linear protein with an axial length to width ratio of 15:1 [22]. The asymmetry allows increased protein-protein interaction and also protein-red cell interaction. This elevated viscosity plays a role in venous stasis which may lead to postoperative thrombosis [23]. Increased viscosity also occurs in infection secondary to coagulation activation with subsequent increases in fibrinogen and fibrin monomers [24]. However, in this situation as in the postoperative state, elevation of normal fibrinogen is insufficient to raise the viscosity into the clinical range of the hyperviscosity syndrome.

Dysfibrinogens are abnormal proteins often resulting in bleeding, but occasionally presenting with thrombosis [25]. The most common acquired form is a cryofibrinogen with a temperature-dependent precipitation leading to increased viscosity, particularly in the peripheral circulation. While small amounts of cryofibrinogen can occur with no apparent significance in normals, amounts greater than 100 mg/L are generally seen only in patients with malignancies [26] or with inflammatory conditions such as ulcerative colitis [27] and vasculitis [28]. These patients differ from those with the serum hyperviscosity syndrome in that Raynaud's phenomenon, cutaneous gangrene, and recurrent thrombophlebitis are the most common symptoms. They do share the common feature of increased bleeding.

The globulins are the major component of the plasma resulting in hyperviscosity and will be discussed collectively for their production of the serum hyperviscosity syndrome.

THE SERUM HYPERVISCOSITY SYNDROME

History

In the 1930s, the first laboratory and clinical observations of increased serum viscosity were made [29,30]. While these patients had myeloma, the association with increased viscosity was later defined in a group of patients described by Waldenström in 1944 with globulins of abnormally high molecular weight [31]. Patients with macroglobulinemia formed the basis for Fahey's description in 1965 of the clinical symptoms of bleeding, ocular disorders, and neurologic signs as the serum hyperviscosity syndrome [32]. Further study of myeloma patients with hyperviscosity led to insight into the determinants of intrinsic protein viscosity [33]. Most recently this syndrome has been recognized in disorders of polyclonal globulin production and immune complex formation [34].

Pathophysiology

The immunoglobulins (Igs) are the serum proteins most frequently involved in the serum hyperviscosity syndrome. Viscosity is determined not only by globulin concentration, but also by the intrinsic properties of the protein (Table II). The differences in these properties result in a wide variation in the relationship of Ig concentration to viscosity (Fig. 3). These curves emphasize relative differences in viscosity properties between Ig classes and subclasses. For any individual monoclonal protein, the intrinsic properties are highly variable, and viscosity can only be accurately determined by measurement. IgM with its high molecular weight of 900,000 daltons and high axial length-to-width ratio has a higher intrinsic viscosity than the other globulins. With increased concentration, it tends to aggregate into macromolecules, presumably due to its pentameric configuration [37]. The degree

TABLE II. Factors Influencing Globulin Viscosity

Concentration
Intrinsic viscosity (IgM > IgA > IgE > IgG)
Aggregation (IgM, IgG_3)
Polymer formation (IgA)
Molecular asymmetry
Cryoprecipitability
Immune complex formation
Interaction with other plasma proteins

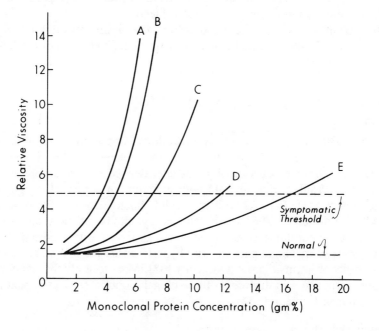

Fig. 3. A composite of several different reported monoclonal proteins and their relationships. A-IgM [32]; B-aggregated IgG_3 [35]; C-polymeric IgA [36]; D-monomeric IgA [36]; E-non-aggregated IgG_1 [41].

of aggregation is variable, but often results in a steep rise in viscosity between 3 and 5 g/dL (Fig. 3, A).

For the other Igs, it is more difficult to predict viscosity relationships because so many subclass and individual variations have been described. IgA accounts for approximately 20% of myeloma patients, but until recently hyperviscosity was thought to be relatively less common than in IgG myeloma [38]. IgA has a higher intrinsic viscosity than IgG, but hyperviscosity syndrome due to massive protein elevation is unusual (Fig. 3, D). Most cases have been seen in the setting of increased polymerization of IgA with the formation of disulfide bonds [36]. Normally 5–15% of IgA exists in polymeric form. This percentage is thought to be limited by the amount of plasma cell J chain that links the IgA monomers. However, in IgA myeloma the degree of polymerization can vary widely. In patients with greater than 50% polymer formation, J chain can be detected in the serum by immunoelectrophoresis with anti J chain serum [39]. Of even greater importance is the degree of polymerization. While patients with 50% dimer may have minimal viscosity elevations, as little as 5–10% of trimer formation or greater is generally associated with hyperviscosity [36]. Thus, the shape of curve C in Figure 3 is highly variable. A monoclonal IgA with a high degree of polymerization has resulted in hyperviscosity at a concentration of 1.5 g/dL [36]. Other than hyperviscosity, there are no clinical features that distinguish patients with polymer formation from those without polymer. The propensity toward hyperviscosity does not bear a relationship to light chain type, IgA subclass, carbohydrate composition, or any known property other than J chain availability [36,38–40]. The degree of polymer formation also may vary during the clinical course of IgA myeloma.

Nonaggregated IgG, generally of the IgG_1 subclass, commonly results in a linear increase in serum viscosity with concentration (Fig. 3, E). Hyperviscosity syndrome has been reported in this situation in the range of 14–18 g/dL [41]. Hyperviscosity syndrome at lower IgG concentrations has been attributed to multiple mechanisms. Reversible and concentration-dependent aggregation can result in hyperviscosity at a protein concentration of 4–6 g/dL (Fig. 3, B) [35]. This usually involves the IgG_3 subclass, although it has been described in an IgG_1 patient [42]. In some cases of IgG_3 aggregation, increased viscosity is provoked at lower temperatures. Between the two curves of the aggregation-dependent and concentration-dependent hyperviscosity states of IgG, a number of other variables may be involved and *hyperviscosity has been described in virtually all intermediate concentration ranges.* Some factors that may be responsible for these situations have included individual proteins with very high molecular asymmetry and high intrinsic viscosity [41], and complexing with other serum proteins such as Igs, albumin, and lipoproteins [43,44]. Similar protein-protein interactions may also be important in rare cases of IgA myeloma [45]. One case of hyperviscosity syndrome has been reported in IgE myeloma at an IgE protein concentration of 7.5 g/dL [46]. No detailed studies of the properties of this protein are available. Disorders of polyclonal Ig production can lead to hyperviscosity syndrome through a concentration-dependent aggregation or polymerization of immune complexes [47]. This will be discussed further in a subsequent section.

An additional property that leads to a temperature-dependent viscosity increase for some IgM, IgG, and IgA proteins and for some immune complexes is cryoprecipitability. Cryoglobulins do not differ consistently in size, shape, net charge, or carbohydrate content from other globulins. They are most commonly associated with κ-light chains, and the Fab fragment may be responsible for self-association and cold precipitation [48]. Clinically this group of patients is distinguished by reduced blood flow to the skin at lower temperatures [49] and the dominant clinical manifestations often are purpura, peripheral gangrene, Raynaud's phenomenon, and arterial thrombosis.

The effect of serum hyperviscosity must always be considered in light of whole blood viscosity and the rheologic parameters previously discussed. Increased Ig concentrations would be expected to increase red cell interaction and rouleaux formation. In addition, monoclonal IgG produces a greater degree of rouleaux formation than comparable amounts of normal IgG [50]. Furthermore, macroglobulins increase rouleaux formation to a much greater degree than do non-IgM myleoma proteins [51]. Thus, increases in plasma viscosity secondary to Ig are magnified in the microcirculation.

Clinical Manifestations

The triad of bleeding, ocular findings, and neurologic alterations initially described by Fahey remain the most constant features of the serum hyperviscosity syndrome [32] (Table III). Patients with a relative serum viscosity of less than 4.0 seldom have hyperviscosity syndrome. Even above 5.0, the appearance of symptoms is very variable. However, for a given patient, the level of relative viscosity at which symptoms are first seen is reproducible. This has been called the "symptomatic threshold" [32]. The fact that a specific serum viscosity does not correlate with clinical symptoms in all patients is probably related to other important rheological variables such as hematocrit and vascular anatomy.

Bleeding is the most common presenting complaint in patients with hyperviscosity syndrome. It is a frequent feature of dysproteinemias in general, and it is not specific for the diagnosis [52]. Hemostatic defects have been described in 15% of IgG myelomas and over 30% of IgA myelomas and macroglobulinemia patients [53]. A multitude of abnormalities have been described, including altered platelet function, depressed clotting factors, and factor inhibitors, all presumably related to the monoclonal protein and its interactions [54]. The most consistent abnormalities seem to be a prolonged bleeding time and decreased platelet adhesiveness. It is unclear how much of the increased bleeding in the hyperviscosity syndrome relates to these protein interactions and how much relates to viscosity itself, resulting in sludging of blood in the microcirculation. In any event, the appearance of new epistaxis, oral or mucosal bleeding, purpura, or ecchymoses in a patient with an established dysproteinemia should be a significant warning signal for the possibility of hyperviscosity syndrome.

TABLE III. Clinical Manifestations

Bleeding—epistaxis, gingival bleeding, purpura, ecchymoses, postoperative bleeding, vaginal hemorrhage, hematuria, melena, hematochezia

Ocular manifestations—distended retinal veins, tortuosity, segmentation (box-car effect), retinal hemorrhage, retinal vein thrombosis with papilledema, diplopia, decreased visual acuity, partial or total blindness

Neurologic manifestations—headache, dizziness, vertigo, nystagmus, stroke, lethargy, stupor, coma, seizures, postural hypotension

Cardiovascular—angina, congestive heart failure, cryoprotein-related symptoms of Raynaud's phenomenon, gangrene, digital ulcers, pulmonary infarction, arterial thrombosis

Renal—renal functional impairment, occasional acute renal failure, proteinuria, tubular defects

General—fatigue malaise, weakness

Lab abnormalities—dilutional anemia secondary to hypervolemia, macrocytosis, hyponatremia, hypokalemia, decreased anion gap

While *ocular symptoms* are not as common as bleeding, the presence of retinopathy is probably the most diagnostic finding for hyperviscosity syndrome. The clinical diagnosis has rarely been made in the absence of retinal changes. At a minimum one would expect to see distended retinal veins with tortuosity. In more severely affected patients retinal hemorrhage, segmentation of the vascular column of blood (box-car or sausage effect), or even papilledema secondary to retinal vein thrombosis may be present (Fig. 4). In one series, the presence of retinopathy was consistently predictive of a relative serum viscosity greater than 4.0 [52].

In contrast to its relationship to the bleeding complications of dysproteinemias, viscosity per se appears to be the major etiologic factor in retinopathy. Retinal changes of increased tortuosity of vessels and hemorrhages have been produced in monkeys by infusion of high molecular weight dextran [55]. Clinically, lowering of viscosity can be expected to improve the retinal circulation time, restore veins to their normal shape and prevent formation of new hemorrhages. Results are often seen within hours or days of initiating plasmapheresis [56]. Conjunctival vessel changes are also present and have provided an opportunity to study flow directly in hyperviscosity states. Using microcinematography, flow can actually be seen to stop and start within these vessels [56,57]. Thus, the clinical description of "sludging" has a correlate with increased red cell aggregation [58].

Neurologic manifestations include headaches, dizziness, nystagmus, seizures, altered mental status, and stroke [95]. The pathophysiology of the neurologic manifestations has been related to intravascular erythrocyte aggregation [60]. While some correlation exists between symptoms and the

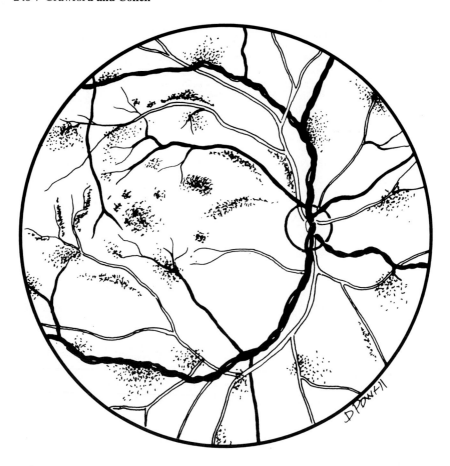

Fig. 4.   Retina with typical changes of hyperviscosity. Note the dilated veins with segmentation and the retinal hemorrhages.

level of serum viscosity, the patient's age and prior status of the cerebro-vascular circulation seem to be very important variables. The differential is especially difficult in myeloma where neurologic symptoms may also be present because of hypercalcemia, renal failure, amyloidosis, infection, or the debilitation of the disease. Response to plasmapheresis has been excellent for those neurologic symptoms related to hyperviscosity syndrome. In some situations, the only method of establishing the role of hyperviscosity in producing the neurologic symptoms is to assess the response to plasma-pheresis. This approach has improved our understanding of the peripheral neuropathy of Waldenström's macroglobulinemia. In Fahey's original article

[32], peripheral neuropathy is listed as a manifestation of hyperviscosity. Since this manifestation seldom improves with plasmapheresis, it is more likely that it, along with pyramidal tract symptoms and hearing loss, are more a part of the disease per se than related to viscosity [59], and in some cases may relate to direct myelin damage from the paraprotein [96].

A feature common to all patients with hyperviscosity, not always apparent clinically, is an *increase in plasma volume*. A relatively linear relationship exists between viscosity and plasma volume expansion. Though this seems to plateau somewhat at higher viscosities, most patients with the hyperviscosity syndrome can be expected to have an increase in plasma volume of at least 50–80% [61]. Given the setting of increased viscosity and expanded plasma volume in a generally elderly population of patients, the most striking aspect of the cardiac manifestations of hyperviscosity is that they are not more common. Congestive heart failure and angina are both described, but are far less common than the neurologic manifestations. With respect to angina, Wells has suggested that the cardiac circulation may be more independent of viscosity than the rest of the microcirculation because of the extravascular compression that occurs during systole [62].

Acute changes in viscosity induced in dogs by dextran injection leads to intravascular aggregation of red cells, decreased cardiac output, and increased vascular resistance [63]. However, the dilutional anemia that accompanies the expanded plasma volume in the clinical setting of the hyperviscosity syndrome may attenuate these effects. The relationship between proteins and red cells should always be remembered in the clinical arena when considering blood transfusions for patients with dysproteinemia and potential hyperviscosity. Sudden increases in blood viscosity may lead to dangerous cardiovascular or neurological complications [61]. Peripheral vascular symptoms are usually only seen if the protein is cryoprecipitable. Raynaud's syndrome, ulceration, and gangrene of the fingertips have been described in such situations. Another surprising feature of the cardiovascular symptoms is the relative infrequency of venous thrombosis. Although no explanation exists for this, the commonly present hemostatic defect may be somewhat protective.

Renal function abnormalities may occur in hyperviscosity syndrome, and include acute renal failure, usually secondary to a cryoglobulin. In most cases of hyperviscosity, creatinine clearance ranges from increased to mildly or moderately decreased [22]. Though other renal function abnormalities such as renal tubular acidosis, proteinuria, concentrating defects, and tubular defects have been reported, it is often difficult to separate these manifestations from those directly related to dysproteinemia in the absence of hyperviscosity [65].

The general symptoms of malaise, weakness, and lassitude cannot be attributed to any one system but are quite commonly part of the hyperviscosity syndrome. Multiple other manifestations have been described including pulmonary infarction, abdominal pain, mesenteric vascular occlusion and priapism [64].

Hyperviscosity can lead to several artifacts of laboratory data. Technical difficulties include drawing blood and preparing blood films. In addition, the blood may clot poorly with insufficient serum available for routine automated chemistries. Furthermore, the increased viscosity may result in aspiration of a smaller than expected volume of serum by many autoanalyzers. This will result in spuriously low sodium and potassium concentrations and a low or negative anion gap. A cationic protein can also decrease the anion gap [66].[2] The effects of the protein on osmolality can also result in hyponatremia. Chronic anemia is common in the diseases that result in hyperviscosity. Because of an expanded plasma volume, a component of dilutional anemia is also present. In addition, electronic counting of aggregated red cells can result in a spuriously elevated mean corpuscular volume [67]. A recent report demonstrated an elevated thyroid panel secondary to hyperviscosity syndrome and binding of thyroxine by the protein [68]. This represents one of an ever-enlarging number of unique properties that these proteins may possess. Therefore, one must be cautious in the interpretation of laboratory data in patients with hyperviscosity.

Diagnosis

The laboratory diagnosis of hyperviscosity syndrome is easily made once the clinical diagnosis has been entertained. In patients with known dysproteinemia one must maintain a level of suspicion of hyperviscosity in view of the many complications that arise in the course of these diseases. Alternatively, the existence of underlying dysproteinemia may not be known. Therefore, in evaluation of epistaxis, postoperative bleeding, or altered mental status, particularly in the elderly, one must keep hyperviscosity in the differential and pay careful attention to the examination of the retina.

When the laboratory diagnosis is made, but the underlying disease is not clear, the clinical examination plus review of the blood film, bone marrow, serum protein electropheresis, and immunoelectrophoresis will usually lead to a diagnosis. To further characterize the protein involved, determination of cryoglobulins, rheumatoid factor, and viscosities performed with serum and whole blood at varying temperatures are helpful. Measuring viscosities at lower shear rates also may lead to insight into the degree of aggregation of proteins and cellular elements.

Table IV reviews the *differential diagnosis* to be considered in the patient presenting with the hyperviscosity syndrome. The past clinical impression that hyperviscosity syndrome was synonymous with Waldenström's disease

[2]Ed. note: See also Chapter 3.

TABLE IV. Differential Diagnosis of Serum Hyperviscosity Syndrome

Monoclonal immunoglobulin disorders
  Waldenström's macroglobulinemia
  Multiple myeloma
Polyclonal immunoglobulin disorders
  Rhematoid arthritis
  Sjögren's syndrome
  Systemic lupus erythematosus
  Other connective tissue diseases
  Chronic active hepatitis
  Angioimmunoblastic lymphadenopathy
  Other lymphoproliferative disorders

has been a disservice to both disorders. The incidence of hyperviscosity syndrome in Waldenström's macroglobulinemia has been reported variously between 30% and 70% [45]. However, in one series the incidence of hyperviscosity syndrome in macroglobulinemia was only 11% [69]. In myeloma the incidence of hyperviscosity syndrome has been reported between 4% and 8%. This has been predominantly in IgG myeloma patients, and it is unclear what the true incidence is among IgA patients. Because the incidence of myeloma is ten-fold greater than the incidence of Waldenström's macroglobulinemia [70], myeloma is probably the most common etiology of hyperviscosity syndrome. With the inability to predict which myeloma patients will become hyperviscous at a given level of Ig, serum viscosities should be a routine part of the initial evaluation of patients with myeloma. If symptoms suggesting hyperviscosity develop during the course of the illness, the serum viscosity should be repeated despite the level of the monoclonal protein. In IgA patients, the degree of polymer formation, and therefore viscosity, can increase significantly at a time when little change may be noted in the M-protein [52].

The polyclonal hyperviscosity syndrome is now well described in connective tissue diseases [97], but its prevalence is not known. In one series, elevated serum viscosity was present in over 90% of rheumatoid arthritis and systemic lupus erythematosus patients, excluding those with severe hypoalbuminemia, but the degree of elevation was not in the range seen in hyperviscosity states [71]. Case reports would suggest that the hyperviscosity syndrome in the presence of polyclonal immunoglobulin disorders is most common in rheumatoid arthritis [47,72,73]. Hyperviscosity in polyarthritis [74], hepatitis [75], Sjögren's syndrome [76,77], and lymphoproliferative diseases [47] has also been reported. These patients have in common diffuse hypergammaglobulinemia of greater than 5 g/dL, a relative viscosity generally greater than 5, and a variably positive rheumatoid factor. Common to all these situations has been the presence of intermediate complexes in the serum. Initially described by Kunkel [78], these are immune complexes intermediate between the sedimentation rates of IgG and IgM. Varieties of intermediate complexes include polymerizing IgG-IgM complexes, polymerizing IgG-IgG complexes, and self-aggregating IgG [47]. In one well-described case of IgG-IgG interaction, a stable dimer formation was created by antigen-antibody binding between Fc and Fab regions of the two IgG molecules. The dimers could then aggregate by the same manner into larger polymers [73]. As in monoclonal hyperviscosity states, these intermediate complexes may be cryoprecipitable. Thus, polyclonal hyperviscosity syndrome may overlap clinically with mixed cryoglobulinemia [79,80].

It is likely that the hyperviscosity syndrome as a result of intermediate complexes can occur in any situation of chronic inflammatory disease resulting in a severe hyperglobulinemic response. The clinical manifestations appear similar to those of patients with Waldenström's macroglobulinemia and myeloma and the response to therapy with plasmapheresis has been equally successful.

Treatment

Plasmapheresis is the mainstay for the successful symptomatic treatment of hyperviscosity. It can be employed both acutely and for chronic maintenance therapy. It should be remembered, however, that optimal control of this syndrome is only attained when the protein production is halted by more specific therapy. Thus, for patients with multiple myeloma and macroglobulinemia, successful control of cellular proliferation with cytotoxic therapy will result in lowering of serum protein levels and viscosity and abrogate the need for symptomatic treatment. Failure to achieve such control or relapse from it would again necessitate symptomatic therapy. Symptomatic and specific therapy should be considered as complementary approaches in the management of such patients.

The procedure of plasmapheresis involves removal of whole blood from a patient, separation of the plasma by centrifugation or sedimentation, and reinfusion of the packed erythrocytes and buffy coat. The manual procedure was first introduced into clinical medicine in the 1950s [81]. It is best performed using the two-bag transfer pack as described by Fahey [82]. Phlebotomy is performed and after the cells are centrifuged or sedimented, the plasma is expressed into the transfer bag and the red cells and buffy layer are then reinfused. With this method 1–4 units of plasma are usually removed on the first day followed by 1–2 U/day. This method can successfully remove 3,000–5,000 M of plasma within a few days to a week. The response of bleeding complications, neurologic symptoms, and retinopathy has already been noted. The major disadvantage is the large amount of nursing and physician time required to perform manual plasmapheresis.

In the last 10 years, experience has grown in the use of a cell separator to perform plasmapheresis. Two models are widely used and have been reviewed [83]. Basically both systems use venous access and return. Blood, anticoagulated with heparin or citrate, is separated directly within the circuit in a centrifuge bowl. The plasma is removed and the cells are then reinfused. One model is a continuous flow system which can remove as much as 1 liter of plasma in an hour. The second model is an intermittant flow system in which the machine's bowl is filled and emptied in a cyclic fashion. While less rapid, this model has the advantage of portability and simplicity. Newer cell separators are being developed to combine advantages of both systems.

Technical difficulties include clogging of the protein within the plasmapheresis equipment. In addition, side effects of the procedure include rigors, paresthesias, nausea and vomiting, and, less commonly, chest pain, dyspnea, abdominal pain, and shock in the hemodynamically unstable patient. Laboratory changes as a result of plasmapheresis may include a rise in hematocrit (secondary to decrease in plasma volume) and often a rise in white count, but platelets decrease.

It was initially suggested that IgG and IgA myeloma patients might not respond successfully to plasmapheresis because the distribution of these proteins normally is largely extravascular, whereas IgM has a largely intravascular distribution. However, plasmapheresis of greater than 80 patients with monoclonal proteins has resulted in successful reversal of hyperviscosity regardless of the Ig class [84,85]. This may relate to a difference between the distribution of monoclonal and normal immunoglobulins. In one study of seven IgG and IgA myeloma patients, 54–80% of the protein was intravascular [86]. These differences in distribution may relate to the tendency toward aggregation or polymerization of the monoclonal protein resulting in hyperviscosity. A similar explanation may apply to the intermediate complexes of the polyclonal hyperviscosity states.

A method has been described for the selective removal of IgG from a patient with myeloma and hyperviscosity [86]. By attaching a filter containing heat-killed *Staphylococcus aureus* to the plasmapheresis unit, monoclonal IgG was immunoadsorbed and the remaining plasma reinfused into the patient. Such selective immunoglobulin removal allows an alternate approach in some hemodynamically unstable patients.

As previously mentioned, red cell transfusion can be hazardous to the patient with hyperviscosity. Reduction in plasma volume by plasmapheresis can alleviate this problem by removing the dilutional component of the anemia and lowering the viscosity, making cautious transfusions possible. A second difficult situation is congestive heart failure in the setting of hyperviscosity.

Conventional therapy with diuretics can lead to dangerous increases in viscosity. Plasmapheresis has been the most successful approach to this situation.

When one carefully considers basic disease pathophysiology, the hyperviscosity syndrome is composed of a group of disorders that can be properly understood, diagnosed, and treated. It also provides a fascinating situation in which to advance our understanding of the forces interacting in determining blood flow, the relationship between the abnormalities of the serum proteins and clinical symptoms, and the unique and interesting properties of the various Ig molecules.

CASE REPORT (See Fig. 5) [87]

A 45-year-old man was well until March 1971, when he noted the onset of gingival bleeding. This continued until 2 months later when he was admitted to the Durham Veterans Administration Hospital complaining of decreased vision and syncopal episodes. He appeared acutely ill and somewhat pale but not jaundiced. His blood pressure was 130/80 mm Hg. Fundoscopic examination showed hemorrhages, exudates, and dilated retinal veins. His gums were swollen and oozing blood. There was no increase in bone tenderness and no enlargement of the superficial lymph nodes, liver, or spleen. Stool

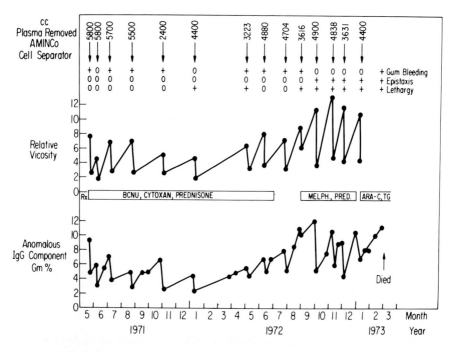

Fig. 5. Multiple myeloma (IgG$_1$-κ-protein) hyperviscosity syndrome, previously reported by Cohen [87].

guiac test was positive. Hematocrit was 17% and white blood cell count was 11,700/mm³. Clot retraction was prolonged, serum was very difficult to obtain for hematologic and other studies. Serum protein concentration was 18 g/dL. On electrophoresis, a large spike was present in the γ-region in a concentration of 10 g/dL. The anomalous serum component was an IgG_1-κ type. Bence Jones protein was not present in the urine. Bone marrow aspirated from the sternum showed a heavy infiltration with plemorphic plasma cells. X-ray films of the skeleton showed no lytic lesions or osteoporosis. The serum viscosity was strikingly elevated to 7.5. Plasmapheresis was begun soon after admission, employing a blood cell separator to remove plasma and reinfuse the patient's own erythrocytes. During the initial plasmapheresis, 12 units of plasma were removed. During this time, the patient's gingival bleeding decreased, and he thought there was some improvement in vision. Fundoscopic examination showed the retinal veins to be smaller in diameter. Changes in serum viscosity and protein concentration following plasmapheresis are shown in Figure 5. Chemotherapy was instituted with the administration of carmustine, 140 mg, and cyclophosphamide 750 mg, IV, every 4 weeks and prednisone 80 mg/day for 7 days each month.

Chemotherapy was maintained subsequently, but the anomalous protein continued to reaccumulate and to require frequent plasmapheresis. The patient's hemorrhagic and other symptoms waxed and waned in parallel with changes in the concentration of anomalous protein. Epistaxis, bleeding of the gums, and lethargy were the most troublesome symptoms. The chemotherapy regimen was later changed to one of melphalan and prednisone and, finally, to one of cytarabine and thioguanine, but the patient continued to reaccumulate the anomalous protein rapidly and died of overwhelming infection on March 1, 1973.

REFERENCES

1. Brobeck JR (ed): "Best and Taylor's Physiological Basis of Medical Practice." Baltimore: Williams and Wilkins, 1979.
2. Barbee JH, Cokelet GR: The Fåhraeus effect. Microvasc Res 3:6, 1971.
3. Dintenfass L: Inversion of the Fåhraeus-Lindqvist phenomenon in blood flow through capillaries of diminishing radius. Nature 215:1099, 1967.
4. Jay AWL, Rowlands S, Skibo L: The resistance to blood flow in the capillaries. Can J Phys Pharmacol 50:1007, 1972.
5. Papenfus HD, Gross JF: The interaction between transmural fluid exchange and blood viscosity in narrow blood vessels. Biorheology 14:217, 1977.
6. Wells R: Syndromes of hyperviscosity. N Engl J Med 283:183, 1970.
7. Stone HO, Thompson HK, Schmidt-Nielsen K: Influence of erythrocytes on blood viscosity. Am J Physiol 214:913, 1968.
8. Mentzer WC: Polycythemia and the hyperviscosity syndrome in newborn infants. Clin Haematol 7:63, 1978.
9. Humphrey PRD, Marshall J, Russell RWR, Wetherley-Mein G, Bonlay GH, Pearson TC, Symon L, Zilkha E: Cerebral blood flow and viscosity in relative polycythemia. Lancet 2:873, 1979.
10. Friedland RP, Grant S: Hematocrit, viscosity, and blood flow. Am Heart J 97:404, 1979.
11. Meiselman HJ: Rheology of shape-transformed human red cells. Biorheology 15:225, 1978.
12. Clark MR, Mohandas N, Shohet SB: Deformability of oxygenated irreversibly sickled cells. J Clin Invest 65:189, 1980.
13. McKee, LC: Intravascular leukocyte thrombi and aggregates as a cause of morbidity and

mortality in leukemia. Medicine 53:463, 1974.

14. Preston FE, Sokol RJ, Lilleyman JS, Winfield DA, Blackburn EK: Cellular hyperviscosity as a cause of neurological symptoms in leukemia. Br Med J 1:476, 1978.

15. Dintenfass L: Clinical applications of blood viscosity factors and functions: Especially in the cardiovascular disorders. Biorheology 16:69–84, 1979.

16. Wu, KK-Y: Platelet hyperaggregability and thrombosis in patients with thrombocythemia. Ann Intern Med 88:7, 1978.

17. Leonhardt H, Arntz H-R, Klemens UH: Studies of plasma viscosity in primary hyperlipoproteinemia. Atherosclerosis 28:29, 1977.

18. Arntz HR, Leonhardt H, Dreykluff HR: Influence of clofibrate on blood viscosity in primary hyperlipoproteinemia. Klin Wochenschr 57:43, 1979.

19. Betteridge DJ, Bakowski M, Taylor KG, Reckless JPD, DeSilva SR, Galton DR: Treatment of severe diabetic hypertriglyceridaemia by plasma exchange. Lancet 1:1368, 1978.

20. Hutchinson RM, Eastham RD: A comparison of the erythrocyte sedimentation rate and plasma viscosity in detecting changes in plasma proteins. J Clin Pathol 30:345, 1977.

21. Bradlow BA, Haggan JM: A comparison of the plasma viscosity and erythrocyte sedimentation rate as screening tests. South Afr Med J 55:415, 1979.

22. Somer T: Hyperviscosity syndrome in plasma cell dyscrasia. Adv Microcirc 6:155, 1975.

23. Dupont PA, Sirs JA: The relationship of plasma fibrinogen, erythrocyte flexibility, and blood viscosity. Thromb Haemost 38:660, 1977.

24. Richardson SGN, Matthews KB, Cruickshank JK, Geddis AM, Stuart J: Coagulation activation and hyperviscosity in infection. Br J Haematol 42:469, 1979.

25. Gralnick HR: Congenital disorders of fibrinogen. In Williams WJ, Beutler E, Erslev AJ, Rundles RW (eds): "Hematology." New York: McGraw-Hill, 1977, p 1423.

26. McKee PA, Kalbfleish JM, Bird RM: Incidence and significance of cryofibrinogenemia. J Lab Clin Med 61:203, 1963.

27. Ball GV, Goldman LN: Chronic ulcerative colitis, skin necrosis, and cryofibrinogenemia. Ann Intern Med 85:464, 1976.

28. Cwazka WF, Sprenger JD, Naguwa SN, Birnberg FA: Cryofibrinogenemia in Henoch-Schönlein purpura. Arch Intern Med 139:592, 1979.

29. Reimann HA: Hyperproteinemia as a cause of autohemagglutination. Observation in a case of myeloma. JAMA 99:1411, 1932.

30. Wintrobe MM, Buell MV: Hyperproteinemia associated with multiple myeloma. Bull Johns Hopkins Hosp 52:156, 1933.

31. Waldenström J: Incipient myelomatosis or "essential" hyperglobulinemia with fibrinogenopenia: A new syndrome? Acta Med Scand 117:216, 1944.

32. Fahey JL, Barth WF, Solomon A: Serum hyperviscosity syndrome. JAMA 192:464, 1965.

33. Smith E, Kochwa S, Wasserman LR: Aggregation of IgG globulin in vivo. Am J Med 39:35, 1965.

34. Pruzanski W: Hyperviscosity and immunoglobulin complexes. Ann Intern Med 80:107, 1974.

35. Capra JD, Kunkel HG: Aggregation of γG_3 proteins: Reference to the hyperviscosity syndrome. J Clin Invest 49:610, 1970.

36. Preston FE, Cooke KB, Foster MD, Winfield DA, Lee A: Myelomatosis and the hyperviscosity syndrome. Br J Haematol 38:517, 1978.

37. Chesebro B, Bloth B, Svehag S-E: The ultrastructure of normal and pathologic IgM immunoglobulins. J Exp Med 127:399, 1968.

38. Roberts-Thomson PJ, Mason DY, MacLennan ICM: Relationship between paraprotein polymerization and clinical features in IgA myeloma. Br J Haematol 33:117, 1976.

39. Mestecky J, Hammock WJ, Kulhany R, Wright GP, Tomana M: Properties of IgA my-

eloma proteins isolated from sera of patients with the hyperviscosity syndrome. J Lab Clin Med 89:919, 1977.

40. Virella G, Preto RV, Graca F: Polymerized monoclonal IgA in two patients with myelomatosis and hyperviscosity syndrome. Br J Haematol 30:479, 1979.

41. MacKenzie MR, Fudenberg HH, O'Reilly RA: The hyperviscosity syndrome I. In IgG myeloma. The role of protein concentration and molecular shape. J Clin Invest 49:15, 1970.

42. Lindsley H, Teller D, Noonan B, Peterson M, Mannik M: Hyperviscosity syndrome in multiple myeloma. Am J Med 54:682, 1973.

43. Pruzanski W, Watt JG: Serum viscosity and hyperviscosity syndrome in IgG multiple myeloma. Ann Intern Med 77:853, 1972.

44. Pruzanski W, Russell ML: Serum viscosity syndrome in IgG multiple myeloma—the relationship to Sia test and to concentration of M component. Am J Med Sci 271:145, 1976.

45. Fudenberg HH, Virella G: Multiple myeloma and Waldenström's macroglobulinemia: Unusual presentations. Semin Hematol 17:63, 1980.

46. Ogawa M, Kochwa S, Smith C, Ishizaka K, McIntyre OR: Clinical aspects of IgE myeloma. N Engl J Med 281:1217, 1969.

47. Hadler NM, Gabriel D, Chung K Su, Teague P, Napier MD: Polyclonal hyperviscosity syndrome. Arthritis Rheum 20:1388, 1977.

48. CPC—Cryoglobulinemia. Am J Med 68:757–766, 1980.

49. McGrath MA, Penny R: Blood hyperviscosity in cryoglobulinemia: temperature sensitivity and correlation with reduced skin flow. Aust J Exp Biol Med Sci 56:127, 1978.

50. Rovel A, Vigneron C, Streiff F: Comparison of in vitro effects of normal IgG and of a monoclonal IgG on the rheological behavior of erythrocytes. Br J Haematol 41:509, 1979.

51. Dintenfass L, Somer T: On the aggregation of red cells in Waldenström's macroglobulinemia and multipe myeloma. Microvasc Res 9:279, 1975.

52. Russell JA, Powles RL: The relationship between serum viscosity, hypervolaemia and clinical manifestations associated with circulating paraprotein. Br J Haematol 39:163, 1979.

53. Perkins HA, MacKenzie MR, Fudenberg HH: Hemostatic defects in dysproteinemias. Blood 35:695, 1970.

54. Lackner H: Hemostatic abnormalities associated with dysproteinemias. Semin Hematol 10:125, 1973.

55. Mausolf FA, Mensher JH: Experimental hyperviscosity retinopathy. Ann Opthalmol 5:205, 1973.

56. Luxenberg MN, Mausolf FA: Retinal circulation in the hyperviscosity syndrome. Am J Ophthalmol 70:588, 1970.

57. Wells R, Edgerton H: Blood flow in the microcirculation of the conjunctival vessels of man. Angiology 18:699, 1967.

58. Goldstone J, Schmid-Schönbein H, Wells R: The rheology of red cell agregates. Microvasc Res 2:273, 1970.

59. Solomon A: Neurological manifestations of macroglobulinemia. In Brain L, Norris F Jr (eds): "The Remote Effects of Cancer in the Nervous System." New York: Grune & Stratton, 1965, p 112.

60. Rosenblum WI: Vasoconstriction, blood viscosity, and erythrocyte aggregation in macroglobulinemia and polycythemic mice. J Lab Clin Med 73:359, 1969.

61. McGrath MA, Penny R: Paraproteinemia. Blood hyperviscosity and clinical manifestations. J Clin Invest 58:1155–1162, 1976.

62. Wells R: Microcirculation and coronary blood flow. Am J Cardiol 29:847, 1972.

63. Gelin L-E, Bergentz S-E, Helander C-G, Linder E, Nilsson NJ, Rudenstom CM: Hemodynamic consequences from increased viscosity of blood. In Copeley AL (ed): International Conference on Hemorheology. New York: Pergammon Press, 1966.
64. Rosenbaum EH, Thompson HE, Glassberg AB: Priapism and multiple myeloma. Urology 12:201, 1978.
65. DeFronzo RA, Cooke CR, Wright JR, Humphrey RL: Renal function in patients with multiple myeloma. Medicine 57:151, 1978.
66. Emmett M, Narins RG: Clinical use of the anion gap. Medicine 56:38, 1977.
67. Nelson DA: Basic methodology. In Henry JB (ed): Todd, Sanford, Davidsohn's "Clinical Diagnosis and Management by Laboratory Methods." Philadelphia: Saunders 1979, p 887.
68. Tamagna E, Hershman J, Premachandra BN: Circulating thyroid hormones in a patient with hyperviscosity syndrome. Clin Chim Acta 93:263, 1979.
69. Krajny M, Pruzanski W: Waldenström's macroglobulinemia, review of 45 cases. Can Med Assoc J 714:899, 1976.
70. Ameis A, Ko HS, Pruzanski W: M components—a review of 1242 cases. Can Med Assoc J 114:889, 1976.
71. Shearn MA, Epstein WV, Engleman EP: Serum viscosity in rheumatic diseases and macroglobulinemia. Arch Intern Med 112:684, 1963.
72. Jaslin HE, LoSpalluto J, Ziff M: Rheumatoid hyperviscosity syndrome. Am J Med 49:484, 1970.
73. Pope RM, Mannik M, Gilliland BC, Teller DC: The hyperviscosity syndrome in rheumatoid arthritis due to intermediate complexes formed by self-association of IgG-rheumatoid factors. Arthritis Rheum 18:97, 1975.
74. Abruzzo, JL, Heimer R, Guiliano V, Martinez J: The hyperviscosity syndrome, polysynovitis, polymyositis, and an unusual 13S serum IgG component. Am J Med 49:258, 1970.
75. Lee WM, Lebwohl O, Chien S: Hyperviscosity syndrome attributable to hyperglobulinemia in chronic active hepatitis. Gastroenterology 74:918, 1978.
76. Blaylock WM, Waller M, Nomansell DE: Sjögren's syndrome: hyperviscosity and intermediate complexes. Ann Intern Med 80:27, 1974.
77. Alarcon-Segovia D, Fishbein E, Abruzzo JL, Heimer R: Serum hyperviscosity in Sjögren's syndrome. Ann Intern Med 80:35, 1974.
78. Kunkel HG, Müller-Eberhard HJ, Fudenberg HH, Tomasi TB: Gammaglobulin complexes in rheumatoid arthritis and certain other conditions. J Clin Invest 40:117, 1961.
79. Meltzer M, Franklin EC: Cryoglobulinemia—a study of 29 patients. Am J Med 40:828, 1966.
80. M'Seffar A, Reynolds J, Weinstein A, Randolph Y, Broder I, Deck JHN: Connective tissue disease and hyperviscosity syndrome with cryoprotein and immune complexes. J Rheum 5:412, 1978.
81. Adams WS, Blahd WH, Bassett SH: A method of human plasmapheresis. Proc Soc Exp Biol Med 80:377, 1957.
82. Solomon A, Fahey JL: Plasmapheresis therapy in macroglobulinemia. Ann Intern Med 58:789, 1963.
83. Isbister JP: Plasma exchange: a selective form of blood letting. Med J Aust 2:167, 1979.
84. Russell JA, Toy JL, Powles RL: Plasma exchange in malignant paraproteinemias. Exp Hematol 5:105, 1977.
85. Isbister JP, Biggs JC, Penny R: Experience with large volume plasmapheresis in malignant paraproteinemias and immune disorders. Aust N Z J Med 8:154, 1978.
86. Ray PK, Besa E, Idicullar A, Rhoads JE, Bassett JG, Cooper DR: Efficient removal of abnormal immunoglobulin G from the plasma of a multiple myeloma patient. Cancer 45:2633, 1980.

87. Cohen HJ, Rundles RW: Managing the complications of plasma cell myeloma. Arch Intern Med 135:177, 1975.
88. Dintenfass L: The clinical impact of the newer research in blood rheology: An overview. Angiology 22:217, 1981.
89. Golde DW, Hocking WG, Koeffler HP, Adamson JW: Polycythemia: Mechanisms and management. Ann Intern Med 95:71, 1981.
90. Wade JPH, Pearson TC, Russell RWR, Wetherley-Mein G: Cerebral blood flow and blood viscosity in patients with polycythaemia secondary to hypoxic lung disease. Br Med J 283:689, 1981.
91. Menon D, York EL, Bornstein RA, Jones RL, Sproule BJ: Optimal hematocrit and blood viscosity in secondary polycythemia as determined from cerebral blood flow. Clin Invest Med 4:117, 1981.
92. Horne MK: Sickle cell anemia as a rheologic disorder. Am J Med 70:288, 1981.
93. Jacob HS, Craddock PR, Hammerschmidt DE, Moldow CF: Complement-induced granulocyte aggregation. N Engl J Med 302:789, 1981.
94. Seplowitz AH, Chien S, Smith FR: Effects of lipoproteins on plasma viscosity. Atherosclerosis 38:89, 1981.
95. Pavy MD, Murphy PL, Virella G: Paraprotein-induced hyperviscosity. Postgrad Med 68:109, 1980.
96. Latov N, Sherman WH, Nemni R, Galassi G, Shyong JS, Penn AS, Chess L, Olarte MR, Rowland LP, Osserman EF: Plasma-cell dyscrasia and peripheral neuropathy with a monoclonal antibody to peripheral-nerve myelin. N Engl J Med 303:618, 1980.
97. Cryer PE, Kissare JM (eds): Rheumatoid arthritis with Felty's syndrome, hyperviscosity and immunologic hyperreactivity (Clinicopathologic correlation). Am J Med 70:89, 1981.
98. Wolf RE, Levin WC, Ritzmann SE: Thermoproteins. In Ritzmann SE, Daniels JC (eds): "Serum Protein Abnormalities: Diagnostic and Clinical Aspects," 2nd printing. New York: Alan R. Liss, Inc., 1982, pp 487–512.

Pathology of Immunoglobulins: Diagnostic and
Clinical Aspects, pages 261–292
© 1982 Alan R. Liss, Inc., 150 Fifth Avenue, New York, NY 10011

10

Bence Jones Proteins

Robert A. Kyle, MD

> Saturday, November 1st, 1845
> Dear Doctor Jones: The tube contains urine of very high specific gravity. When boiled it becomes slightly opaque. On the addition of nitric acid, it effervesces, assumes a reddish hue, and becomes quite clear; but as it cools, assumes the consistence and appearance which you see. Heat reliquefies it. What is it? [5]

This cryptic message and a urine sample were sent by a leading physician of London, Dr. Thomas Watson, to Henry Bence Jones, a 31-year-old physician at St. George's Hospital who had already established a reputation as a chemical pathologist. Born in Suffolk in 1814, he attended Harrow and graduated from Trinity College, Cambridge, in 1836. Jones then studied medicine at St. George's Hospital of London, and chemistry at Giessen under Liebig. Although Henry Bence Jones gained eponymic fame for his description of the unusual properties of the urine [4,6], the credit actually belongs to Dr. William Macintyre [72]. A well-known Harley Street consultant, Dr. Macintyre had been called by Dr. Watson on October 30, 1845, to examine a patient, Thomas Alexander McBean, "a highly respectable tradesman," who complained of excruciating bone pain.

Because edema had been observed during the patient's illness, the astute Macintyre personally examined the urine, but he found no evidence of sugar. When heated, the urine was seen to "abound in animal matter . . . ." The urine became clear with addition of nitric acid, but developed a precipitate after an hour. This precipitate "underwent complete solution on the application of heat, but again consolidated on cooling" [72]. After Macintyre's visit, Watson sent the foregoing note and a sample of the urine to Jones.

Having received specimens of the patient's urine from both Watson and Macintyre on November 1, Jones corroborated the finding of a protein that was precipitated by heating, dissolved by boiling, and reprecipitated by cooling. He calculated that the patient excreted 60 g daily. Jones concluded that the protein was an oxide of albumin, specifically "hydrated deutoxide of albumen" [6]. Although the heat properties of the urinary protein he described were not his own discovery, Jones certainly deserves credit for emphasizing its place in the diagnosis of myeloma, for he said, "I need hardly remark on the importance of seeking for this oxide of albumen in other cases of mollities ossium" [5].

Henry Bence Jones was an accomplished physician and acquired a large and remunerative practice. Among his patients was the great naturalist Charles Darwin, whom Bence Jones treated with a diet that "half-starved him to death." Interestingly, although Bence Jones's obituary in 1873 described his work on renal stones, diabetes mellitus, malignant and tuberculous involvement of the kidney—and his emphasis on the value of microscopic analysis of the urine—there was no mention of his papers on the unique urinary protein that bears his name [81].

Actually, J. F. Heller in 1846 described a protein in the urine which precipitated when warmed a little above 50°C and then disappeared upon further heating. Although he did not recognize the precipitation of the protein when the urine was cooled, it is nearly certain that this was Bence Jones protein. He distinguished this new protein from albumin and casein [41].

DESCRIPTION OF BENCE JONES PROTEIN[1]

More than a century later, it was found that the urinary proteins that evoked such interest from Macintyre and Jones were the light (L) chain components of the immunoglobulin (Ig) molecule. In 1962, Edelman and Gally [29] demonstrated that the L chains prepared from a serum IgG myeloma protein and the Bence Jones protein (BJP) from the same patient's urine had the same amino acid sequence, similar spectrofluorometric behavior, the same molecular weight, identical appearance on chromatography with carboxymethylcellulose and on starch gel electrophoresis after reduction and alkylation, and the same ultracentrifugal pattern—as well as the same thermal solubility. They precipitated when heated to between 40 and 60°C, dissolved on boiling, and reprecipitated when cooled to between 40 and 60°C.

Two distinct groups of BJPs (group I and group II) were recognized by Bayne-Jones and Wilson [3] in 1922. In 1956, two major classes of BJPs were described by Korngold and Lipari [50]; and these have been designated

---

[1]Ed. note: See also Hahn GS in Ritzmann SE (ed): "Physiology of Immunoglobulins: Diagnostic and Clinical Aspects" [118]. Also, Ritzmann SE in Ritzmann SE, Daniels JC (eds): "Serum Protein Abnormalities: Diagnostic and Clinical Aspects" [119].

κ and λ. Approximately 70% of serum IgG monoclonal proteins are of the κ-type, and the remainder are λ. In patients with Waldenström's macroglobulinemia (MW), 80% are κ; in IgD myeloma 90% are λ.

BJPs (L chains) have a molecular weight of 22,500 daltons and contain 210 to 220 amino acids. Analyses of amino acid sequence in individual L chains have disclosed that the region of the chain from amino acid 107 to the carboxy terminus at position 210 to 220 is very similar in chains of the same type (κ or λ), and it has been designated the constant region (C_L)— although amino acid substitutions have been found at a dozen different positions in the constant region of human λ-chains [67]. The region from the amino (NH_2) terminus (position 1) to approximately position 107 has been different in every L chain thus far analyzed and is called the variable region (V_L). It is the variable half of the L chain that contains the unique thermal solubility characteristics of BJPs (101).

The amino acid differences in the constant portions of the L chains can be related to certain markers. In κ-chains, if the amino acid leucine is at position 191, the protein is Inv(1) or Inv(2); whereas if valine is at this position, the L chain is Inv(3). Inv(1) has valine at position 153; the others have alanine. Of Caucasians who have the Inv(1) antigen, 98% also have the Inv(2) antigen. In contrast, no genetic factors have been identified for human λ-chains. The isotypic markers in these chains include Oz(+) if lysine is at position 193, whereas if arginine is present, it is Oz(−). Another marker in λ-chains has been designated Kern(+) when glycine is present at position 156 and Kern(−) when serine is there; and another variant, Mcg, has been reported which has threonine at position 103 instead of glycine [33,99]. The human λ-chain genes are carried on chromosome 22 [30].

Amino acid sequence studies have revealed four basic subtypes of κ-L chains, designated κI, κII, κIII, and κIV [109]. The frequency of occurrence of these subclasses is approximately 60, 10, 28, and 2%, respectively; and as one would expect, this reflects the proportion of κI, κII, κIII, and κIV L chains in Igs of normal serum [100]. The λ-L chains have not been so well delineated, but six subtypes of λ-chains have been reported [31,38].

Ordinarily, κ-chains are in the monomeric form (22,500 daltons); but they may exist as noncovalently linked dimers or as a mixture of monomers and dimers, whereas λ-chains occur as dimers (45,000 daltons), linked covalently by their penultimate cysteinyl residues [99]. In addition, κ-L chains precipitate maximally over a narrower range of pH than λ-L chains [90]. Recognition of L chains as κ or λ by monospecific antisera depends on the variable and constant domains as well as the interdomain "switch" region between the variable and constant regions [100].

Three regions of "hypervariability" have been identified in V_L: positions 24 to 34, 50 to 56, and 89 to 97 [115]. This hypervariability and the existence of similar hypervariable regions in the variable portion of the H chain (V_H) in positions 30 to 37, 51 to 68, 84 to 91, and 101 to 110 [14] permit the formation of many different antigen-combining sites.

BJPs may exhibit cryoproperties, i.e., form a precipitate at 4°C but redissolve at 37°C. The cryoprecipitation is done by BJ dimers but not by monomers [77]. Conformational changes in BJP occur as the temperature is lowered. Stabilization of the dimer by formation of an interchain disulfide bond between two monomers prevents both the conformational change and cryoprecipitation [48]. The cause of cryoprecipitation is probably complex and not the result of identical amino acid sequences in the hypervariable regions [78]. In one case, cryoprecipitation depended upon the variable portion of the BJP [117].

METABOLISM OF BENCE JONES PROTEINS

BJPs are synthesized de novo *in plasma cells and are not degradation products of the complete immunoglobulin in the serum.* Putnam and Hardy [91] showed that ^{13}C-labeled glycine is incorporated promptly into BJP and cannot be the result of breakdown of serum or other tissue protein.

L chains clearly are catabolized by the kidney. After injection into mice, ^{131}I-labeled BJPs of humans were cleared rapidly from the circulation. Ligating and severing the ureters lengthened the disappearance time only slightly, but removal of the kidneys greatly prolonged the survival of L chains. Human IgG was not cleared by the kidney in the same experiments [113].

BJ proteinemia may occur in the absence of BJ proteinuria. This paradox is due to the formation of tetramers (88,000 daltons) of BJP in the serum. Bence Jones proteinuria is absent [52]. Tetramers of κ have been reported in the serum, and monomers of κ-L chains have been found in the urine [36].

ROLE OF BENCE JONES PROTEIN IN RENAL INSUFFICIENCY

The role of BJP in renal insufficiency is not clear. When injected intraperitoneally in mice, these proteins produced extensive cast formation in the distal renal tubules. The casts contained BJP but Tamm-Horsfall protein appeared after 5 days. Giant cells appeared around many casts, and atrophy, degeneration, and regeneration of the renal tubules occurred [51]. This experimental model of BJ nephropathy is very similar to "myeloma kidney" in man.

The degree of renal insufficiency correlates best with tubular atrophy and degeneration. The amount of BJ proteinuria may also be a factor. The 20 patients studied by DeFronzo and associates [27] included 11 who excreted more than 1 g of BJP daily. Eight of the 11 had creatinine clearance less than 50 mL/min, and 7 of the 8 had advanced tubular atrophy. Of the nine patients without BJ proteinuria, all had creatinine clearance greater than 50 mL/min; and light microscopy revealed no diagnostic morphologic changes in any.

My colleagues and I have seen several patients who excreted 1–10 g of BJP daily for 5–20 years without developing significant renal insufficiency. Van Geelen and Mulder [105] described a patient with multiple myeloma (MM) who excreted 18 g of monoclonal λ-L chain (BJP) daily. The patient's renal function was normal and a renal biopsy revealed minimal changes [105]. Apparently some Bence Jones proteins have a nephrotoxic effect and others do not.

The mechanism of nephrotoxicity of BJPs is unknown. Clyne et al. [17], injecting Sprague-Dawley rats with BJPs, found that renal function and morphology became abnormal if the injected protein had an isoelectric point above 5.7 and that the toxicity was greater when the isoelectric range of the BJP exceeded the urinary pH. They also found that mixing Tamm-Horsfall mucoprotein with BJP of pH 5.5 or less resulted in precipitation, and they postulated that the interaction between positively charged BJP and negatively charged Tamm-Horsfall protein lining the distal nephron may be important in the initiation of acute renal failure [16]. However, it is apparent that the nephrotoxicity of BJPs is more complex than the isoelectric point [110]. The pathophysiology of BJPs on the kidney has recently been reviewed [18].

Preuss et al. [89] reported that ammoniagenesis and gluconeogenesis by rat kidney slices were significantly less during incubation with urine proteins from patients with myeloma than during incubation with urine proteins from patients with the nephrotic syndrome. Their findings suggest that proteins in the urine of patients with myeloma have a part in disturbing tubular function.

MONOCLONAL PROTEINS
Relationship to Normal Immunoglobulins

Although monoclonal proteins have long been thought of as abnormal, studies conducted over the past several years have disclosed strong indications that they occur normally in small amounts. The striking feature of monoclonal proteins that led investigators to consider them as abnormal is their homogeneity. Whereas normal IgG in human serum is electrophoretically heterogeneous and is distributed from the α_2- to the slow γ-regions, IgG monoclonal proteins are localized sharply in their electrophoretic migration.

Kunkel [53] showed that each L chain type and H chain subclass in monoclonal proteins has its counterpart among normal Igs and also among antibodies. After the discovery of two types of L chains (κ and λ) in myeloma proteins in a ratio of approximately 2:1, these same L chains were detected in essentially the same ratio among normal immunoglobulins. Similarly, the IgG and IgA subclasses and IgD class were discovered among myeloma proteins and then found as normal serum components. These identifications have gradually weakened the belief that the monoclonal proteins of MM and MW are abnormal and suggest that they represent the overproduction of a normal product by an abnormally functioning cell. However, many of the H chains found in the H chain diseases (HCDs) show significant deletions of amino acids; thus they are abnormal Igs.

As illustrated in Figure 1, the normal collection of Ig molecules comprises minute amounts of highly homogeneous but not identical proteins from many diverse single clones of plasma cells and thus is polyclonal. If a single clone escapes the normal control over its multiplication, it reproduces excessively and synthesizes an excess of monoclonal protein with a single H chain class and subclass and a single L chain type. Sometimes only light chains are secreted, with resultant BJ proteinemia and proteinuria. *The presence of a monoclonal light chain is usually associated with a neoplastic or potentially neoplastic process.*

Patterns of Overproduction

Normally, plasma cells produce H chains and a slight excess of L chains that spill over into the urine. In IgG myeloma, about three fourths of patients have an excess of L chains that may be excreted in the urine (BJ proteinuria) or catabolized [13]. This small excess of L chain production could be due to imbalance in translation or transcription within occasional clones or a possible suppression of H chain synthesis in such clones. In other instances, no H chain is excreted by the plasma cell and only excessive quantities of L chains are detected ("light chain disease" [LCD]) [102]. Finally, in a small proportion of myeloma patients the plasma cells do not secrete either H or L chains to excess, whether because of simple failure of production [46] or blocking of secretion; this type of myeloma is called "nonsecretory" [87].

LABORATORY METHODS FOR STUDY OF IMMUNOGLOBULINS IN URINE

Analysis of Igs in urine requires sensitive, rapid, dependable screening to detect the presence of protein and a specific assay to identify the type of protein and to determine whether it is polyclonal or monoclonal [60].

Although there are many qualitative tests—use of heat with acetic acid, nitric acid (Heller's test), potassium ferrocyanide, sulfosalicylic acid, magnesium sulfate (Roberts' test), and the biuret reaction—we prefer Exton's test (sulfosalicylic acid and sodium sulfate) [32].

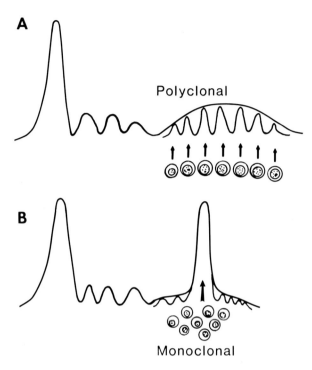

Fig. 1. Polyclonal and monoclonal electrophoretic patterns. A. Broad outline comprising small peaks of many different proteins (each represented here in normal amount, related by an arrow to its peak) that have been produced by many different plasma cell clones—polyclonal. B. Tall, narrow peak of homogeneous protein (single H chain and single L chain type), which represents excessive output of single clone—monoclonal. (From Kyle and Greipp [60].)

Exton's Test: Indicator of Presence of Urine Protein

A fresh morning urine specimen should be collected without a preservative.

REAGENT

Dissolve 200 g of sodium sulfate in 750 mL of deionized water in a volumetric flask with heating. Cool the solution and add 50 g of sulfosalicylic acid and dilute to 1 L with deionized water. This 5% sulfosalicylic acid solution is stable indefinitely and can be stored at room temperature.

PROCEDURE

1) Centrifuge 15 mL of urine for 5 minutes at 2000 rpm.
2) Put 1.5 mL of 5% sulfosalicylic acid in a 15 × 150-mm Pyrex tube.
3) Add 1.5 mL of supernatant fluid from a centrifuged urine specimen to the 1.5 mL of sulfosalicylic acid and mix well.
4) Warm to about 70°C.

Interpretation

Grade	Description	Amount of protein (est. mg/dL)
1	Faint trace	5–20
2	Definite precipitate (finger is visible behind tube)	30–50
3	"Cannot see finger behind tube"	60–90
4	"Thick with curdle"	>100

If the urine specimen is turbid after centrifugation, this may be due to the presence of phosphates or urates. If the urine is alkaline, phosphates will disappear when it is acidified with 10% acetic acid. Urates will disappear when the specimen is heated to 41°C. Turbidity from chyluria will not clear, and the degree of turbidity should be subtracted from that obtained with the addition of Exton's reagent.

Sulfosalicylic acid precipitates protein in urine and produces turbidity that is approximately proportional to the concentration of protein in the solution. Sulfosalicylic acid detects albumin and globulin as well as BJP, polypeptides, and proteases. False-positive reactions may be induced by penicillin (and its derivatives, nafcillin and oxacillin), tolbutamide metabolites, sulfisoxazole metabolites, and certain organic roentgenologic contrast media [70]. This reaction usually disappears with subsequent boiling.

Dipstick tests are used in many laboratories to screen for protein. The dipstick is impregnated with a buffered indicator dye that binds to protein in the urine and produces a color change proportional to the amount of protein bound to it. However, the dipsticks are often insensitive to BJP [43,94] and should not be used when a possibility of BJ proteinuria exists.

Normal persons excrete less than 150 mg of protein/d in the urine, the mean value being 40–80 mg/d. The protein content of normal urine is 2–8 mg/dL [93].

Identification of Bence Jones Protein: Heat Test

Almost from the time of the discovery of the unique thermal properties of urinary L chains by MacIntyre and Jones, screening tests for their detection have been in use. All have shortcomings, but the heat test of Putnam et al. [90] is the simplest and is generally satisfactory. The sulfosalicylic acid test (Exton's) [32] should be performed first; if its result is negative, the heat test will not detect BJP.

REAGENT

The reagent used for the heat test is an acetate buffer consisting of 17.5 g of sodium acetate trihydrate and 4.1 mL of glacial acetic acid. First, put the sodium acetate trihydrate in a 100 mL volumetric flask and add the glacial acetic acid; then add water to 100 mL (pH 4.9, 2 M).

PROCEDURE

1) Add 1.0 mL of 2 M acetate buffer of pH 4.9 to 4.0 mL of filtered urine and mix. The pH should be 4.9 ± 0.1.
2) Heat the mixture at 56°C in an incubation bath for 15 minutes. Precipitation suggests BJP.
3) Heat the same tube for 3 minutes at 100°C and observe while the tube is in the boiling bath. Any decrease in the amount of precipitate or clearing of the opacity is suggestive of BJ proteinuria.
4) Filter the contents of the tube taken directly from the boiling water. If the filtrate is clear and then becomes cloudy as it cools, Bence Jones protein is present.

Interpretation. Turbidity of urine or large amounts of albumin will obscure the dissolution of any BJP with heating. The urine specimen should be fresh or refrigerated, because BJP may denature if the urine is left at room temperature for prolonged periods. A large amount of BJP precipitating at 56°C may not redissolve upon boiling, so the test should be repeated with diluted urine. With the Putnam heat test, a protein concentration of 145 mg/dL is required for a positive result [68].

We have encountered false-positive results with the heat test (no localized globulin band on electrophoresis of concentrated urine and no monoclonal L chain on immunoelectrophoresis [IEP]). The most frequent cause was connective-tissue diseases, and then chronic renal insufficiency, nonmyelomatous malignancies, and fever of undetermined origin [85]. The results of urine electrophoreses performed in the cases with false-positive results were nearly evenly divided between normal and polyclonal patterns. It appears that the heat test detected an increased quantity of κ- and λ-chains—a polyclonal effect often seen in connective tissue diseases and neoplasia. Chronic renal insufficiency may cause lessening of the catabolism of L chains by the renal tubules and thus increase the amounts of κ- and λ-polyclonal chains in the urine. Therefore, the lack of a dense localized band on electrophoresis of adequately concentrated urine and a reaction to both κ- and λ-antisera on IEP indicates that the positive result of the BJ heat test is false.

On the other hand, the BJ heat test results have been negative in some cases where urinary electrophoresis has shown a dense globulin band or spike and where IEP has demonstrated a monoclonal L chain. In a study of urines with a monoclonal protein and either positive or negative response to the BJ heat test, we were unable to demonstrate the presence of a substance inhibiting the formation of dimer L chains from monomers. Both positive and negative groups had gel electrophoretic patterns with bands corresponding to the molecular weights of dimer and monomer species. Neither free sulfhydryl groups nor carbohydrates were demonstrable. Isoelectric focusing revealed similar values for both positive and false-negative BJPs. Other studies disclosed similar amino acid compositions. There was no correlation between the L chain type or subtype and the thermal properties. The most likely explanation for the false-positive heat test results is an atypical BJP with differences in amino acid sequence that change the conformation of the variable portion of the L chain [84].

Not all precipitates that form with heating of urine are BJP. In one instance when a precipitate formed after heating of the urine and the possibility of BJ proteinuria was suggested, electrophoresis showed a sharp band of α_2 mobility. This band was red-brown when stained with toluidine and subsequently was identified as hemoglobin, which is insoluble at 57°C at a pH of 5.2. Therefore, one must remember that hemoglobinuria can result in a dense band on electrophoresis and can produce a positive response to the heat test [83].

It is obvious that the heat test for BJP has many shortcomings and can be used only as a rough screening test. The presence of BJ proteinuria depends upon the demonstration of a monoclonal L chain by electrophoresis and IEP of an adequately concentrated urine specimen.

Identification and Typing of Bence Jones Protein

Electrophoresis and IEP of urine should be performed in all cases with a monoclonal protein in the serum. In addition, both tests should be applied to urine in all instances of MM, MW, amyloidosis, monoclonal gammopathy of undetermined significance, H chain diseases, or suspicion of these entities. In addition, IEP should be performed on a concentrated urine specimen from all adults older than 40 years of age with an apparently idiopathic nephrotic syndrome, because the detection of a monoclonal L chain strongly suggests the diagnosis of primary systemic amyloidosis.

First, a 24-hour collection of the urine must be made for determination of the total amount of protein excreted per day. This is most important when following the course of a patient with a monoclonal L chain in the urine, because the amount of protein correlates directly with the amount of tumor burden.

MEASUREMENT OF TOTAL PROTEIN

The biuret solution is prepared by adding 900 mL of 23% NaOH to 300 mL of $CuSO_4$ · 5 H_2O. Add tungstic acid (prepared by adding 100 mL of 10% Na_2WO_4 · 2 H_2O to 800 mL of 0.083 N H_2SO_4), and then add 0.1 mL of H_3PO_4. Add 1 mL of filtered and centrifuged urine to 5 mL of tungstic acid and allow to sit for 5 minutes; then centrifuge. Dissolve the precipitate in 5 mL of saline and 5 mL of biuret solution. After 10 minutes, read at 545 nm in a Beckman Model 34 spectrophotometer. The concentration mode of the instrument is set to match a standard of known protein concentration.

Electrophoresis. In 1937, Tiselius [103] used electrophoretic techniques to separate serum globulins into three components that he designated α, β, and γ. Electrophoresis was applied to the study of MM by Longsworth et al. [71], who demonstrated the tall, narrow-based "church-spire" peak. The method was cumbersome and difficult, so electrophoresis was not readily available until the early 1950s, when filter paper was introduced as a supporting medium (zone electrophoresis). Cellulose acetate now has largely supplanted filter paper in this use [49].[2] The advantages of cellulose acetate membrane for electrophoresis include decreased absorption of urine on the supporting medium, less tailing, and sharper separation of protein bands. This technique also allows for a smaller amount of urine to be applied and is much faster.

The basic principle of electrophoresis is that charged particles in solution migrate according to their charge—for example, albumin migrates toward the anode (positive pole). Since electrophoresis is performed at pH 8.8, where most proteins have a negative charge, the vast majority of Igs migrate toward the anode. The size of the molecule and the viscosity of the electrophoresis medium have little or no influence when the supporting medium is a cellulose acetate membrane.

Many instruments are available for electrophoresis of urinary protein. We use a Zip Zone electrophoresis chamber (Helena Laboratories, Beaumont, TX), Super Z applicator, Drummond microdispenser, Titan III cellulose polyacetate electrophoresis strips, Ponceau S protein stain, tris (hydroxymethyl) aminomethane-barbital-sodium-barbital buffer (pH 8.8), and a Cliniscan densitometer (Helena Laboratories).

ELECTROPHORESIS OF URINE

For electrophoresis of urine, it is usually necessary first to concentrate a sample of the 24-hour urine specimen. The ideal concentration of protein for electrophoresis is 3 g/dL. Urine may be concentrated by dialysis against polyvinylpyrrolidine or dextran or by vacuum. We prefer ultrafiltration with a Minicon-B15 concentrator (Amicon Corp., Lexington, MA). First, 5 mL of urine are added to the concentrator; when the volume has decreased, 3 mL more of urine are added. The volume of urine is reduced to 0.1 mL ($\times$ 80) or to 0.04 mL ($\times$ 200). All substances with a molecular weight greater than 15,000 are retained.

Details for the performance of electrophoresis of urine have been published [56]. Ordinarily, controls are not needed for the performance of electrophoresis; if the laboratory does need them, it is advisable to run a specimen known to contain a large amount of monoclonal protein and one known to have a normal pattern. Quality control should be maintained by utilizing sera or urine in which amounts of component proteins are agreed upon by several laboratories. Instrument standardization is also important, and linearity of

---

[2]Ed. note: See also Kohn J, Riches PG, in Ritzmann SE (ed): "Physiology of Immunoglobulins: Diagnostic and Clinical Aspects" [118]. Also, Ritzmann SE, Daniels JC, in Ritzmann SE, Daniels JC (eds): "Serum Protein Abnormalities: Diagnostic and Clinical Aspects" [121].

response may be checked by use of densitometric standards, such as a step wedge.

In normal persons albumin constitutes about a third of urinary protein, and α_1- and α_2-globulins constitute almost half. The remainder are β- and γ-components [10]. These proteins consist of α_2- and β_2-microglobulins as well as both κ- and λ-L chains [65]. In a study of normal individuals, 15% of the γ-globulins had the characteristics of an Fc fragment. More than half of the γ-globulins were κ- and λ-L chains [106]. The mean normal urinary excretion of IgG is 2.9 mg and for IgA is 2.0 mg/24 h [42]. In most normal individuals the cellulose acetate tracing shows no bands or only a small albumin band (Fig. 2).

Urinary monoclonal protein appears as a dense, localized band on the cellulose acetate strip or a tall, narrow, homogeneous peak on the densitometer tracing (Fig. 3). In general, a monoclonal protein in urine produces a wider band than a monoclonal protein in serum, so IEP must be done. Occasionally two discrete globulin bands may be seen in the cellulose acetate tracing of the urine. These bands may represent a monoclonal L chain plus a monoclonal Ig fragment from the serum, or they may represent monomers and dimers of the monoclonal L chain (Fig. 4). Rarely, two monoclonal L chains (κ and λ) have been reported in the urine [24].

A polyclonal increase of L chains is seen as a very broad band extending through most of the γ-area; it has fuzzy, indistinct advancing and trailing borders. The densitometer tracing is broad-based and IEP shows both κ- and λ-arcs (Fig. 5). In the nephrotic syndrome, one sees a reduction of the albumin level and prominent α_2- or β-bands but minimal amounts of α_1- and γ-globulins in the serum electrophoretic pattern and mainly albumin in the urine (Figs. 6,7).

The electrophoretic pattern signifying tubular abnormality is characterized by a small amount of albumin (10 to 20% of total protein), with the remainder being globulin fractions. Significant amounts of L chains are always present. The pattern representing glomerular abnormalities is characterized by a large amount of albumin (more than 50% of the total) and modest amounts of globulin [74].

Immunoelectrophoresis. IEP *establishes the presence or absence of L chains and determines whether they are monoclonal or polyclonal.* It should be performed on concentrated urine in all cases with a sharp peak or band in the globulin region of the cellulose acetate tracing, in all cases with a monoclonal protein in the serum, and in all cases where MM, MW, amyloidosis, or a related disorder is known or suspected.

The concentrated urine specimen is placed in a well on a microscope slide covered with 1% agar or agarose and is subjected to electrophoresis to separate the various components. A trough is cut into the agar, parallel to the line of migration of the components, and

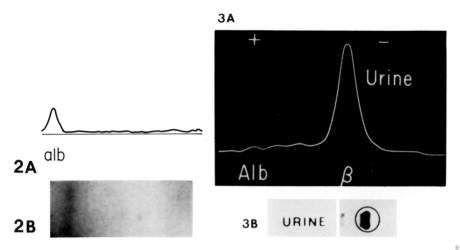

Fig. 2. Normal urine. A. Densitometer tracing (alb = albumin). B. Cellulose acetate electrophoretic pattern (anode toward left): only a small amount of albumin is seen. (From Kyle RA: Analysis of immunoglobulins in urine. In Durarte CG (ed): "Renal Function Tests: Clinical Laboratory Procedures and Diagnosis." Boston: Little, Brown & Co., 1980, pp 291–326.)

Fig. 3. Urine of patient with monoclonal protein (Alb = albumin). A. Densitometer tracing. Tall, narrow-based monoclonal peak of β-mobility. B. Cellulose acetate electrophoretic pattern. Dense band of β-mobility represents monoclonal L chain. (From Kyle and Greipp [60].)

the trough is filled with a specific antiserum. Proteins from the sample that has undergone electrophoresis (antigen) and from the antiserum (antibody) are allowed to diffuse toward each other and to form precipitin lines or arcs along the line of contact between antigen and antibody [56]. It is essential to use monospecific antisera to determine whether the L chains consist of either κ or λ or both (polyclonal). It would be best to use antisera that recognize only free κ- or λ-Igs rather than L chain antisera that recognize L chains in an intact Ig, but such antisera are not readily available. We recently evaluated a κ-antiserum that was considered to be specific for free κ-chains. It recognized 9 of 10 urines with free κ-chains, but also gave a positive reaction to 5 of 17 urines containing only λ-chains; in addition, it reacted with 5 sera containing an intact monoclonal Ig. Thus the κ-antisera recognized almost all free monoclonal κ-chains but also reacted to several serum and urine specimens without monoclonal free κ-proteins, so it was less specific than one would wish. A λ-antiserum from the same source gave no reaction to any of the 9 κ-urines but recognized only 5 of 15 urines containing free λ-chains. None of the sera containing complete Igs reacted with the λ-antiserum. Thus the λ-antiserum exhibited excellent specificity but was not potent enough for general use. Consequently, we use κ- and λ-antisera that recognize both free and combined L chains but are monospecific and potent.

A monoclonal protein forms an arc that is bowed locally or restricted, whereas a polyclonal increase of L chain causes elongation and fuzziness of

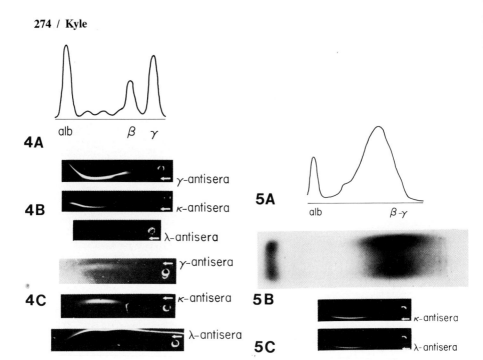

4A

alb   β γ

4B

← γ-antisera

← κ-antisera

λ-antisera

5A

alb   β-γ

4C

← γ-antisera

← κ-antisera

← λ-antisera

5B

5C

← κ-antisera

← λ-antisera

Fig. 4. A. Densitometer tracing of urine showing albumin (alb), β-peak, and γ-peak. The two peaks at right may represent a monoclonal immunoglobulin plus free L chain, or monomers and dimers of a monoclonal L chain. B. Immunoelectrophoresis of concentrated urine has produced dense IgG arc (top); double bowing of κ-arc corresponding to monoclonal IgG protein and another arc representing free monoclonal κ-chains (middle); and small amount of polyclonal λ (bottom). This pattern is indicative of IgG κ-monoclonal protein plus free monoclonal κ in urine. C. Immunoelectrophoresis of urine, with antisera to IgG (top), showing no localized arc; with anitsera to κ (middle), showing normal-appearing κ-arc; and with antisera to λ (bottom), showing a dense, doubly bowed λ-arc overwhelming the antisera. This pattern is consistent with monomers and dimers of a monoclonal λ-L chain. (From Kyle and Greipp [60].)

Fig. 5. Urine with polyclonal excess of light chains. A. Densitometer tracing (alb = albumin). Note broad-based β-γ-peak. B. Electrophoretic pattern on cellulose acetate. Note small albumin band and broad β-γ-band with advancing and trailing edges diffuse and fading into background. C. Result of immunoelectrophoresis with κ- and λ-antisera, showing both κ- and λ-arcs, which appear to be normal and represent polyclonal excess of L chains. (From Kyle and Greipp [60].)

the arc. Most importantly, a monoclonal L chain in the urine produces a characteristic heavy, bowed, or restricted arc of a monoclonal protein, whereas the other L chain type produces a faint, fuzzy, elongated arc. Because of the arc configurations, therefore, we have had little difficulty in distinguishing monoclonal from polyclonal L chains in the urine.

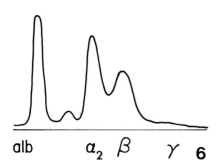

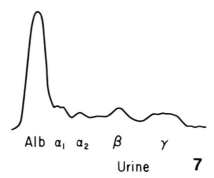

Fig. 6. Nephrotic syndrome. Serum electrophoretic pattern showing decreased albumin (alb) (0.95 g/dL) and γ-globulin with increased α_2- and β-globulin. (From Kyle and Greipp [60].)

Fig. 7. Nephrotic syndrome. Urine electrophoretic pattern; most of protein is albumin (Alb). (From Kyle RA, Bieger RC, Gleich GJ: Diagnosis of syndromes associated with hyperglobulinemia. Med Clin North Am 54:917, 1970. With permission.)

PRACTICAL DIFFICULTIES

Various difficulties are encountered in IEP. The agar must be free from bubbles and impurities, because they produce distortions in the precipitin arcs. Since unequal depth of agar can cause aberrations of the arcs, the agar must be of uniform depth throughout the plate. Drying or freezing of the agar plates will prevent satisfactory electrophoresis and diffusion of the samples in the agar. In removing the agar from the wells and cutting the troughs, great care must be taken to avoid any irregularity or splitting of the agar because this may allow artifactual bowing or asymmetry of the arcs, suggesting a monoclonal protein. One must avoid pulling the agar away from the microscope slide, since this would allow antiserum to run under the agar. During electrophoresis, the wicks must maintain good contact between the slide holder and the microscope slides and the buffer, or electrophoresis of the protein will be irregular. Inadvertent dropping of antiserum on the agar slide will produce artifactual distortion of the arcs and make interpretation very difficult.

Interpretation. Potent monospecific antisera to κ- and λ-chains are essential. It is most important for each laboratory to test its antisera. For example, to ascertain the specificity and strength of κ-antiserum, it should be run against known IgA-κ, IgA-λ, IgM-κ, IgM-λ, IgG-κ, and IgG-λ sera as well as several urines containing only κ- or λ-monoclonal L chains. It is always useful to have antisera of various sources available when typing monoclonal proteins, because the antigenic determinants of some monoclonal proteins are so restricted that they will not be recognized by all antisera.

A monoclonal protein forms an arc (with κ- or λ-antisera) that is bowed or restricted locally, whereas a polyclonal increase of L chain causes elongation and fuzziness of both κ- and λ-arcs. In cases of renal insufficiency, one often sees faint, fuzzy, or normal-appearing κ- and λ-arcs; but in the event of an underlying MM or amyloidosis, one may see an additional bowed or restricted arc with either κ- or λ-antisera. Because of the arc configurations, we have had little difficulty in distinguishing monoclonal from polyclonal L chains in the urine.

Occasionally, a thickened monoclonal arc appears as if cut off abruptly near the trough. This "break off" phenomenon may result from overwhelming of the antiserum by the antigen or from formation of a soluble antigen-antibody complex (antigen excess). Consequently, immunoelectrophoresis should then be repeated with unconcentrated urine. Sometimes the monoclonal L chain content of the urine is so high that the unconcentrated urine must be diluted to make an arc visible. Occasionally the concentrated urine needs to be diluted for detection of a localized arc. Lesser concentrations of antigen will produce an arc near the well. Most precipitin arcs form within 24 hours. If the diffusion is allowed to continue longer than 24 hours, the arcs become diffuse and exaggerated, making interpretation very difficult.

If electrophoresis of the urine reveals a localized globulin spike but IEP does not demonstrate a monoclonal L chain, one must suspect the presence of γ-H chain disease. Then concentrated urine should be tested by IEP with antisera to IgG (γ-H chains) (Fig. 8).

IEP should be performed on the urine of a patient with suspected monoclonal gammopathy, even if the sulfosalicylic acid test is negative for protein. We have seen a number of cases in which the urine osmolality was normal or elevated and the reaction for protein negative, yet electrophoresis of concentrated urine revealed a small, localized globulin band and IEP demonstrated a monoclonal L chain. As stated previously, these findings may be the first clue to amyloidosis.

IEP with monospecific L chain antisera should be performed on the urine of every adult who develops a nephrotic syndrome in which the cause is not evident. We have seen a number of cases in which electrophoresis of urine showed a large amount of albumin and insignificant amounts of globulin, but the urine contained a monoclonal L chain also. Most of the patients had primary amyloidosis, though a few had MM. A monoclonal L chain in the urine is sometimes the first clue that a nephrotic syndrome is due to amyloidosis rather than idiopathic.

Immunofixation may be helpful in detecting monoclonal BJPs. Various concentrations of urine are electrophoresed on agarose gel. The protein is overlayed with monospecific L chain antisera. The presence of a localized band characterizes the presence of a monoclonal L chain. This technique is more sensitive than electrophoresis [111]. We have found that immunofixation is most helpful when a monoclonal L chain occurs in the presence of a polyclonal increase in L chains.

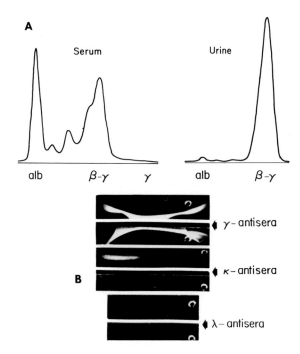

Fig. 8. γ-Heavy-chain disease. A. Densitometer tracings (alb = albumin). Serum: Note tall peak of β-γ-mobility. Urine: Note dense β-γ-band. B. Immunoelectrophoresis. Top well in each immunoelectrophoretic pattern contained serum, bottom well contained concentrated urine. With γ-antisera, a dense, thickened, asymmetric arc is seen in both serum and urine. With κ-antisera, a faint, fuzzy arc is seen in serum and no arc in urine. With λ-antisera, there is a faint, fuzzy λ-arc in serum and none in urine. This pattern represents a monoclonal γ-chain in scrum and urine (γ-heavy-chain disease). (From Kyle and Greipp [60].)

The need for collection of a 24-hour urine specimen cannot be overemphasized. First, it allows one to measure the amount of the monoclonal protein excreted in the urine, which is an excellent indication of the effect of chemotherapy or evidence of progression of the disease and is also very useful in following the course of a patient with amyloidosis and nephrotic syndrome.

Immunodiffusion. All urine specimens studied by IEP should also be examined by immunodiffusion utilizing a neat (unconcentrated) specimen as well as specimens concentrated 80- to 200-fold [56].

Interpretation. The presence of a dense precipitin band confirms the presence of protein of that class (Fig. 9). Again, the concentrated urine may overwhelm the antisera without forming a band. Conversely, a very faint band suggests the possibility of a monoclonal protein; then IEP should be

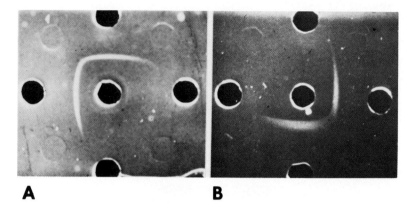

A   **B**

Fig. 9. Immunodiffusion (Ouchterlony) of urine. Sample from different patient in each of four outer wells. A. With antisera to κ in center well, κ-band appears between center well and top and left wells. B. With antisera to λ in center well, dense λ-band appears between center well and bottom and right wells.

performed with a more concentrated urine specimen to determine whether the band on Ouchterlony double immunodiffusion represents an excess of monoclonal light chain or merely polyclonal L chain.

Immunodiffusion is more sensitive than IEP and is a useful screening test, but it reacts to both monoclonal and polyclonal L chains; therefore, IEP must always be performed to prove that the protein detected is monoclonal.

Radioimmunodiffusion utilizing antisera for free κ- and free λ-L chains has been used to quantitate free serum L chain (BJ proteinemia) and the amount of monoclonal L chain in the urine [19].

Although the heat test for BJP is useful as a clinical screening test, one must remember the previously mentioned shortcomings of this test. For demonstrating a monoclonal protein in the urine, electrophoresis and IEP of an adequately concentrated specimen are the methods of choice.

DIFFERENTIAL DIAGNOSIS OF MONOCLONAL PROTEINS IN URINE (BENCE JONES PROTEINURIA)

The presence of BJ proteinuria suggests the following possibilities:

Malignant Monoclonal Gammopathies

Multiple myeloma (IgG, IgA, IgD, IgE, and free L chains)
1) Overt multiple myeloma
2) Smoldering multiple myeloma

3) Plasma cell leukemia
4) Acquired Fanconi syndrome in adults
5) L chain nephropathy (systemic L chain deposition)

Plasmacytoma

1) Solitary plasmacytoma of bone
2) Extramedullary plasmacytoma, solitary and multiple (with a plasmacytoma, BJ proteinuria is strong evidence of multiple myeloma)

Malignant lymphoproliferative diseases

1) Waldenström's macroglobulinemia (MW) (primary macroglobulinemia, IgM)
2) Malignant lymphoma

μ-Heavy chain disease

Amyloidosis

1) Primary or with myeloma (AL) (secondary, localized, and familial amyloidosis are not associated with BJ proteinuria)

Monoclonal Gammopathy of Undetermined Significance

1) *With small amounts of monoclonal light chains*
2) *Idiopathic BJ proteinuria*

Malignant Monoclonal Gammopathies

Multiple myeloma. Overt *MM* is the most common cause of a monoclonal L chain in the urine (BJ proteinuria). At the Mayo Clinic, 658 of 869 myeloma patients seen between 1960 and 1971 were tested for the presence of BJ proteinuria by the heat test [54]. Of the 658 tested, 47% were positive, 48% negative, and 5% equivocal.

Electrophoresis of the urine in 551 myeloma cases at the Mayo Clinic revealed a globulin peak in 75% and an albumin peak in 10%. No albumin or globulin peak was seen in 15%. In that series, the incidence of globulin peaks in the urine is higher than expected; but it would be lower if urine electrophoresis had been performed in all 869 cases (since globulin peaks would be less likely in the cases where electrophoresis was omitted because routine urinalysis had shown no proteinuria). Of the 551 patients, 9% excreted more than 10 g of BJP daily. We have had one patient who regularly produced more than 50 g of BJP daily. A MM patient described by Hayes et al. [40] secreted between 31 and 70 g of monoclonal κ-protein daily.

IEP of concentrated urine and immunodiffusion of neat urine were performed in 198 cases and showed a monoclonal L chain in 80%. Of those patients with a monoclonal protein in the urine, 58% had κ-L chains.

The finding of BJP in the urine of patients with MM and renal insufficiency is of interest. All of our patients with MM whose creatinine or urea was measured initially were divided into two groups on the basis of normality or insufficiency of renal function (creatinine > 1.2 mg/dL in males and > 0.9 mg/dL in females, or blood urea > 50 mg/dL in either males or females). BJ proteinuria was present (by heat test) in 58% of our 299 patients with renal insufficiency and in 43% of the 317 with normal renal function; this difference is of borderline statistical significance. Of the patients with renal insufficiency (elevated creatinine or urea), 80 had a monoclonal L chain in the urine, which was κ in 54% and λ in 46%. Of the patients with normal renal function, 79 had a monoclonal L chain in the urine—κ in 63% and λ in the remainder [59]. The presence of a single L chain class was not associated with an excessive incidence of renal insufficiency.

Among our 64 patients with κ-monoclonal protein in their urine, the mean serum creatinine concentration was lower than among the 55 with λ, but the difference was not significant [59]. The same was true of the amount of urinary globulin excretion (Table I). The serum creatinine was 2 mg/dL or more in 20% of the patients with κ-monoclonal protein in the urine and in 29% of those with λ. We found no convincing evidence that a monoclonal λ-protein was significantly more nephrotoxic than κ.

Whether the prognosis is related to the type of Ig abnormality is not clear. A report stating that patients producing only the λ-type of BJP did not respond to melphalan, whereas those producing only κ-BJP did respond [8], was later refuted [66,82]. It has been said that patients with λ-L chains have shorter survival than those with κ-L chains, and that those producing only BJP survive for the shortest period [2]; and in one reported study [1], patients with λ-BJP did not survive as long as those with κ. In another study the median survival from diagnosis was 30 months for 52 patients with κ-L chain disease and 10 months for 45 patients with λ-L chain disease [97]. It has been reported that the measured myeloma cell mass was significantly higher than predicted from clinical staging in patients with λ-BJ myeloma [28]. This could be partially responsible for the shorter survival in these patients. The controversy continues. Cornell et al. [20] reported that, among a group of patients with IgG myeloma, 43% of 44 with κ-BJ proteinuria responded to therapy, whereas only 3 (13%) of 24 with λ-BJ proteinuria had a good response. In a recent series of 173 patients with IgG, IgA, or L chain myeloma, no significant difference in survival appeared between the L chain types [79].

Since the discovery of IgD immunoglobulin in 1965 [45] more than 130 cases of IgD myeloma have been reported. Bence Jones proteinuria is present in more than 90% of cases. Monoclonal λ-L chains have been reported in 90%, contrasting with 30% in IgA and IgG myeloma.

Smoldering Multiple Myeloma. We have seen six patients who fulfilled the criteria for diagnosis of multiple myeloma (≥ 10% atypical plasma cells in the bone marrow and > 3.0 g/dL of monoclonal protein in the serum) but

TABLE I. Multiple Myeloma: Serum Creatinine and Urinary Globulin (Within One Month of Diagnosis) in Patients With Monoclonal Light Chains in Urine

	Urinary protein	
Parameters	Kappa	Lambda
Serum creatinine (mg/dL)	(N = 64)	(N = 55)
Mean	1.9	2.3
≥2.0	20%	29%
Urinary globulin (g/24 h)	(N = 60)	(N = 53)
Mean	3.8	4.2
≥2.0	45%	55%
≥4	32%	32%
≥6	20%	25%
≥10	10%	11%

From Kyle RA, Bayrd ED: "The Monoclonal Gammopathies: Multiple Myeloma and Related Plasma-Cell Disorders." Springfield, Illinois: Charles C. Thomas, Publisher, 1976. By permission.

did not exhibit anemia, hypercalcemia, renal insufficiency, or lytic bone lesions during a follow-up period of 5 years or more. Five of these patients had a small quantity of monoclonal L chains in the urine (≤ 0.5 g/24 h). We have designated these cases smoldering myeloma [61].

Plasma Cell Leukemia. Increased numbers of plasma cells in the peripheral blood characterize plasma cell leukemia (> 20% plasma cells and an absolute plasma content of at least 2000/mm^3). Plasma cell leukemia should be considered a form of MM and not a separate entity [64].

Acquired Fanconi Syndrome in Adults. Adult patients with acquired Fanconi syndrome have dysfunction of the proximal renal tubules, which produces glycosuria, aminoaciduria, phosphaturia, and acidosis. Of 17 cases in the literature, 11 involved BJ proteinuria; and typing in 7 cases showed that the BJP was of the κ-type [73]. The amount of monoclonal L chain in the urine must be determined periodically, because patients with acquired Fanconi syndrome may develop symptomatic MM or amyloidosis. One of the three patients with adult Fanconi syndrome in our initial report developed MM, and amyloidosis was found in another, after 17 years.

Since that report, we have encountered eight other patients with acquired Fanconi syndrome. Altogether, we have seen several patients with BJ proteinuria stable for more than 5 years, a patient with stable monoclonal proteinuria and proteinuria for more than 15 years, a patient with a monoclonal protein in the serum and BJ proteinuria for 15 years before the recognition of amyloidosis, a patient with monoclonal gammopathy of undetermined significance in the serum and urine who developed symptomatic MM 10 years later, and several patients who presented with pain from lytic bone lesions due to typical MM.

In a case reported by Gailani et al. [35], successful treatment of myeloma with radiation, melphalan, prednisone, and vincristine produced a marked reduction of BJ proteinuria and improvement in the Fanconi syndrome. Smithline et al. [98] described a patient with monoclonal κ-protein in his urine who had proximal renal tubular dysfunction (glycosuria, phosphaturia, uricosuria, aminoaciduria, and proximal renal tubular acidosis)—which is characteristic of the adult Fanconi syndrome—but this patient also had distal tubular dysfunction manifested by distal renal tubular acidosis and nephrogenic diabetes insipidus.

Light-Chain Nephropathy. Deposition of BJPs in multiple organs can produce serious problems. Randall et al. [92] described a patient with MM who had renal failure from widespread deposition of κ-L chains in the basement membranes and adjacent areas. This resulted in hepatic dysfunction, bilateral facial nerve paralysis, and a Guillain-Barré-like polyneuropathy. Their second patient also had widespread deposits of monoclonal κ-L chains, which produced renal insufficiency, hepatomegaly, cardiac fibrosis, hypothyroidism, gastrointestinal dysfunction, and multiple neurologic abnormalities. Neither patient had amyloidosis.

Tubbs et al. [104] described 11 patients with L chain nephropathy. All had presented with renal insufficiency. Deposits of monoclonal L chains— more often κ than λ—were found in the glomerular and tubular basement membranes. Electron microscopy showed no evidence of amyloid fibrils. Despite the tissue deposition of a monoclonal L chain in every case, only six patients had circulating free serum or urine monoclonal light chains. Surprisingly, only 4 of the 11 patients had clinically evident MM. Other investigators have emphasized the presence of nodular glomerular lesions [96]. Widespread deposits of monoclonal λ-L chains may produce death from an arrhythmia [37]. Preud'homme et al. [88] found abnormally short or large monoclonal L chains in patients with L chain deposition.

Plasmacytoma

Solitary plasmacytoma of bone. The diagnosis of solitary plasmacytoma depends on histologic proof that the tumor consists of plasma cells identical to those seen in myeloma and on absence of any other evidence of MM. Meyer and Schulz [80] reported that 9 of their 12 patients with solitary myeloma showed dissemination 2 to 10 years after diagnosis. In another series of 12 patients, 5 developed MM in a median period of 9 years after diagnosis [114]. Electrophoresis and IEP of an adequately concentrated urine specimen are helpful in recognizing the development of multiple myeloma. Although BJ proteinuria has been reported with solitary plasmacytoma [7], its occurrence strongly suggests MM.

Extramedullary plasmacytoma. These plasma cell tumors arise outside the bone marrow. They may be extensions of already existing MM, or they may appear to be primary and disseminate later to produce widespread disease. Their most frequent location is the upper respiratory tract—including the nasal cavity and sinuses, nasopharynx, and larynx [112]. In a group of 12 cases, MM developed in only 2 during a follow-up period of 14–320 months [21]. Periodic testing of the urine for monoclonal L chains is helpful in monitoring extramedullary plasmacytoma.

Malignant Lymphoproliferative Disease

Waldenström's macroglobulinemia. MW is a malignant lymphoplasmo-proliferative disorder characterized by a large amount of monoclonal IgM protein in the serum. Approximately one fourth of the patients have BJ proteinuria [22,75,86]; but in one series of 33 cases, the proportion with BJ proteinuria was 78% [76].

Malignant lymphoma. Although urinary L chain excretion may be increased in lymphoma, the protein usually is polyclonal. In a study of 30 patients with non-Hodgkin's lymphoma, Lindström and co-workers [69] found that 7 excreted more than 100 mg of L chains/24 h. None of these were monoclonal.

A monoclonal κ-protein was found in the serum and urine of a patient with atypical lymphoma [15]. In another case of malignant lymphoproliferative disorder, acute renal failure was the first manifestation but there was also marked BJ proteinuria (25 g/L). It is difficult to differentiate this case from a lymphoid myeloma, because the malignant lymphocytes had a plasmacytoid appearance and lytic bone lesions were noted [9]. In addition, the patient had no hepatosplenomegaly or lymphadenopathy. Yoon [116] reported urinary monoclonal L chains in five patients with non-Hodgkin's lymphoma. Synthesis of monoclonal L chains has been reported in non-Hodgkin's lymphoma and chronic lymphocytic leukemia (CLL) [39]. BJ proteinuria has been found in CLL [47,76]. We have seen a few patients with the histologic and clinical features of non-Hodgkin's lymphoma who excreted large amounts of monoclonal L chain in the urine.

μ-Heavy Chain Disease

Of the first seven reported cases of μ-HCD, six had CLL [34]; but lymphoma has been present in several more recent cases. BJ proteinuria has been noted in two thirds of cases [11].

Amyloidosis

Primary. The diagnosis of primary amyloidosis (AL) is based on histologic proof of amyloidosis without preceding or coexisting disease. Recognition of amyloidosis is facilitated by the presence of a monoclonal protein in the serum or urine. Indeed, the presence of a monoclonal protein in a patient with a nephrotic syndrome, congestive heart failure, carpal tunnel syndrome, peripheral neuropathy, or orthostatic hypotension requires the exclusion of amyloidosis. Since adopting this policy, we have doubled the number of new cases of amyloidosis recognized at our institution.

Almost half of patients with primary amyloidosis have renal insufficiency when the diagnosis is made, and 90% have proteinuria. Electrophoresis of the urine frequently shows a large albumin peak, because almost a third of patients with primary amyloidosis have nephrotic syndrome. Not infrequently, a small monoclonal L chain is found in the urine of these patients. The globulin spike in these instances is usually very small and easily overlooked. IEP of a concentrated urine specimen is recommended for every patient with nephrotic syndrome of undetermined etiology. When a monoclonal protein has been sought in both serum and urine of our patients with primary amyloidosis, it has been found in 90% of cases. Monoclonal λ-L chains are twice as common as κ in amyloidosis [58] Although it has been said that a λVI subtype is often associated with amyloidosis, we found λVI subtype in only 7 of 49 cases of primary systemic amyloidosis with a monoclonal λ-L chain (test performed by Dr. Alan Solomon, University of Tennessee Center for the Health Sciences, Knoxville, TN).

Monoclonal Gammopathy of Undetermined Significance (MGUS)

We have followed 241 cases in which there was a monoclonal protein in the serum but initially no evidence of MM, MW, amyloidosis, or lymphoma [55]. After a follow-up of 10 years, the patients were classified as follows: group 1, patients without significant increase in monoclonal protein, 38%; group 2, patients with more than 50% increase in monoclonal serum protein or development of monoclonal urine protein, 9%; group 3, patients who had died without myeloma or related diseases, 35%; and group 4, patients in whom MM, MW, or amyloidosis developed, 18% [57].

Retrospective analysis by age, sex, presence of organomegaly, hemoglobin level, amount and type of serum monoclonal protein, presence of small amounts of monoclonal L chain in the urine, serum albumin level, levels of uninvolved Igs, IgG subclass, and level of plasma cells in the bone marrow did not show how to distinguish initially between stable benign disease and progressive disease.

IEP demonstrated a monoclonal L chain in the urine of 12 of 45 patients in group 1 (no significant increase of monoclonal protein) [55]. BJ proteinuria was recognized in six cases at the time when the serum monoclonal protein was diagnosed; and the monoclonal urine protein disappeared from one after removal of a parathyroid adenoma, but remained stable in the other five. In the six other cases where the urinary monoclonal protein was discovered during the period of observation, the monoclonal serum protein diminished in four, increased 0.1 g/dL in one, and remained the same in one. Among all 12 of these patients, 8 had 24-hour urinary excretion of 0.5 g or less. In three of the cases with greater excretion, the amount of urinary L chain remained stable for more than 10 years, and in the fourth it disappeared after removal of a parathyroid adenoma.

Urine studies in 17 cases of group 2 (more than 50% increase of monoclonal serum protein from initial value, or appearance of monoclonal urine protein), demonstrated a monoclonal L chain in 8, although the amount exceeded 0.5 g/24 h in only 1 [55]. The urinary protein was discovered at the same time as the serum monoclonal protein in two cases and the BJ proteinuria increased during the observation period in one of these. The serum monoclonal protein increased in the other seven; thus, either the urinary protein peak or the serum protein peak increased in all eight. During the subsequent 5-year follow-up (total 10 years), 10 patients of group 2 developed MM or related diseases.

Association of Bence Jones proteinuria with a monoclonal serum protein usually indicates a neoplastic process. Waldenström [108] stated that excretion of a demonstrable amount of BJP in the urine of a patient with a monoclonal serum protein was strong evidence of malignancy. Hobbs [44] said that BJ proteinuria of more than 1.0 mg/dL (10 mg/L) was of "sinister significance" and suggestive of malignant plasmacytic disease. Seligmann and Basch [95] noted that a BJP level of 30 mg/dL (300 mg/L) or more in a patient with a pathologic serum Ig and decreased normal Igs strongly suggested malignant proliferation. Dammacco and Waldenström [25], from a study of 42 patients with benign monoclonal gammopathy, reported weakly positive results of the heat test for BJP in 1 case and small amounts of L chains in 10. None of these patients had more than 60 mg/L of BJP. The presence of a monoclonal L chain in the urine is very suggestive of a neoplastic process, and a patient with this finding must be followed closely for the development of MM, amyloidosis, or other serious disease. However, in our experience there are exceptions to this usual course.

Idiopathic Bence Jones Proteinuria (Benign Monoclonal L Chain Gammopathy)

Despite the fact that BJ proteinuria is a recognized feature of MM, MW, primary amyloidosis, and occasionally lymphoma, the possibility of a benign monoclonal gammopathy of the L chain type must be considered.

Cronstedt et al. [23] described a patient in whom decreased IgG and IgA protein had persisted for 5 years and then BJ proteinuria appeared (175 mg/L), without evidence of myeloma. Virella et al. [107] described two patients with "idiopathic" BJ proteinuria, but the follow-ups were only 2 and 7 months. Therefore, appreciable BJ proteinuria may be benign or the patients may develop MM or amyloidosis only after many years.

BJ proteinuria has been found in children with immunodeficiency and repeated infections. Danon and Seligmann [26] described a child with primary immune deficiency and BJ proteinuria. In another report, a child with type I dysgammaglobulinemia and repeated infections had multiple monoclonal proteins in the serum and one κ- and two λ-monoclonal proteins in the urine [12].

We have followed two patients who have maintained a stable serum concentration of monoclonal protein and excreted 0.8 g or more of BJP daily for more than 15 years without evidence of multiple myeloma, amyloidosis, or similar malignant disease. One of these patients had documented proteinuria for 10 years before the recognition of BJ proteinuria, making a total of 25 years of proteinuria [63].[3]

We have reported on seven additional patients who presented with BJ proteinuria (> 1 g/24 h) but who had no monoclonal protein in the serum and no evidence of MM or related diseases. Three patients developed symptomatic MM after 8, 15, and 21 years and have been treated. One of them had a carpal tunnel syndrome from systemic amyloidosis. One patient had marked but stable renal insufficiency after two episodes of acute renal failure. Because he had small kidneys and a history of hypertension and coronary artery disease, it was felt that his renal insufficiency was more likely due to the acute renal failure or nephrosclerosis rather than myeloma kidney or amyloidosis. One patient probably had a slowly evolving MM, but he died without overt myeloma. The two remaining patients both fulfilled the criteria for benign BJ proteinuria after a follow-up period of 7 to 12 years. Thus, BJ proteinuria comprises a wide variety of manifestations. *Patients with apparently benign BJ proteinuria should be followed indefinitely, because multiple myeloma or amyloidosis often develops [62].*

ACKNOWLEDGMENTS

This investigation was supported by Research Grants CA 16835 and NS-14304-K from the National Institutes of Health, U.S. Public Health Service.

REFERENCES

1. A Cooperative Study by Acute Leukemia Group B: Correlation of abnormal immunoglobulin with clinical features of myeloma. Arch Intern Med 135:46, 1975.

[3]Ed. note: See also section on Presence of Bence Jones Proteins (concerning benign course in patient with IgA (λ) and BJP (λ) monoclonal gammopathy for more than 6 years), Ritzmann SE in Ritzmann SE, Daniels JC (eds): "Serum Protein Abnormalities: Diagnostic and Clinical Aspects" [122].

2. Alexanian R, Haut A, Khan AU, Lane M, McKelvey EM, Migliore PJ, Stuckey WJ Jr, Wilson HE: Treatment for multiple myeloma: Combination chemotherapy with different melphalan dose regimens. JAMA 208:1680, 1969.
3. Bayne-Jones S, and Wilson DW: Immunological reactions of Bence-Jones proteins. II. Differences between Bence-Jones proteins from various sources. Bull Johns Hopkins Hosp 33:119, 1922.
4. Bence Jones H: On a new substance occurring in the urine of a patient with mollities ossium (abstract). Proc R Soc Lond [Biol] 5:673, 1847.
5. Bence Jones H: Papers on chemical pathology: Lecture III. Lancet 2:88, 1847.
6. Bence Jones H: On a new substance occurring in the urine of a patient with mollities ossium. Philos Trans R Soc Lond [Biol], p 55, 1848.
7. Benedict KT Jr: Destructive lesion of the proximal radius. JAMA 212:464, 1970.
8. Bergsagel DE, Migliore PJ, Griffith KM: Myeloma proteins and the clinical response to melphalan therapy. Science 148:376, 1965.
9. Berkel J, Granillo-Bodansky C, van der Borne AEGK: Acute renal failure associated with a malignant lymphoproliferative disorder with monoclonal light chain immunoglobulin production: Report of a case. Scand J Haematol 20:377, 1978.
10. Boyce WH, Garvey FK, Norfleet CM Jr: Proteins and other biocolloids of urine in health and in calculous disease. I. Electrophoretic studies at pH 4.5 and 8.6 of those components soluble in molar sodium chloride. J Clin Invest 33:1287, 1954.
11. Brouet J-C, Seligmann M, Danon F, Belpomme D, Fine J-M: μ-Chain disease: Report of two new cases. Arch Intern Med 139:672, 1979.
12. Bushell AC, Whicher JT, Yuille T: The progressive appearance of multiple urinary Bence-Jones proteins and serum paraproteins in a child with immune deficiency. Clin Exp Immunol 38:64, 1979.
13. Buxbaum JN: The biosynthesis, assembly, and secretion of immunoglobulins. Semin Hematol 10:33, 1973.
14. Capra JD, Kehoe JM: Hypervariable regions, idiotypy, and the antibody-combining site. Adv Immunol 20:1, 1975.
15. Chenais F, Virella G, Young CD, Liu P, Whittle TS Jr: Atypical B cell dyscrasia with Bence-Jones proteinuria and intracellular retention of γ-chains. Acta Haematol (Basel) 58:166, 1977.
16. Clyne DH, Kant KS, Pcscc AJ, Pollack VE: Nephrotoxicity of low molecular weight serum proteins: Physicochemical interactions between myoglobin, hemoglobin, Bence-Jones proteins and Tamm-Horsfall mucoprotein. Curr Prob Clin Biochem 9:299, 1979.
17. Clyne DH, Pesce AJ, Thompson RE: Nephrotoxicity of Bence Jones proteins in the rat: Importance of protein isoelectric point. Kidney Int 16:345, 1979.
18. Clyne DH, Pollak VE: Renal handling and pathophysiology of Bence Jones proteins. Contrib Nephrol 24:78, 1981.
19. Cole PW, Durie BGM, Salmon SE: Immunoquantitation of free light chain immunoglobulins: Applications in multiple myeloma. J Immunol Methods 19:341, 1978.
20. Cornell CJ Jr, McIntyre OR, Kochwa S, Weksler BB, Pajak TF: Response to therapy in IgG myeloma patients excreting lambda or kappa light chains: CALGB experience. Blood 54:23, 1979.
21. Corwin J, Lindberg RD: Solitary plasmacytoma of bone vs. extramedullary plasmacytoma and their relationship to multiple myeloma. Cancer 43:1007, 1979.
22. Creyssel R: Diagnostic value of Bence-Jones protein. In Manuel Y, Revillard JP, Betuel H (eds): "Proteins in Normal and Pathological Urine." Basel: S. Karger, 1970, pp 100–110.
23. Cronstedt J, Carling L, Östberg H: Idiopathic light chain dyscrasia—a new distinct entity? Report of a case. Acta Med Scand 196:445, 1974.
24. Dalal FR, Winsten S: Double light-chain disease: A case report. Clin Chem 25:190, 1979.

25. Dammacco F, Waldenström J. Bence Jones proteinuria in benign monoclonal gamma-pathies: Incidence and characteristics. Acta Med Scand 184:403, 1968.
26. Danon F, Seligmann M: Serum monoclonal immunoglobulins in childhood. Arch Dis Child 48:207, 1973.
27. DeFronzo RA, Cooke CR, Wright JR, Humphrey RL: Renal function in patients with multiple myeloma. Medicine (Baltimore) 57:151, 1978.
28. Durie BGM, Cole PW, Chen H-SG, Himmelstein KJ, Salmon SE: Synthesis and metabolism of Bence Jones protein and calculation of tumour burden in patients with Bence Jones myeloma. Br J Haematol 47:7, 1981.
29. Edelman GM, Gally JA: The nature of Bence-Jones proteins: Chemical similarities to polypeptide chains of myeloma globulins and normal γ-globulins. J Exp Med 116:207, 1962.
30. Erikson J, Martinis J, Croce CM: Assignment of the genes for human λ immunoglobulin chains to chromosome 22. (Letter to the editor.) Nature 294:173, 1981.
31. Eulitz M: A new subgroup of human L-chains of the λ-type: Primary structure of Bence-Jones protein DEL. Eur J Biochem 50:49, 1974.
32. Exton WG: A simple and rapid test for albumin and other urinary proteins. JAMA 80:529, 1923.
33. Fett JW, Deutsch HF: Primary structure of the Mcg chain. Biochemistry 13:4102, 1974.
34. Franklin EC: μ-Chain disease. Arch Intern Med 135:71, 1975.
35. Gailani S, Seon B-K, Henderson ES: κ Light chain—myeloma associated with adult Fanconi syndrome: Response of the nephropathy to treatment of myeloma. Med Pediatr Oncol 4:141, 1978.
36. Gallango ML, Suinaga R, Ramirez M: Bence Jones myeloma with a tetramer of kappa-type globulin in serum. Clin Chem 26:1741, 1980.
37. Ganeval D, Noël LH, Droz D, Leibowitch J: Systemic lambda light-chain deposition in a patient with myeloma. Br Med J 282:681, 1981.
38. Glenner GG: Amyloid deposits and amyloidosis. The β-fibrilloses. N Engl J Med 302:1283, 1980.
39. Gordon J, Howlett AR, Smith JL: Free light chain synthesis by neoplastic cells in chronic lymphocytic leukaemia and non-Hodgkin's lymphoma. Immunology 34:397, 1978.
40. Hayes JS, Jankey N, Cuthbert AL, Das PM: Massive proteinuria in light chain disease. Arch Intern Med 138:785, 1978.
41. Heller JF: Die mikroskopisch-chemisch-pathologische untersuchung. In von Gaal G (ed): "Physikalische Diagnostik und deren Anwendung in der Medicin, Chirurgie, Oculistik, Otiatrik und Geburtshilfe, enthaltend: Inspection, Mensuration, Palpation, Percussion und Auscultation, nebst einer kurzen Diagnose der Krank-heiten der Athmungs und Kreis-laufsorgane." Wein: Braumüller & Seidel, 1846, p 576.
42. Hicks EJ, Nordschow CD, Griep JA: Multiple myeloma and macrogammaglobulinemia. I. Urinary protein excretions and serum interrelationships. Am J Clin Pathol 64:1, 1975.
43. Hinberg IH, Katz L, Waddell L: Sensitivity of in vitro diagnostic dipstick tests to urinary protein. Clin Biochem 11:62, 1978.
44. Hobbs JR: Paraproteins, benign or malignant? Br Med J 3:699, 1967.
45. Jancelewicz Z, Takatsuki K, Sugai S, Pruzanski W: IgD multiple myeloma: Review of 133 cases. Arch Intern Med 135:87, 1975.
46. Joyner MV, Cassuto J-P, Dujardin P, Schneider M, Ziegler G, Euller L, Masseyeff R: Non-excretory multiple myeloma. Br J Haematol 43:559, 1979.
47. Kim H, Heller P, Rappaport H: Monoclonal gammopathies associated with lymphopro-liferative disorders: A morphologic study. Am J Clin Pathol 59:282, 1973.
48. Klein M, Kells DIC, Tinker DO, Dorrington KJ: Thermodynamic and conformational

studies on an immunoglobulin light chain which reversibly precipitates at low temperatures. Biochemistry 16:552, 1977.

49. Kohn J: A cellulose acetate supporting medium for zone electrophoresis. Clin Chim Acta 2:297, 1957.

50. Korngold L, Lipari R: Multiple-myeloma proteins. III. The antigenic relationship of Bence Jones proteins to normal gamma-globulin and multiple-myeloma serum proteins. Cancer 9:262, 1956.

51. Koss MN, Pirani CL, Osserman EF: Experimental Bence Jones cast nephropathy. Lab Invest 34:579, 1976.

52. Kozuru M, Benoki H, Sugimoto H, Sakai K, Ibayashi H: A case of lambda type tetramer Bence-Jones proteinemia. Acta Haematol 57:359, 1977.

53. Kunkel HG: The "abnormality" of myeloma proteins. Cancer Res 28:1351, 1968.

54. Kyle RA: Multiple myeloma: Review of 869 cases. Mayo Clin Proc 50:29, 1975.

55. Kyle RA: Monoclonal gammopathy of undetermined significance: Natural history in 241 cases. Am J Med 64:814, 1978.

56. Kyle RA: Classification and diagnosis of monoclonal gammopathies. In Rose NR, Friedman H (eds): "Manual of Clinical Immunology." 2nd ed. Washington, D.C.: American Society for Microbiology, 1980, pp 135–150; 1105.

57. Kyle RA: Monoclonal gammopathy of undetermined significance (MGUS): A review. Clin Haematol 11:123, 1982.

58. Kyle RA, Bayrd ED: Amyloidosis: Review of 236 cases. Medicine (Baltimore) 54:271, 1975.

59. Kyle RA, Elveback LR: Management and prognosis of multiple myeloma. Mayo Clin Proc 51:751, 1976.

60. Kyle RA, Greipp PR: The laboratory investigation of monoclonal gammopathies. Mayo Clin Proc 53:719, 1978.

61. Kyle RA, Greipp PR: Smoldering multiple myeloma. N Engl J Med 302:1347, 1980.

62. Kyle RA, Greipp PR: "Idiopathic" Bence Jones proteinuria: Long-term follow-up in seven patients. N Engl J Med 306:564, 1982.

63. Kyle RA, Maldonado JE, Bayrd ED: Idiopathic Bence Jones proteinuria—a distinct entity? Am J Med 55:222, 1973.

64. Kyle RA, Maldonado JE, Bayrd ED: Plasma cell leukemia: Report on 17 cases. Arch Intern Med 133:813, 1974.

65. Laurell C-B: Composition and variation of the gel electrophoretic fractions of plasma, cerebrospinal fluid and urine. Scand J Clin Lab Invest 29 (Suppl 124):71, 1972.

66. Lee BJ, Korngold L, Weiner MJ: Melphalan and antigenic type of Bence Jones proteins in myeloma. Science 149:564, 1965.

67. Lieu T-S, Deutsch HF, Tischendorf FW: Human λ-chain sequence variations and serologic associations. Immunochemistry 14:429, 1977.

68. Lindström FD, Williams RC Jr, Swaim WR, Freier EF: Urinary light-chain excretion in myeloma and other disorders—An evaluation of the Bence-Jones test. J Lab Clin Med 71:812, 1968.

69. Lindström FD, Williams RC Jr, Theologides A: Urinary light chain excretion in leukaemia and lymphoma. Clin Exp Immunol 5:83, 1969.

70. Line DE, Adler S, Fraley DS, Burns FJ: Massive pseudoproteinuria caused by nafcillin. JAMA 235:1259, 1976.

71. Longsworth LG, Shedlovsky T, MacInnes DA: Electrophoretic patterns of normal and pathological human blood serum and plasma. J Exp Med 70:399, 1939.

72. Macintyre W: Case of mollities and fragilitas ossium, accompanied with urine strongly charged with animal matter. Med Chir Trans R Med Chir Soc Lond 33:211, 1850.

73. Maldonado JE, Velosa JA, Kyle RA, Wagoner RD, Holley KE, Salassa RM: Fanconi syndrome in adults: A manifestation of a latent form of myeloma. Am J Med 58:354, 1975.
74. Manuel Y, Revillard JP: Study of Urinary Proteins by Zone Electrophoresis: Methods and Principles of Interpretation. In Manuel Y, Revillard JP, Betuel H (eds): "Proteins in Normal and Pathological Urine." Basel: S. Karger, 1970, pp 153–171.
75. McCallister BD, Bayrd ED, Harrison EG Jr, McGuckin WF: Primary macroglobulinemia: Review with a report on thirty-one cases and notes on the value of continuous chlorambucil therapy. Am J Med 43:394, 1967.
76. McLaughlin H, Hobbs JR: Clinical significance of Bence-Jones proteinuria. Protides Biol Fluids 20:251, 1973.
77. Meinke GC, Sigrist PH, Spiegelberg HL: The NH_2-terminal amino acid sequence of a κ and a λ Bence-Jones cryoglobulin. Immunochemistry 11:457, 1974.
78. Meinke GC, Spiegelberg HL: Amino acid sequence of the first hypervariable region of 2 κ and a λ Bence Jones cryoglobulin. Immunochemistry 13:915, 1976.
79. Merlini G, Waldenström JG, Jayakar SD: A new improved clinical staging system for multiple myeloma based on analysis of 123 treated patients. Blood 55:1011, 1980.
80. Meyer JE, Schulz MD: "Solitary" myeloma of bone: A review of 12 cases. Cancer 34:438, 1974.
81. Obituary: Dr. Henry Bence Jones. Lancet 1:614, 1873.
82. Osserman EF: Melphalan and antigenic type of Bence Jones proteins in myeloma. Science 149:564, 1965.
83. Payne RB: A red herring in the detection of Bence-Jones protein (letter to the editor). J Clin Pathol 25:183, 1972.
84. Perry MC: Personal communication, 1978.
85. Perry MC, Kyle RA: The clinical significance of Bence Jones proteinuria. Mayo Clin Proc 50:234, 1975.
86. Pinoteau A, Cassuto JP, Quaranta JF, Audoly P, Masseyeff R: Bence-Jones proteinuria revisted (abstract). "Medical Oncology." Abstracts of the 4th Annual Meeting of the Medical Oncology Society and the Biannual Meeting of the Immunology and Immunotherapy Group, Nice, France, December 2–4, 1978. New York: Springer-Verlag, 1978, pp 1–29.
87. Preud'homme JL, Hurez D, Danon F, Brouet JC, Seligmann M: Intracytoplasmic and surface-bound immunoglobulins in 'nonsecretory' and Bence-Jones myeloma. Clin Exp Immunol 25:428, 1976.
88. Preud'homme JL, Morel-Maroger L, Brouet JC, Cerf M, Mignon F, Guglielmi P, Seligmann M: Synthesis of abnormal immunoglobulins in lymphoplasmacytic disorders with visceral light chain deposition. Am J Med 69:703, 1980.
89. Preuss HG, Weiss FR, Iammarino RM, Hammack WJ, Murdaugh HV Jr: Effects on rat kidney slice function in vitro of proteins from the urines of patients with myelomatosis and nephrosis. Clin Sci Mol Med 46:283, 1974.
90. Putnam FW, Easley CW, Lynn LT, Ritchie AE, Phelps RA: The heat precipitation of Bence-Jones proteins. I. Optimum conditions. Arch Biochim Biophys 83:115, 1959.
91. Putnam FW, Hardy S: Proteins in multiple myeloma. III. Origin of Bence-Jones protein. J Biol Chem 212:361, 1955.
92. Randall RE, Williamson WC Jr, Mullinax F, Tung MY, Still WJS: Manifestations of systemic light chain deposition. Am J Med 60:293, 1976.
93. Relman AS, Levinsky NG: Clinical examination of renal function. In Strauss MB, Welt LG (eds): "Diseases of the Kidney." 2nd ed, Vol 1. Boston: Little Brown and Company, 1971, pp 87–137.

94. Scarpioni L, Ballocchi S, Bergonzi G, Cecchettin M, Dall'Aglio P, Fontana F, Gandi U, Pantano C, Poisetti PG, Zanazzi MA: Glomerular and tubular proteinuria in myeloma. Relationship with Bence Jones proteinuria. Contrib Nephrol 26:89, 1981.

95. Seligmann M, Basch A: The clinical significance of pathological immunoglobulins. In: XII Congress of the International Society of Hematology, Plenary Session Papers. New York, 1968, pp 21–31.

96. Seymour AE, Thompson AJ, Smith PS, Woodroffe AJ, Clarkson AR: Kappa light chain glomerulosclerosis in multiple myeloma. Am J Pathol 101:557, 1980.

97. Shustik C, Bergsagel DE, Pruzanski W: κ and λ light chain disease: Survival rates and clinical manifestations. Blood 48:41, 1976.

98. Smithline N, Kassirer JP, Cohen JJ: Light-chain nephropathy: Renal tubular dysfunction associated with light-chain proteinuria. N Engl J Med 294:71, 1976.

99. Solomon A: Bence-Jones proteins and light chains of immunoglobulins (Parts 1 and 2). N Engl J Med 294:17, 91, 1976.

100. Solomon A: Bence Jones proteins and light chains of immunoglobulins. XIV. Conformational dependency and molecular localization of the kappa (κ) and lambda (λ) antigenic determinants. Scand J Immunol 5:685, 1976.

101. Solomon A, McLaughlin CL: Bence-Jones proteins and light chains of immunoglobulins. I. Formation and characterization of amino-terminal (variant) and carboxyl-terminal (constant) halves. J Biol Chem 244:3393, 1969.

102. Stone MJ, Frenkel EP: The clinical spectrum of light chain myeloma: A study of 35 patients with special reference to the occurrence of amyloidosis. Am J Med 58:601, 1975.

103. Tiselius A: Electrophoresis of serum globulin. II. Electrophoretic analysis of normal and immune sera. Biochem J 31:1464, 1937.

104. Tubbs RR, Gephardt GN, McMahon JT, Hall PM, Valenzuela R, Vidt DG: Light chain nephropathy. Am J Med 71:263, 1981.

105. Van Geelen JA, Mulder AW: Histology and function of the kidney in marked Bence Jones paraproteinuria. Neth J Med 22:158, 1979.

106. Vaughan JH, Jacox RF, Gray BA: Light and heavy chain components of gamma globulins in urines of normal persons and patients with agammaglobulinemia. J Clin Invest 46:266, 1967.

107. Virella G, Lopes-Virella MF, Levine J, Ogawa M, Gonzalez J: 'Idiopathic' Bence-Jones proteinuria. Acta Haematol 60:269, 1978.

108. Waldenström JG: "Diagnosis and Treatment of Multiple Myeloma." New York: Grune & Stratton, 1970.

109. Wang AC, Fundenberg HH, Wells JV, Roelcke D: A new subgroup of the kappa chain variable region associated with anti-Pr cold agglutinins. (Letter to the editor.) Nature 243:126, 1973.

110. Weiss JH, Williams RH, Galla JH, Gottschall JL, Rees ED, Bhathena D, Luke RG: Pathophysiology of acute Bence-Jones protein nephrotoxicity in the rat. Kidney Int 20:198, 1981.

111. Whicher JT, Hawkins L, Higginson J: Clinical applications of immunofixation: A more sensitive technique for the detection of Bence Jones protein. J Clin Pathol 33:779, 1980.

112. Wiltshaw E: The natural history of extramedullary plasmacytoma and its relation to solitary myeloma of bone and myelomatosis. Medicine 55:217, 1976.

113. Wochner RD, Strober W, Waldmann TA: The role of the kidney in the catabolism of Bence Jones proteins and immunoglobulin fragments. J Exp Med 126:207, 1967.

114. Woodruff RK, Malpas JS, White FE: Solitary plasmacytoma. II. Solitary plasmacytoma of bone. Cancer 43:2344, 1979.

The basic difficulty in defining amyloid better biochemically was its insolubility. Franklin's [10] and Glenner's [11] initial work in solubilization, isolation, and purification led to an explosive growth in the knowledge and understanding of amyloid over the last decade. It is now well recognized that the protein we call amyloid is different biochemically in different clinical disorders [182,183].

HISTOLOGIC BASIS OF AMYLOID PROTEIN

The gross description of amyloid infiltration has changed little since the time of Virchow. Involved organs are often enlarged with a rubbery firm consistency and a waxy pink or gray appearance. By light microscopy, amyloid appears as an amorphous pink refractile material with hematoxylin and eosin staining. However, this stain may not be sensitive enough to detect minimal quantities [12]. Crystal violet stain produces a reddish purple color with amyloid, but has the problem of variable staining with different batches of dye. Under ultraviolet light, Thioflavin-T will create a yellow fluorescence

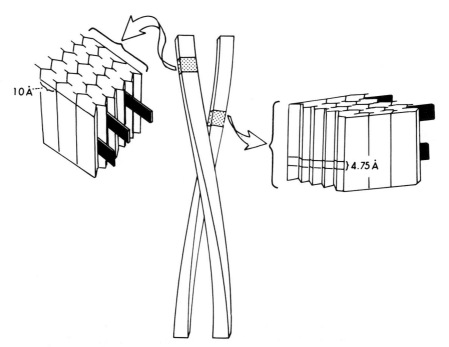

Fig. 1. An amyloid fibril demonstrating the twisted β-pleated sheet configuration of its polypeptide filaments. The dark blocks represent the alignment of Congo red dye molecules. (Modified from Cooper [17]).

and is very sensitive for amyloid, but probably not specific. Congo red staining of amyloid yields a pink color on light microscopy and pink fluorescence in ultraviolet light, but both can result in false positives. The most constant and specific feature of amyloid is its characteristic green birefringence when stained with Congo red and examined under a polarizing microscope [184].

When amyloid deposits are examined under the electron microscope, the protein has a fibrillar structure composed of rigid fine non-branching fibrils, 100 Å in width [13]. Each fibril, in turn, is composed of aggregates of two to five filaments arranged in a twisted ribbon appearance. X-ray diffraction studies suggest that these amyloid filaments are polypeptide chains that fold back and forth on themselves with an axis perpendicular to the axis of the fibril [14]. This structure is known as the β-pleated sheet configuration (Fig. 1). This configuration is not normally found in mammalian tissues, but can be assumed by a variety of polypeptide chains under pathologic conditions [15]. This β-pleated sheet configuration is credited for the property of insolubility in physiologic solutions and the relative resistance of amyloid to proteolytic enzymes. In addition, it is this configuration that provides the lattice for the binding of Congo red dye molecules parallel to the long axis of the amyloid fibrils, resulting in the optical properties by which amyloid is defined histologically [16,17]. Since all amyloid deposits share this common structure, Glenner has recently suggested reclassifying amyloidosis as the β-fibrilloses [18].

BIOCHEMISTRY OF AMYLOID PROTEIN

Table I lists the current nomenclature for the amyloid fibrils that have thus far been defined biochemically. The first amyloid protein to be char-

TABLE I. Defined amyloid fibrils

Amyloid fibril	Related serum protein	Clinical disorder
AL	L, immunoglobulin light chains	Primary amyloidosis
		Multiple myeloma—associated amyloidosis
AA	SAA, an HDL apoprotein	Secondary amyloidosis
		Familial Mediterranean fever-associated amyloidosis
$AF_{p,s,j}$	Prealbumin	Familial amyloidotic polyneuropathy
AE_t	Calcitonin (local deposition)	Medullary carcinoma of thyroid
AS_{c_1}		Senile cardiac amyloidosis

acterized was that associated with amyloidosis in multiple myeloma and primary amyloidosis. In 1971, Glenner was able to show sequence homology between the amino terminal segment of an amyloid protein and the Ig L chain produced by the patient's plasma cells [19]. These AL (i.e., Amyloid Light chain) fibrils can be created from some but not all human Bence Jones proteins (BJP) by proteolytic digestion under physiologic conditions [20]. In other experiments, human kidney lysosomal enzymes have caused the formation of amyloid fibrils from BJP [21]. κ_1-, κ_2-, and λ-L chain subtypes of amyloid fibrils have all been described [22]. The amyloid proteins that have been chemically characterized from patients with primary amyloidosis and myeloma-associated amyloidosis have had molecular weights ranging from 8,000 to 25,000 daltons. The major component contains the variable portion of an Ig L chain, the intact L chain, or a fusion of the two.

A second group of amyloid fibril proteins share a common amino-terminal amino acid sequence distinct from the L chains of Igs. These amyloid proteins have been designated as amyloid A (AA) fibrils and are found largely in amyloid depositions secondary to inflammatory diseases and familial Mediterranean fever. The characteristic component of these proteins, protein AA, appears to be unique, consisting of 76 amino acids in a single chain with a molecular weight of 8,500 daltons [23,24]. Serum AA (SAA), a substance antigenically related to AA protein, has been found to be elevated in the serum of patients with secondary amyloidosis but also in a variety of other diseases [25]. It has a molecular weight between 60,000 and 120,000 daltons and appears to function as the apoprotein for high-density lipoprotein [26]. Fractionation under mildly acidic conditions yields a 12,000 to 14,000 dalton fragment which contains a portion homologous with tissue protein AA. It has been suggested that SAA is, thus, a circulating precursor of the tissue component AA [27].

An amyloid fibril protein (AF_p) distinct from AA and AL has been described in familial amyloid polyneuropathy of the Portugese variety [28]. This protein has an apparent molecular weight of 14,000 daltons and shares common antigenic determinants with human prealbumin. The amyloid protein of familial amyloid polyneuropathy of the Swedish variety also appears to be related to a serum prealbumin precursor [185,186], as is the Japanese variety [187]. Thus, all geographic variants of type I familial polyneuropathy probably share a common biochemical as well as clinical basis [188]. Table II lists the other clinical familial amyloidoses that await biochemical characterization.

In medullary carcinoma of the thyroid, localized amyloid deposition is characteristic and also appears to be secondary to a unique fibrillar protein thought to be related to the prohormone of calcitonin [29]. This may be one type of amyloid protein in a class termed APUD-amyloid [30]. Many of the endocrine glands share the ability for amino acid precursor uptake and decarboxylation (APUD). Within these glands, localized amyloid deposition can occur in the setting of polypeptide tumors producing insulin, calcitonin, and growth hormone [31], and in gastrinomas and parathyroid adenomas [32]. Since insulin, calcitonin, and other polypeptide hormones can assume a β-pleated sheet configuration *in vitro* when subjected to acid treatment or proteolytic treatment [17,33], it has been proposed that APUD-amyloid may represent biochemically distinct proteins created by alteration of various polypeptide hormones.

At least one amyloid protein associated with aging has been shown to be biochemically distinct from the other proteins thus far characterized. In senile cardiac amyloidosis, a unique protein, ASc_1, has been described that shares common antigenic properties in affected patients [34,35]. It is not known whether ASc_1 is derived from alteration of a circulating substance or a result of local secretion. Recently, another form of amyloid has been described that affects only the atria in the aging heart [36]. Another example of localized amyloid deposition is seen in the adenomatoid odontogenic tumor in which enamel protein is thought to be the precursor [37]. Further biochemical studies of these and other clinical disorders will undoubtedly lead to the description

TABLE II. Generalized and localized hereditary amyloid deposits

GENERALIZED HEREDITARY AMYLOIDOSIS

Neuropathic forms
   Amyloid neuropathy type I (Portuguese or Andrade type)
   Amyloid neuropathy type II (Indiana or Rukavina type)
   Amyloid neuropathy type III (Iowa or Van Allen type)
   Amyloid neuropathy type IV (Finland or Meretoja type)

Nonneuropathic forms
   Amyloid neuropathy of Ostertag
   Amyloidosis of familial Mediterranean fever
   Amyloid nephropathy with deafness, urticaria, and limb pains (Muckle-Wells syndrome)
   Amyloid cardiomyopathy (Denmark)
   Amyloid cardiomyopathy with persistent atrial standstill

LOCALIZED HEREDITARY AMYLOID DEPOSITS
   Hereditary cerebral hemorrhage (Iceland)
   Lattice dystrophy of the cornea
   Hereditary amyloid deposits of the cornea
   Gingival hyperplasia, conjunctivitis, and mental retardation with amyloid infiltration (?)
   Papular cutaneous amyloid infiltration
   Poikilodermal cutaneous amyloid infiltration
   Bullous cutaneous amyloid infiltration
   Medullary carcinoma of the thyroid in MEA 2 with amyloid deposits

of many more proteins that can assume the β-fibrillar pattern of amyloid [189].

The P component is a protein, distinct from amyloid fibrillar proteins thus far described, that has been found in association with a variety of amyloid subtypes [38]. It has a pentagonal structure and its binding to amyloid fibrils appears to be calcium dependent and relatively selective [39]. A serum component, SAP, has been described, but levels in patients with amyloidosis do not differ from normal [40]. Immunofluorescence studies suggest that P components may be derived from human fibroblasts. Although P component appears to be an integral part of many types of amyloid, its role in pathogenesis of amyloidosis remains unclear [41]. Amyloid P component has been located in elastic fiber microfibrils of normal human tissue and basement membranes [190]. It is interesting that these elastic fiber microfibrils and amyloid fibrils are closely associated *in vivo*.

PATHOGENESIS OF AMYLOID DEPOSITION

Although the biochemical basis of amyloidosis of the AL type is now better understood, the pathogenesis remains in question. In both primary amyloidosis and multiple myeloma associated amyloidosis, a basic plasma cell dyscrasia has been well identified. However, only 5 to 15% of myeloma patients have clinical amyloid deposition [42]. In the case of L chain myelomas, the incidence is approximately 20 to 25% [43,44]. In an effort to define why only a subgroup of patients with plasma cell dyscrasias develop amyloidosis, Osserman showed that fluorescein-conjugated BJP from amyloidosis patients have a much greater tissue binding affinity than nonamyloidosis-related BJP [9]. Glenner has developed the concept that specific properties of L chains make them amyloidogenic [22]. Support for this theory comes from his studies that some BJP will form β-pleated sheets while others will not. In addition, the κ-type amyloid proteins share antigenic determinants among themselves, but will not cross-react with many nonamyloid κ-BJP. A similar relationship exists for λ-type amyloid proteins [191]. All AL proteins thus far sequenced have included an intact variable portion of the L chain with a generally absent or deficient constant region. Thus, it is likely that the *variable portion determines the amyloidogenic properties of the L chain* [45]. However, little is known about the possible additional contribution of abnormal metabolism of L chains at the end-organ level, such as altered proteolysis or phagocytic function.

In secondary amyloidosis, there is also evidence to suggest that differences in SAA, the AA protein precursor, may relate to amyloid deposition [192]. Studies have shown that there is polymorphism of mouse AA and SAA proteins [46] as well as human SAA proteins [193]. Another study in humans suggested that SAA from amyloidosis patients was more resistant to dissociation than SAA from normals [47]. Additionally, many investigations have revolved around possible alterations in the metabolism of amyloid precursors. SAA is the apoprotein for high density lipoprotein in man [26] and has also been described in the rabbit and mouse [48,49]. In addition to this carrier function, SAA behaves as an acute phase reactant and is elevated in a variety of acute and chronic inflammatory states [50]. An elevated SAA level may distinguish amyloidosis secondary to inflammatory disease or familial Mediterranean fever, from heredofamilial amyloidosis, where its level is usually normal. However, confusion arises because of SAA elevation in amyloidosis of the primary or myeloma associated variety. In fact, because of the wide variety of inflammatory diseases without amyloidosis in which SAA levels are elevated, its role as a precursor to AA deposition has been questioned [25]. However, others have suggested that SAA elevation represents the first phase of the biphasic development of secondary amyloidosis [51]. In this model, the second phase of amyloid deposition is dependent upon the way in which the AA precursor is metabolized. In casein-injected CBA/J mice, amyloidosis develops secondary to the inflammatory response generally within 2 weeks. If A/J mice are injected on the same schedule, amyloidosis does not appear before 7 weeks [52]. In both settings, similar elevations of SAA exist, suggesting a genetic basis for the predisposition to amyloid development, expressed through the structure and/or metabolism of SAA. The amyloid resistance in A/J mice has been explained on the basis of a single gene [53]. If these two strains of mice are injected with bovine serum albumin instead of casein, both develop an elevated SAA level, but neither develop amyloidosis [52]. Therefore, not only do host factors play a role in the development of amyloidosis, but the inciting stimulus to SAA production may be more or less amyloidogenic.

Several studies in this murine model suggest a role for immune dysfunction. Neonatal thymectomy and immunosuppressive therapy enhance amyloid formation, while thymosin, which restores T-cell function, seems to retard it [27]. An increased response to polyclonal B-cell activators also suggests a decrease in suppressor T-cell activity in this model. This B-cell hyperfunction may explain some of the confusion that exists over the elevated SAA levels in amyloidosis associated with myeloma. In this regard, it has been suggested that normally SAA provides an immunoregulatory function by indirectly suppressing B-cell response either through the lymphocyte or macrophage [54]. This interrelationship can also be seen in Balb/c mice, where intraperitoneal injections of mineral oil result in serum M-components, elevated SAA, and amyloidosis. These deposits are composed of the AA rather than the AL protein [55].

SAA has been reported to be derived from connective tissue or fibroblasts [56], stimulated B-cell lymphocytes [57], monocytes and macrophages [58], and polymorphonuclear leukocytes [59]. However, recent information suggests that the major site of synthesis is the liver [60–62]. In the acute phase response, SAA synthesis accounts for 2.5% of total hepatic protein synthesis [194]. Moreover, in a murine model of amyloid deposition, selective inhibition of liver protein synthesis prevents the usual SAA elevation and splenic amyloid deposition [61].

The reticuloendothelial system (RES) bears a close spatial relationship to amyloid deposits [63]. The lysosomes of these cells have been shown to be one site of amyloid formation [64] and breakdown [65]. Amyloidogenesis has been demonstrated in monolayer mouse spleen explants consisting predominantly of macrophages [66]. In humans, blood monocytes have been shown to possess surface-associated enzymes capable of degrading SAA protein [67]. In these studies, the degree of SAA degradation differed among individuals. Thus, some patients' monocytes completely degraded the protein, others degraded it only to AA protein and others had an intermediate step in which AA was formed temporarily before further degradation occurred. In ten patients with amyloidosis, all followed the last pattern. This variability in handling of SAA provides one possible explanation for the presence or absence of amyloid in patients with the same underlying inflammatory disease. Family studies of the amyloid patients are underway to see if this enzyme activity has a genetic basis [68].

Despite the diverse clinical and biochemical backgrounds for AL and AA, certain common features exist in their pathogenesis and are outlined in Figure 2. In this hypothetical model, chronic antigenic stimulation provides the environment for decreased suppressor T-cell activity and B-cell hyperactivity. On one hand, this can lead to plasma-cell dyscrasias, resulting in the production of amyloidogenic L chains and tissue deposition of AL proteins. On the other hand, SAA is produced as an immunologic modulator of the B-cell hyperactivity. Because of heredity or acquired alterations in the production and/or metabolism of SAA, tissue deposition of AA proteins occurs. From this model, it is not surprising that the coexistence in tissues of protein AA and Ig L chain fragments has been described [69]. Future studies will hopefully resolve the question of what role the RES plays in the genesis of AL protein. In addition, detailed biochemical studies of various SAA proteins are needed to evaluate the frequency of polymorphism and its relationship to amyloidogenesis.

DISORDERS OF AMYLOID DEPOSITION

Despite the advances in our understanding of the protein chemistry of amyloid, the most useful classification of disorders of amyloid deposition remains a clinical one (See Table III). In any series of patients with amyloidosis, the frequency of the various forms will depend upon the population being studied. In certain parts of the Mediterranean, familial amyloidosis is most common [70]. In areas with a high prevalence of chronic inflammatory disease, secondary amyloidosis may rank first. However, in the largest American series, primary amyloidosis and amyloidosis associated with multiple myeloma represent the two most common presentations for systemic amyloid deposition [195].

Plasma Cell Dyscrasia-Related Amyloidosis

The clinical diagnosis of primary amyloidosis is based upon the absence of underlying inflammatory disease, family history, or overt myeloma by the criteria of less than 20% plasma cells in the bone marrow, no lytic bone

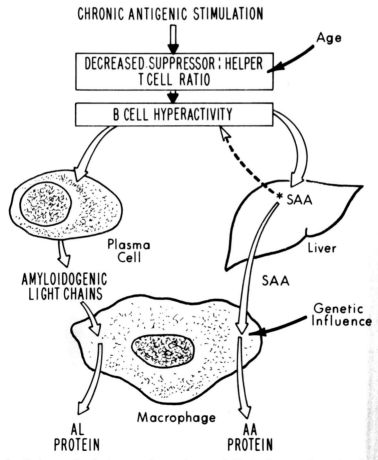

Fig. 2. Pathogenesis of primary and secondary amyloidosis. See text for explanation.

TABLE III. Disorders of amyloid deposition

Plasma-cell dyscrasia related amyloidosis	AL
1° Amyloidosis	
systemic	
organ-limited	
Myeloma-associated amyloidosis	
Secondary amyloidosis	AA
systemic	
organ-limited	
Heredofamilial amyloidosis	
FMF	AA
Familial amyloid polyneuropathy	AF_p, AF_s, AF_j
Other	
Amyloidosis of endocrine glands	
Medullary cancer of thyroid	AE_t
Other	
Amyloidosis of aging	
Senile cardiac amyloidosis	AS_{c_1}
Other	

lesions, and in some series the absence of an excessively large M-protein. In primary amyloidosis, however, there is almost invariably evidence of plasma cell dyscrasia with mild plasmacytosis of bone marrow or a monoclonal protein in the serum or urine of almost 90% of patients [71,72]. Thus, the distinction between multiple myeloma-associated amyloidosis and primary amyloidosis is one of degree. It remains valid nonetheless, since the former group seems to have a somewhat worse prognosis and such patients often die of myeloma-related complications [71,72]. In addition, patients with primary amyloidosis tend not to develop overt myeloma later in their course. Both disorders are clearly separated from multiple myeloma without amyloidosis in that they carry a uniformly poor prognosis with a generally poor response to chemotherapy. Amyloidosis has also been reported in heavy (H) chain disease [73] and in Waldenström's macroglobulinemia [74]. However, few of these cases have had specific biochemical determinations, and in at least one case of macroglobulinemia, the protein was determined to be AA rather than AL [75].

There is a subgroup of primary amyloidosis patients who present with organ-limited disease. In Kyle's series this comprised less than 10% [71]. The usual sites of involvement include the skin, the urinary tract, the respiratory tract, and the adnexal structures surrounding the eye. The natural history of the few patients that have been followed suggests that most do not develop systemic disease. There have been few biochemical studies performed; but in one case of nodular pulmonary amyloidosis, biochemical determination revealed the protein to be of the AL type [76]. The clinical manifestations of organ-limited amyloidosis will be considered here, while manifestations of systemic amyloidosis will be considered subsequently.

Amyloidosis localized to the *skin* occurs most commonly in lichen amyloidosis or nodular amyloidosis, although other clinical presentations are described [196]. The first disorder is quite rare and is characterized by a chronic pruritic eruption, usually of the lower extremities [77]. The deposition of amyloid in this disorder is unique in that it involves the epidermis and can involve the dermal papillae, but not the subcutaneous layer of the skin. The protein associated has not been biochemically determined. It has been suggested that the epidermis may be involved in the pathogenesis of this amyloid protein [78]. Treatment with topical corticosteroids relieves the pruritus, but has no effect on the amyloid deposition [79]. Nodular amyloidosis appears similar to the skin involvement that occurs in primary systemic amyloidosis [80]. Patients present with nonpruritic, but often purpuric, nodules or plaques with involvement commonly occurring on the extremities, trunk, genitals, and face. In this situation, no amyloid deposition appears in the epidermis; involvement is present in the deep parts of the corium and within blood vessels. In nodular amyloidosis in contrast to systemic amyloidosis, plasma-cell infiltration of the lesions is present [78]. This suggests that these plasma cells may be responsible for the local AL deposition.

Within the *urinary tract,* the most common site of localized amyloidosis is within the bladder. These patients generally present with hematuria [81]. The gross appearance is often similar to that of an infiltrating neoplasm with thickening of the bladder wall and a roughened, nodular, or ulcerated mucosal surface. On histologic examination, the deposits are largely found in the submucosa and the inner layers of the muscularis with involvement of vessel walls, but to a lesser extent than is usually seen in systemic amyloidosis. Immunohistochemical studies suggest that most of these deposits are of the AL type [197]. Other reported sites of involvement include the renal pelvis [82], ureters [83] urethra [84], seminal vesicles [85], and prostate [82]. With proper surgical excision, recurrence is unusual in this primary form.

Amyloidosis localized to the *lower respiratory tract* can present with involvement of the tracheobronchial tree, single or multiple pulmonary parenchymal nodules, or diffuse pulmonary amyloidosis [86]. Plasma cells, lymphocytes, and multinucleated giant cells are often seen in biopsies of these lesions. While resection has been highly successful for the nodular form, the tracheobronchial form has been more difficult to approach. The clinical course is variable, but these patients may develop symptoms of airway obstruction. Resection of an obstructing lesion may occasionally be successful [198], but patients often die of respiratory insufficiency. In addition, bleeding during surgical resection, particularly when attempted through the bronchoscope, has been difficult to control in this subgroup. In the few cases of documented diffuse amyloidosis limited to the lungs, eventual progression to respiratory failure and death has occurred [86]. In the limited follow-up that exists of the nodular form, local recurrence has been described, but systemic involvement is probably unusual [87]. Amyloidosis localized to the upper respiratory tract is well described and often involves the larynx [88] or the false vocal cords [89]. Symptoms are generally those of hoarseness. Occasionally amyloid deposition in the upper respiratory tract has been associated with plasmacytomas, particularly in the sinus, pharynx, and tonsils [90].

Localized involvement of the *orbit* and *conjunctiva* has been described and seems to be associated with plasma-cell infiltration [91]. If the skin of the eyelids is also involved, primary systemic amyloidosis is generally present.

Secondary Amyloidosis

Secondary amyloidosis has been described in the setting of a wide variety of diseases. Table IV presents a list of some of the more common associations.

TABLE IV. Diseases associated with secondary amyloidosis

CHRONIC GRANULOMATOUS AND SUPPURATIVE DISEASES

Tuberculosis
Leprosy
Granulomatous bowel disease
Bronchiectasis
Osteomyelitis
Pyelonephritis
Paraplegia

CHRONIC INFLAMMATORY DISEASES

Rheumatoid arthritis
Juvenile rheumatoid arthritis
Ankylosing spondylitis
Other collagen vascular diseases

NEOPLASTIC DISEASES

Hodgkin's disease
Non-Hodgkin's lymphoma
Renal cell carcinoma
Other carcinomas

IMMUNE DEFICIENCY STATES (with recurrent infections)

Hypogammaglobulinemia
Cyclic neutropenia

OTHER CHRONIC ANTIGENIC STIMULATION

Multiple blood transfusions
Parenteral drug abusers

These situations are similar to the animal models of amyloidosis in that the host appears to be presented with some form of chronic antigenic stimulus. Other factors must also be present, however, since other "antigenic" diseases such as sarcoidosis only rarely are associated with amyloidosis [92]. The incidence of amyloidosis secondary to inflammatory disease varies widely with the population studied [93]. For example, among leprosy patients in Carrville, Louisiana, amyloidosis has an incidence of 30% and is the major cause of death. However, in Mexico, only 8% of leprosy patients develop amyloidosis. This difference has been attributed to dietary differences in protein intake between the two populations [94]. In the casein model of murine amyloidosis, protein deficiency decreases the incidence of amyloidosis [22].

With the advent of antibiotics, the number of cases of amyloidosis secondary to tuberculosis or the chronic suppurative diseases such as osteomyelitis and bronchiectasis has declined. However, they remain commonly associated in series of secondary amyloidosis [95,96]. Special note should be made of the paraplegic patient who has a compound susceptibility to amyloidosis because of chronic pyelonephritis, decubitus ulcers, and chronic osteomyelitis secondary to such ulcers. In one autopsy series, the incidence of associated amyloidosis was 25% [97].

While rheumatoid arthritis is one of the most frequent causes of secondary amyloidosis, the reported incidence of amyloidosis in rheumatoid arthritis has varied widely [98]. In one series amyloidosis, determined by rectal biopsy, was present in 5% of patients with rheumatoid arthritis [99]. In another series, no difference in amyloidosis was noted between rheumatoid arthritis patients and age-matched controls [100]. However, most rheumatologists feel that the association is real. When amyloidosis is diagnosed clinically, rheumatoid arthritis has been present for a mean of 16 years [101]. Amyloidosis has been described in ankylosing spondylitis, other rheumatoid variants, and other collagen vascular diseases such as Behçet's disease and systemic lupus erythematosus [199]. The association with inflammatory bowel disease is often complicated by coexistant spondyloarthropathy [102]. Juvenile rheumatoid arthritis is the most frequent cause of secondary amyloidosis in childhood, followed by the suppurative diseases [103].

The most frequently reported neoplastic diseases associated with amyloidosis are Hodgkin's disease [104] and renal-cell carcinoma [105]. In one autopsy series of 4,000 cancer patients, the overall incidence of amyloidosis was 0.4% [106]. In this series non-Hodgkin's lymphomas, gastrointestinal carcinomas and bronchogenic carcinomas were also commonly associated with amyloidosis.

The categories of immune deficiency states with recurrent infections and other chronic antigenic stimulation in Table IV represent uncommon causes of amyloidosis. However, they are important in a conceptual framework because of the similarity of these situations to the animal models of amyloidosis. Hypogammaglobulinemic patients have sometimes been classified with primary amyloidosis because of occasional associated plasma-cell dyscrasias. However, the unifying feature in these patients appears to be recurrent infection [107]. The one reported case of cyclic neutropenia [108] is of great interest because of the gray-collie model of cyclic neutropenia where amyloidosis is the rule if the dog survives multiple recurrent infections [109]. Blood transfusions have been implicated in the few case reports of amyloidosis in association with hemophilia [110]. Amyloidosis has been reported with increasing frequency in drug abuse where chronic skin suppuration and repeated "antigenic" stimulation have been implicated [111].

All of the secondary forms of amyloidosis may present in a systemic or organ-limited pattern. In the organ-limited form, the sites are similar to those of primary organ-limited amyloidosis in that skin, bladder, ocular, adnexae, and the upper respiratory tract have all been involved. However, it has been claimed that lung involvement in localized secondary amyloidosis is rare [86].

Familial Amyloidosis

Amyloidosis in a familial setting has presented a wide variety of clinical forms which are well reviewed elsewhere [32,112,113]. Table II lists Glenner's classification, divided by clinical presentation with systemic or localized amyloid deposition [32]. The systemic group is subdivided into neuropathic and non-neuropathic forms. The two forms of familial amyloidosis that have been biochemically defined are those associated with familial Mediterranean fever and the type I polyneuropathy. Tissue deposition of AA protein occurs in amyloidosis secondary to familial Mediterranean fever. SAA levels are also elevated while they have been found to be normal in other inherited amyloidoses [114]. Although many ethnic groups develop familial Mediterranean fever, only Turks and Sephardic Jews seem predisposed to amyloidosis [115]. The biopsy-proven incidence is 60% in Turks and has ranged from 12 to 42% in Sephardic Jews. The Portugese form of familial amyloid polyneuropathy has been characterized as having a unique amyloid protein with an associated serum component thought to be prealbumin [28]. Further biochemical definition of heredofamilial amyloidoses will undoubtedly uncover other amyloid proteins.

Amyloid Deposition in Endocrine Glands

Organ-limited amyloid deposition has been described generally within glands involved in the overproduction of polypeptide hormones. The best-characterized example is medullary cancer of the thyroid, as discussed in the pathogenesis section. There seems to be no association with a systemic form of amyloid deposition.

Amyloid Deposition and Aging

The most common and least well understood disorder of amyloid deposition is that associated with aging. Deposits in the aorta, heart, and brain increase significantly with age after the age of 60 [116]. By age 90, 95% of subjects have histopathologic evidence of amyloid deposition [117]. The origin of these deposits may be diverse. Senile plaques have been related to APUD-amyloid [118] but have also been found to contain Igs [119,120]. Others have favored an association of senile amyloid with the AA protein because levels of SAA seem to rise with age reaching very high levels in the eighth and ninth decades [25]. In at least one form of age-related amyloid deposition, senile cardiac amyloid, a unique protein, ASc_1, has been described [36].

Pathogenetic factors leading to amyloid deposition in the aged are equally numerous. Age predisposes to amyloid deposition in the murine model and to monoclonal gammopathies in man, perhaps secondary to a decrease in suppressor T lymphocytic function. Vascular damage has been implicated, particularly in cerebral amyloid angiopathy [121,122,200]. In addition, senile plaques are found in close relationship with capillaries with amyloid angiopathy, and it has been postulated that local secretion of amyloid by the endothelial cell may be a factor [123]. Another model that has been studied for amyloidosis in the aged is the LAF_1 mouse, which spontaneously develops amyloidosis with aging. This can be inhibited by the use of antioxidants, suggesting that free radicals may play a role in the amyloidosis of the aged [124].

From a clinical standpoint, the role of amyloid in senile plaques and dementia is unclear [125], but in some cases of cerebral vessel amyloid deposition, intracerebral hemorrhage has clearly resulted [126]. Senile cardiac amyloidosis with diffuse involvement of the heart has been described in 10–25% of patients over 60 [127,128]. While it has been difficult to separate the clinical symptoms secondary to amyloidosis from the usual coexisting coronary atherosclerosis, patients with senile cardiac amyloidosis appear to have a higher incidence of congestive heart failure and atrial fibrillation [127]. In one series, seven cases of fatal senile cardiac amyloidosis after a prolonged course of refractory congestive heart failure were described [201]. Involvement of the aorta generally precedes and coexists with cardiac amyloidosis. With more extensive disease, extravascular deposits have been described in other organs and pulmonary involvement also is present in 10–20% of senile cardiac amyloidosis patients over age 80 [129]. Whether this represents the same ASc_1 protein or not remains to be determined.

Thus, suggestive evidence exists that amyloid deposition in the aged can play an important clinical role in selected patients. These patients can generally be separated from primary and secondary amyloidosis patients by their age and pattern of clinical involvement. Further biochemical characterizations are necessary to sort out the number of amyloid proteins associated with aging and their pathogenetic significance to disorders such as Alzheimer's disease [202].

CLINICAL FEATURES OF SYSTEMIC AMYLOIDOSIS

Osserman has proposed that amyloidosis can be classified according to the pattern of organ involvement [130]. Pattern I represents principle involvement of the tongue, heart, gastrointestinal tract, skeletal, and smooth muscles, skin, ligaments, and nerves. Pattern II includes principle involvement of the liver, spleen, kidneys and adrenals. A mixed pattern represents overlapped Pattern I and Pattern II. While primary amyloidosis often follows Pattern I and secondary amyloidosis often follows Pattern II, Kyle found the overlap to be large [71]. In addition, this classification also distorts the biochemical separation that exists in Table III. However, because of the myriad of findings that have been reported in systemic amyloidosis, it is helpful to keep in mind the *more common presenting features of both primary and secondary amyloidosis.*

In Kyle's series, fatigue, weight loss, edema, and dyspnea were common presenting features in approximately 50% of the patients [71]. On physical examination, hepatomegaly was present in more than 40% and congestive heart failure was present in approximately one third. The "classic" manifestations of purpura, macroglossia, and orthostatic hypotension are present in only 10–20% of patients. Among laboratory abnormalities, the most consistent findings are elevated liver enzymes in 50%, hypoalbuminemia in 70%, increased creatinine in 50%, and proteinuria in greater than 90% [71,72].

In systemic amyloidosis of both the primary and secondary types, renal failure is a leading cause of death. If a major difference exists between the clinical course of secondary and primary amyloidosis, it is that the secondary form has an even higher incidence of nephrotic syndrome. The pyelogram may reveal the classic picture of enlarged kidneys; but in the majority of cases the kidneys will be normal sized, and with advanced renal disease the kidneys may even be small [131]. Histologically the glomerulus is generally affected, but interstitial, peritubular, and vascular amyloid may be prominent.

When the urine is examined, cellular casts are uncommon but microscopic hematuria and pyuria are present in over 50% [131]. The proteinuria is largely albumin in the primary and secondary groups. In the myeloma-associated group over 80% have urinary Ig L chains, whereas one third will have Ig L chains in the primary group and virtually none in the secondary group [71]. Nephrotic syndrome is less common in the myeloma-associated group, but the adult Fanconi syndrome with tubular dysfunction is more often described. Progression of nephrotic syndrome to renal failure often occurs within a few years of diagnosis, although in some cases renal disease has remained stable for many years.

Kyle's series of amyloidosis of the AL type suggested that cardiac disease occurred in one third of the patients [71]. In other series [132,133] over 90% of primary amyloid patients showed clinical, EKG, or radiographic evidence of heart disease while only 50% of those with secondary amyloidosis had these findings. The most common manifestation has been congestive heart failure, although some patients present with dominant features of constriction. This can be confusing, particularly when the EKG shows low voltage. *M-mode and two-dimensional* echocardiograms can help separate an infiltrative cardiomyopathy from constrictive pericarditis [133,203]. Left ventricular filling can also be helpful in this differential diagnosis [204]. However, endomyocardial biopsy is sometimes necessary to confirm the presence of amyloid [134]. Amyloid infiltration can result in Q-waves in the anterior leads of the EKG which can simulate an old myocardial infarction. Sudden death is common [201]. Cardiac arrhythmias are well described, particularly varying degrees of atrioventricular block, atrial flutter, and fibrillation. Amyloid involvement of the conduction system is often quite spotty [135] and conduction abnormalities often occur in the absence of direct amyloid infiltration. Digitalis has been implicated as a cause of sudden death in these patients secondary to worsening of underlying conduction disease [136], and direct binding of digoxin to amyloid fibrils *in vitro* has been described as a possible mechanism. A less common manifestation of amyloid heart disease is ischemia secondary to coronary vessel involvement [137].

Pulmonary involvement is present pathologically in 25% of all amyloid patients and usually parallels cardiac involvement [138]. It may include nodular parenchymal involvement, vascular amyloid, or severe diffuse parenchymal involvement. Clinical symptoms are generally not present, but occasionally patients may have a progressive respiratory course, particularly in the tracheobronchial or diffuse forms. Pulmonary involvement is quite unusual in secondary amyloidosis.

Hepatic and gastrointestinal involvement are not common modes of death in amyloidosis, but are of great importance in terms of presentation and diagnosis because of the frequency of involvement. Liver involvement with hepatomegaly or increased enzymes is present in over 50% of patients. Amyloid is present by biopsy in over 90%. Jaundice is uncommon except for rare reports of obstructive jaundice [139]. Generally, clinical symptoms from hepatic involvement are unusual. Splenic involvement is present in about 10–20% and is seldom clinically evident in the absence of hepato-megaly.

Gastrointestinal tract involvement has been reported to occur from the tongue to the rectum. The roentgenolographic picture is one of "stiff intes-tines" [140] associated with evidence of disordered motility such as esoph-ageal reflux, gastric retention, or intestinal dilatation. Motility dysfunction may be secondary to diffuse muscle invasion or on a neuropathic basis [141]. The radiologic findings are similar to those seen in scleroderma and vascular insufficiency, and malabsorption has been reported in about 5% of patients [71]. Gastrointestinal bleeding appears to be more common and was reported in 25% of patients in one series [96].

Neurologic involvement with peripheral neuropathy is present in less than 20% of patients, and is usually characterized by a painful, distal, symmetrical sensorimotor neuropathy [142]. It is progressive in nature and autonomic features are often prominent, particularly orthostatic hypotension. Apart from this neuropathy carpal tunnel syndrome is a frequent manifestation and may be seen in 15–30% of patients of primary amyloidosis [71]. It is less common in secondary amyloidosis. Subclinical skin involvement was present in one series in approximately 40% of both primary and secondary amyloidosis [143]. When clinical symptoms are present, the amyloid infiltrates result in purpura or nodules, plaques, or papules [80]. One unusual, but almost di-agnostic feature, of amyloidosis is involvement of the eyelids, which leads to periorbital purpura [144] particularly after procedures, such as procto-scopy, which raise venous pressure.

Amyloid joint disease can simulate rheumatoid arthritis or present as an asymmetrical arthritis secondary to local amyloid deposition within a large joint such as the hip [145]. When present, the physical finding of massively enlarged shoulders with a rubbery consistency, the "shoulder pad sign," strongly suggests amyloid arthropathy [146].

Lymphadenopathy is not commonly present. Unusual manifestations are factor X and occasionally factor IX deficiencies, secondary to direct binding of the factors by intravascular amyloid fibrils [147,148]. Splenectomy has corrected the deficiency, presumably by removal of a large volume of intra-vascular amyloid [149]. Other unusual presentations of systemic amyloidosis exist in innumerable case reports. For the most part, however, other more common features will also be present to alert the clinician to the diagnosis.

DIAGNOSIS

Although there are clinical and laboratory features suggestive of amyloi-dosis, none are diagnostic. Attempts to develop a noninvasive screening test have been unsuccessful. One such test, Congo red staining of urinary sediment for amyloid, has been found to have unacceptable false-negative and false-positive rates [150]. By definition, the diagnosis of amyloidosis rests on demonstration of tissue amyloid deposition, as discussed in the section on historical aspects.

In order to obtain tissue for the diagnosis of systemic amyloidosis, skin, gingiva, and/or rectal biopsies are often done initially because of their simplicity and yield. If any clinical evidence of skin involvement is present, a punch or excisional biopsy should yield the diagnosis almost 100% of the time. Even in clinically uninvolved skin, the yield is greater than 40% for both primary and secondary amyloidosis [143]. The gingival biopsy yields a diagnosis more than 50% of the time in most series [12]. The rectal biopsy can be done by suction or punch biopsy under sigmoidoscopic visualization. An adequate specimen should contain submucosa. Most deposits will be found in this area or in vessel walls [155]. The yield is generally 70% or better [71,155].

Negative biopsies from these areas do not exclude the diagnosis, and beyond these sites the physician should be directed to sites of suspected organ involvement. Liver biopsies have a greater than 90% yield [71]. Reports exist of excessive bleeding after liver biopsy, particularly in the setting of massive hepatomegaly [12]. However, most hepatologists do not feel the complications are significantly increased. Renal biopsy can be successful more than 90% of the time, but here bleeding may be a more serious problem. Opinion conflicts as to whether open or percutaneous biopsy should be done. Bronchial biopsies may be helpful to clinical diagnosis, but are also complicated by bleeding which is difficult to control locally. If cardiac involvement is important to document, endomyocardial biopsy can be successfully performed [156]. Small bowel biopsies have had a 50% yield when symptoms are present. If carpal tunnel syndrome occurs secondary to amyloidosis, examination of surgically removed tissue should yield a diagnosis in 90% of cases [71].

After establishing a diagnosis of amyloid deposition, ideally one would like to know the biochemical type of amyloid protein, as clinical classification and biochemical analysis may differ [151]. Immunofluorescence assays may eventually be available routinely to identify common amyloid types [152,197].

One method for the separation of amyloid AA from other forms is currently applicable to routine laboratory use. When tissue sections from patients with secondary amyloidosis or amyloidosis associated with familial Mediterranean fever are preincubated with potassium permanganate, the property of green bi-refringence with Congo red staining is lost [153]. On the other hand, amyloid depositions not of the AA type such as myeloma-associated amyloidosis, familial amyloidotic polyneuropathy, medullary carcinoma of the thyroid, pancreatic islet amyloid, and cerebral amyloidosis are not affected and are, therefore, potassium-permanganate resistant. However, the clinical classification has not always agreed with the potassium-permanganate reaction. In one series of 67 patients, a few patients thought to have secondary amyloidosis were reclassified as senile amyloidosis and a few others were shown to have deposits that were sensitive in one organ and resistant in another [153]. In a second series of 56 patients, the major discrepancy was in seven patients who were clinically classified as having primary amyloidosis in whom the potassium-permanganate reaction suggested the AA subtype [154]. These discrepancies may simply represent the imprecision of our clinical stratification. More biochemical correlation is needed, but it would seem that the potassium-permanganate reaction may be a useful adjunct to the methods that currently exist for the classification of amyloidosis patients [201].

PROGNOSIS AND TREATMENT

Patients with amyloidosis in association with multiple myeloma have a median survival of 6–9 months, while patients with primary amyloidosis have a median survival of 12–15 months [71], although a mean survival as long as 28 months for primary amyloidosis has been reported [72]. In the latter report as well, myeloma in association with amyloidosis carried a worse prognosis. Since these diseases both show evidence of plasma-cell dyscrasia, it has been hoped that chemotherapy would be of benefit as for myeloma patients. Isolated case reports have suggested that combinations of alkylating agents and prednisone may occasionally lead to remission of amyloidosis and apparent prolonged survival (157–160). Such therapy has been related to actual tissue amyloid regression in one patient with *in vitro* evidence that excessive L chain synthesis was halted by chemotherapy [161]. However, other patients treated by the same regimen have shown no response [162]. In the only double-blind study of placebo versus melphalan-prednisone, the chemotherapy group was able to continue treatment longer and two patients had disappearance of nephrotic syndrome, while eight others had a 50% reduction in protein excretion. However, survival was not significantly affected [163]. Thus, isolated patients may benefit from chemotherapy, but at this point there are no criteria to suggest who is likely to respond.

Secondary amyloidosis is a more heterogeneous group. Survival after diagnosis has been quite variable, but generally has been 1–5 years, with reports of patients stable 7–8 years after diagnosis. In addition, clinical symptoms have often been present for years prior to diagnosis in this group [96]. Patients with nephrotic syndrome as an isolated manifestation often have a longer survival, and spontaneous remissions have been described [164]. Generally proteinuria may improve while amyloid deposits remain the same or worsen, but in one case secondary to burn injury, actual tissue amyloid regression was documented [165]. In this regard, others have reported improvement in clinical manifestations and occasionally decreased tissue amyloid deposition with control of the underlying disease such as rheumatoid arthritis [166]. In another patient, with tumor-associated amyloidosis secondary to a paraganglioma, the nephrotic syndrome resolved following surgical removal of the tumor and did not recur during four years of follow-up [167]. Thus, the main goal of therapy of secondary amyloidosis has been directed at treatment of the underlying disease.

In familial Mediterranean fever-associated amyloidosis, the disease is predominantly nephropathic. The mean time from the development of proteinuria to uremia is 7 years [32]. At this point, further survival depends upon dialysis or transplantation. Renal transplantation has been performed in selected patients with familial Mediterranean fever and amyloidosis and in secondary amyloidosis, since 1971 [168]. Although amyloid deposits have been documented 2.5–4 years after transplantation (169–172), graft function does not seem to be adversely effected. In one series of predominantly secondary amyloidosis [173], the mean survival was 48 months after transplantation. In a group of 10 patients with familial Mediterranean fever, five of ten had functioning cadaver grafts 1.5–5.5 years posttransplant, similar to a control group [174]. However, in the control group, the majority of patients with nonfunctioning grafts survived, while in the amyloidosis group none survived without functioning grafts. With multiorgan involvement, amyloidosis patients may have difficulty with hemodialysis, but in one series of ten familial Mediterranean fever patients, the complications and survival were equivalent to controls [175]. Thus, in selected patients with uremia as a major manifestation of amyloidosis, both dialysis and transplantation offer reasonable means to prolong survival.

Two other drugs have received attention for their possible therapeutic benefit in amyloidosis, colchicine and dimethyl sulfoxide (DMSO). Colchicine has been shown to inhibit amyloid formation in the casein-induced murine amyloidosis model [176]. It is thought to interfere with the first phase of amyloid production, namely, the generation of SAA. Thus, it is of interest that colchicine has been found to be effective in the prophylaxis of attacks of familial Mediterranean fever [177]. In three patients with amyloidosis associated with familial Mediterranean fever and one with apparent primary amyloidosis, colchicine in a dose of 1.5 mg/day led to an eventual remission of nephrotic syndrome in all four patients [170]. This was interpreted as colchicine blockade of further amyloid formation with eventual resorption of tissue amyloid by the RES.

Dimethyl sulfoxide has received attention because of its ability to cause urinary excretion of amyloid material in animals [178] and in human amyloid nephropathy [179]. In the human situation, only a single intravenous or oral dose was given. In the animal model of casein-induced amyloidosis, repeated injection of DMSO led to partial or complete disappearance of amyloid deposits. In another animal study, DMSO was shown to cause resorption of splenic amyloid deposition, while colchicine was ineffective [181]. Two patients with rheumatoid arthritis and amyloidosis, who showed recovery of renal function after daily DMSO therapy over several months, have been reported [180]. Other trials of daily DMSO have been less conclusive [206]. The mechanism is not clear. It has been suggested that DMSO can partially destroy the β-pleated sheet configuration and allow degradation of the amyloid fibrils and subsequent phagocytosis or urinary excretion.

All of these studies should be considered preliminary, and hopefully further clinical trials will clarify the utility of these agents in treating the various forms of amyloidosis.

CASE REPORT

A 55-year-old postmaster from Swansboro, North Carolina, was admitted to the Durham VA Medical Center on August 4, 1975. Approximately 6 months prior to admission he developed burning dysesthesias over the soles of his feet. Subsequently, a progressive sensory loss developed to the midthigh bilaterally. In addition, episodic, severe shortness of breath without chest pain developed. One episode of syncope was also described. The patient had lost approximately 10 kg. Physical exam revealed a well-developed man with a blood pressure of 100/70 mm Hg without a postural change. The results of head and neck, skin, lymph node, lung and abdominal examinations were normal. Cardiovascular exam revealed a loud S4 and a grade 2/6 apical systolic ejection murmur. Pitting pedal edema was present. Neurologic examination showed a paralysis of upper gaze and a decrease in light touch, pin prick, and vibration over the ulnar distribution of both arms and over a stocking distribution in both legs. Deep tendon reflexes were 2 + in the upper extremities, but absent in the lower extremities. Admission laboratory data included a hematocrit of 36%, normal electrolytes and liver enzymes, a normal urinalysis (by dipstick), a chest x-ray with cardiomegaly, and an electrocardiogram with first degree AV block, left anterior hemi-block, and right bundle branch block. A sural nerve biopsy revealed amyloid deposition. A bone marrow revealed less than 5% plasma cells, a serum protein electrophoresis was normal and a urine immunoelectrophoresis revealed a λ-BJP. Twenty-four-hour urine protein excretion was 1 g and the creatinine clearance was 55 mg/min. A His bundle study revealed delayed sinus node recovery time and a pacemaker was recommended, but the patient declined. The patient was considered to have primary amyloidosis and was treated with a regimen including melphalan, penicillamine, prednisone, and fluoxymesterone, along with lasix. A subjective improvement in sensation and paresthesias occurred after one course of therapy, but sudden death occurred 2 weeks later.

REFERENCES

1. Rokitansky KF: "Handbuch der Pathologischen Anatomie, Vol. 3." Braumüller and Seidel, 1842.

2. Virchow R: Ueber den Gang der amyloiden Degeneration. Arch Pathol Anat Physiol Klin Med 8:364, 1855.
3. Friedrich N, Kekule A: Zur Amyloidfrage. Arch Pathol Anat Physiol Klin Med 16:50, 1859.
4. Krakow NP: Ueber bei Thieren experimentell hervorgerufenes Amyloid. Zentralbl Allg Pathol 6:337, 1895.
5. Kuczynski MH: Neue Beiträge zur Lehre vom Amyloid. Klin Wochenschr 2:727, 1923.
6. Willis S: Cases of lardaceous disease and some allied affections. With remarks. Guy's Hosp Rep 17:103, 1856.
7. Hildebrand O: Ueber Corpora amylacea und locales Amyloid in einem endostalen Sarcom des Brustbeins. Arch Pathol Anat Physiol Klin Med 140:249, 1895.
8. Magnus-Levy A: Bence-Jones-Eiweiss Protein und Amyloid. Z Klin Med 116:510, 1931.
9. Osserman EF, Takatsuki K, Talal N: The Pathogenesis of "Amyloidosis." Semin Hematol 1:3, 1964.
10. Pras M, Schubert M, Zucker-Franklin D, Rimon A, Franklin EC: The characterization of soluble amyloid prepared in water. J Clin Invest 47:924, 1968.
11. Glenner GG, Cuatrecasas P, Isersky C, Bladen HA, Eanes ED: Physical and chemical properties of amyloid fibers. J Histochem Cytochem 17:769, 1969.
12. Cohen AS: "The diagnosis of amyloidosis, in Laboratory Diagnostic Procedures in the Rheumatic Diseases." Boston: Little, Brown and Co., 1975.
13. Cohen AS, Calkins E: Electron microscopic observations on a fibrous component in amyloid of diverse origins. Nature 183:1202, 1959.
14. Eanes ED, Glenner GG: X-ray diffraction studies on amyloid filaments. J Histochem Cytochem 16:673, 1968.
15. Glenner GG, Eanes ED, Bladen HA, Linke RP, Termine JD: β-Pleated sheet fibrils: A comparison of native amyloid with synthetic protein fibrils. J Histochem Cytochem 22:1141, 1974.
16. Puchtler H, Sweat F, Levine M: On the binding of congo red by amyloid. J Histochem Cytochem 10:355, 1962.
17. Cooper JH: Selective amyloid staining as a function of amyloid composition and structure. Lab Invest 17:232, 1974.
18. Glenner GG: Amyloid deposits and amyloidosis: The β-fibrilloses. N Engl J Med 302:1283, 1333, 1980.
19. Glenner GG, Terry W, Harada M, Isersky C, Page D: Amyloid fibril proteins: Proof of homology with immunoglobulin light chains by sequence analyses. Science 172:1150, 1971.
20. Glenner GG, Ein D, Eanes ED, Bladen HA, Terry W, Page DL: Creation of "amyloid" fibrils from Bence Jones proteins in vitro. Science 174:712, 1971.
21. Epstein WV, Tan M, Wood IS: Formation of "amyloid" fibrils in vitro by action of human kidney lysosomal enzymes on Bence Jones proteins. J Lab Clin Med 84:107, 1974.
22. Glenner GG, Page DL: Amyloid, amyloidosis, and amyloidogenesis. Int Rev Exp Path 15:1, 1976.
23. Gruys E: A comparative approach to secondary amyloidosis: Minireview. Dev Comp Immunol 3:23, 1979.
24. Levin M, Franklin EC, Frangione B, Pras M: The amino acid sequence of a major nonimmunoglobulin component of some amyloid fibrils. J Clin Invest 51:2773, 1972.
25. Rosenthal CJ, Franklin EC: Variation with age and disease of an amyloid A protein-related serum component. J Clin Invest 55:746, 1975.
26. Benditt EP, Eriksen N: Amyloid protein SAA is associated with high density lipoprotein from human serum. Proc Natl Acad Sci USA 74:4025, 1977.

27. Scheinberg MA, Wohlgethan JR, Cathcart ES: Humoral and cellular aspects of amyloid disease: present status. Prog Allergy 27:250, 1980.
28. Costa PP, Figueira AS, Bravo FR: Amyloid fibril protein related to prealbumin in familial amyloidotic polyneuropathy. Proc Natl Acad Sci USA 75:4499, 1978.
29. Sletten K, Westermark P, Natvig JB: Characterization of amyloid fibril proteins from medullary carcinoma of the thyroid. J Exp Med 143:993, 1976.
30. Pearse AGE, Ewen SWB, Polak JM: The genesis of apud-amyloid in endocrine polypeptide tumours: Histochemical distinction from immunamyloid. Virchow's Arch 10:93, 1972.
31. Westermark P, Grimelius L, Polak JM, Larsson L-I, Van Noorden S, Wilander E, Everson AG: Amyloid in polypeptide hormone-producing tumors. Lab Invest 37:212, 1977.
32. Glenner GG, Ignaczak TF, Page DL: The inherited systemic amyloidoses and localized amyloid deposits. In Stanbury JB, Wyngaarden JB, Fredrickson DF (eds): "Metabolic Basis of Inherited Disease." 4th ed. New York: McGraw-Hill, 1978, p 1308.
33. Kedar (Keizman) I, Ravid M, Sohar E: In vitro synthesis of "amyloid" fibrils from insulin, calcitonin and parathormone. Is J Med Sci 12:1137, 1976.
34. Westermark P, Natvig JB, Johansson B: Characterization of amyloid fibril protein from senile cardiac amyloid. J Exp Med 146:631, 1977.
35. Cornwell III GG, Natvig JB, Westermark P, Husby G: Senile cardiac amyloid: Demonstration of a unique fibril protein in tissue sections. J Immunol 120:1385, 1978.
36. Westermark P, Johansson B, Natvig JB: Senile cardiac amyloidosis: Evidence of two different amyloid substances in the ageing heart. Scand J Immunol 10:303, 1979.
37. Smith RRL, Olson JL, Hutchins GM, Crawley WA, Levin LS: Adenomatoid odontogenic tumor: Ultrastructural demonstration of two cell types and amyloid. Cancer 43:505, 1979.
38. Skinner M, Cohen AS, Shirahama T, Cathcart ES: P-component (pentagonal unit) of amyloid: Isolation, characterization, and sequence analysis. J Lab Clin Med 84:604, 1974.
39. Pepys MB, Dyck RF, DeBeer FC, Skinner M, Cohen AS: Binding of serum amyloid P-component (SAP) by amyloid fibrils. Clin Exp Immunol 38:284, 1979.
40. Skinner M, Vaitukaitis JL, Cohen AS, Benson MD: Serum amyloid P-component levels in amyloidosis, connective tissue diseases, infection, and malignancy as compared to normal serum. J Lab Clin Med 94:633, 1979.
41. Holck M, Husby G, Sletten K, Natvig JB: The amyloid P-component (protein AP): An integral part of the amyloid substance? Scand J Immunol 10:55, 1979.
42. Kyle OA: Multiple Myeloma: Review of 869 cases. Mayo Clin Proc 50:29, 1975.
43. Shustik C, Bergsagel DE, Pruzanski W. κ and λ light chain disease: Survival rates and clinical manifestations. Blood 48:41, 1976.
44. Stone MJ, Frenkel EP: The clinical spectrum of light chain myeloma. Am J Med 58:601, 1975.
45. Linke RP, Tischendorf FW, Zucker-Franklin D, Franklin EC: The formation of amyloid-like fibrils in vitro from Bence Jones proteins of the VλI subclass. J Immunol 111:24, 1973.
46. Gorevic PD, Levo Y, Frangione B, Franklin EC: Polymorphism of tissue and serum amyloid A (AA and SAA) proteins in the mouse. J Immunol 121:138, 1978.
47- Sipe JD, McAdam KPWJ, Torain BF, Glenner GG: Conformational flexibility of the serum amyloid precursor SAA. Br J Exp Pathol 57:582, 1976.
48. Skogen B, Borresen AL, Natvig JB, Berg K, Michaelsen TE: High-density lipoprotein as carrier for amyloid-related protein SAA in rabbit serum. Scand J Immunol 10:39, 1979.
49. Benditt EP, Eriksen N, Hanson RH: Amyloid protein SAA is an apoprotein of mouse plasma high density lipoprotein. Proc Natl Acad Sci USA 76:4092, 1979.

50. Benson MD, Cohen AS: Serum amyloid A protein in amyloidosis, rheumatic, and neoplastic diseases. Arthritis Rheum 22:36, 1979.
51. Sipe JD, McAdam KPWJ, Uchino F: Biochemical evidence for the biphasic development of experimental amyloidosis. Lab Invest 3:110, 1978.
52. Benson MD, Scheinberg MA, Shirahama T, Cathcart ES, Skinner M: Kinetics of serum amyloid protein A in casein-induced murine amyloidosis. J Clin Invest 59:412, 1977.
53. Wohlgethan JR, Cathcart ES: Amyloid resistance in A/J mice is determined by a single gene. Nature 278:453, 1979.
54. Benson MD, Aldo-Benson M: Effect of purified protein SAA on immune response *in vitro:* Mechanisms of suppression. J Immunol 122:2077, 1979.
55. Baumal R: Similarity of casein- and endotoxin-induced, myeloma-associated and aged SJL/J amyloid in various strains of mice. Int Arch Allergy Appl Immunol 59:20, 1979.
56. Linder E, Anders RF, Natvig JB: Connective tissue origin of the amyloid-related protein SAA. J Exp Med 144:1336, 1976.
57. McAdam KPWJ, Elin RJ, Sipe JD, Wolff SM: Changes in human serum amyloid A and C-reactive protein after etiocholanolone-induced inflammation. J Clin Invest 61:390, 1978.
58. Sipe JD, Vogel SN, Ryan JL, McAdam KPWJ, Rosenstreich DL: Detection of a mediator derived from endotoxin-stimulated macrophages that induces the acute phase serum amyloid A response in mice. J Exp Med 150:597, 1979.
59. Rosenthal CJ, Sullivan L: Serum Amyloid A: Evidence for its origin in polymorphonuclear leukocytes. J Clin Invest 62:1181, 1978.
60. Benson MD, Scheinberg MA, Shirahama T, Cathcart ES, Skinner M: Kinetics of serum amyloid protein A in casein-induced murine amyloidosis. J Clin Invest 59:412, 1977.
61. Kisilevsky R, Benson MD, Axelrod MA, Boudreau L: The effect of a liver protein synthesis inhibitor on plasma SAA levels in a model of accelerated amyloid deposition. Lab Invest 41:206, 1979.
62. Benson MD, Kleiner E: Synthesis and secretion of serum amyloid protein A (SAA) by hepatocytes in mice treated with casein. J Immunol 124:495, 1980.
63. Shirahama T, Cohen AS: An analysis of the close relationship of lysosomes to early deposits of amyloid. Am J Pathol 73:97, 1973.
64. Shirahama T, Cohen AS: Intralysosomal formation of amyloid fibrils. Am J Pathol 81:101, 1975.
65. Shirahama T, Cohen AS: Lysosomal breakdown of amyloid fibrils by macrophages. Am J Pathol 63:463, 1971.
66. Baumal R, Sklar S, Wilson B, Laskov R: Casein-induced murine amyloidosis: Amyloidogenesis *in vitro* by monolayer spleen explants of casein-injected mice. Lab Invest 39:632, 1978.
67. Lavie G, Zucker-Franklin D, Franklin EC: Degradation of serum amyloid A protein by surface-associated enzymes of human blood monocytes. J Exp Med 148:1020, 1978.
68. Franklin EC: Some unsolved problems in the amyloid diseases. Am J Med 66:365, 1979.
69. Westermark P, Natvig JB, Anders RF, Sletten K, Husby G: Coexistence of protein AA and immunoglobulin light-chain fragments in amyloid fibrils. Scand J Immunol 5:31, 1976.
70. Cohen AS: Amyloidosis. N Eng J Med 277:574, 1967.
71. Kyle RA, Bayrd ED: Amyloidosis: Review of 236 cases. Medicine 54:271, 1975.
72. Pruzanski W, Katz A: Clinical and laboratory findings in primary generalized and multiple-myeloma-related amyloidosis. Can Med Assoc J 114:906, 1976.
73. Frangione B, Franklin EC: Heavy chain diseases: Clinical features and molecular significance of the disordered immunoglobulin structure. Semin Hematol 10:53, 1973.

74. Forget BG, Squires JW, Sheldon H: Waldenström's macroglobulinemia with generalized amyloidosis. Arch Intern Med 118:363, 1966.
75. Husby G, Sletten K, Michaelsen TE, et al: Amino acid analysis of AA in macroglobulinemia. Scand J Immunol 2:395, 1973.
76. Page DL, Isersky C, Harada M, Glenner GG: Immunoglobulin origin of localized nodular pulmonary amyloidosis. Res Exp Med 159:75, 1972.
77. Shapiro L, Kurban AK, Azar HA: Lichen amyloidosis: a histochemical and electron microscopic study. Arch Path 90:499, 1970.
78. Westermark P: Amyloidosis of the skin: A comparison between localized and systemic amyloidosis. Acta Derm Venereol 59:341, 1979.
79. Moschella SL, Pillsbury DM, Hurbey HJ: "Dermatology." Philadelphia: Saunders, 1975.
80. Breathnach SM, Black MM: Systemic amyloidosis and the skin: A review with special emphasis on clinical features and therapy. Clin Exp Derm 4:517, 1979.
81. Malek RS, Greene LF, Farrow GM: Amyloidosis of the urinary bladder. Br J Urol 43:189, 1971.
82. Dias R, Fernandes M, Patel RC, De Shadarevian J-J, Lavengood RW: Amyloidosis of renal pelvis and urinary bladder. Urology 14:401, 1979.
83. Mariani AJ, Barrett DM, Kurtz SB, Kyle RA: Bilateral localized amyloidosis of the ureter presenting with anuria. J Urol 120:757, 1978.
84. Ordonez NG, Ayala AG, Gresik MV, Bracken RB: Primary localized amyloidosis of male urethra (amyloidoma). Urology 14:617, 1979.
85. Farah RN, Benson DO, Fine G, Dorman PJ: Primary localized amyloidosis of bladder. Urology 13:200, 1979.
86. Rubinow A, Celli BR, Cohen AS, Rigden BG, Brody JS: Localized amyloidosis of the lower respiratory tract. Am Rev Resp Dis 118:603, 1978.
87. Lipper S, Kahn LB: Amyloid tumor. Am J Surg Path 2:141, 1978.
88. Hellquist H, Olofsson J, Sökjer H, and Ödkvist LM: Amyloidosis of the larynx. Acta Otolaryngol 88:443, 1979.
89. Michaels L, Hyams VJ: Amyloid in localized deposits and plasmacytomas of the respiratory tract. J Path 128:29, 1979.
90. Wiltshaw E: The natural history of extramedullary plasmacytoma and its relation to solitary myeloma of bone and myelomatosis. Medicine 55:217, 1976.
91. Knowles II DM, Jakobiec FA, Rosen M, Howard G: Amyloidosis of the orbit and adnexae. Surv Ophthalmol 19:367, 1975.
92. Bar-Meir S, Topilsky M, Kessler H, Pinkhas J, de Vries A: Coincidence of sarcoidosis and amyloidosis. Chest 71:542, 1977.
93. Kuhlbäck B, Wegelius O: Secondary amyloidosis: A study of clinical and pathological findings. Acta Med Scand 180:737, 1966.
94. Williams RC Jr, Cathcart ES, Calkins E, Fite GL, Rubio JB, Cohen AS: Secondary amyloidosis in lepromatous leprosy: Possible relationships of diet and environment. Ann Intern Med 62:1000, 1965.
95. Kennedy AC, Burton JA, Allison MEM: Tuberculosis as a continuing cause of renal amyloidosis. Br Med J 3:795, 1974.
96. Brandt K, Cathcart ES, Cohen AS: A clinical analysis of the course and prognosis of forty-two patients with amyloidosis. Am J Med 44:955, 1968.
97. Malament M, Friedman M, Pschibul F: Amyloidosis of paraplegia. Arch Phys Med Rehabil 46:406, 1965.
98. Hurd ER: Extraarticular manifestations of rheumatoid arthritis. Semin Arthritis Rheum 8:151, 1979.
99. Arapakis G, Tribe CR: Amyloidosis in rheumatoid arthritis investigated by means of rectal biopsy. Ann Rheum Dis 22:256, 1963.

100. Ozdemir AI, Wright JR, Calkins E: Influence of rheumatoid arthritis on amyloidosis of aging: Comparison of 47 rheumatoid patients with 47 controls matched for age and sex. N Engl J Med 285:534, 1971.
101. Cohen AS: Amyloidosis associated with rheumatoid arthritis. Med Clin N A 52:613, 1968.
102. Shorvon PJ: Amyloidosis and inflammatory bowel disease. Dig Dis 22:209, 1977.
103. Strauss RG, Schubert WK, McAdams AJ: Amyloidosis in childhood. J Ped 74:272, 1969.
104. Falkson G, Falkson HC: Amyloidosis in Hodgkin's disease. South Afr Med J 47:62, 1973.
105. Penman HG, Thomson KJ: Amyloidosis and renal adenocarcinoma; a post-mortem study. J Pathol 107:45, 1972.
106. Kimball KG: Amyloidosis in association with neoplastic disease. Ann Intern Med 55:958, 1961.
107. Gaffney EF, Lee JCK: Systemic amyloidosis and hypogammaglobulinemia. Arch Pathol Lab Med 102:558, 1978.
108. Shiomura T, Ishida Y, Matsumoto N, Sasaki K, Ishihara T, Miwa S: A case of generalized amyloidosis associated with cyclic neutropenia. Blood 54:628, 1979.
109. Machado EA, Gregory RS, Jones JB, Lange RD: The cyclic hematopoietic dog: A model for spontaneous secondary amyloidosis. Am J Pathol 92:23, 1978.
110. Sharma HM, Geer JC: Multiple transfusions with sensitization associated with amyloidosis. Arch Pathol 89:473, 1970.
111. Novick DM, Yancovitz SR, Weinberg PG: Amyloidosis in parenteral drug abusers. Mt Sinai J Med 46:163, 1979.
112. Thomas PK: Genetic factors in amyloidosis. J Med Gen 12:317, 1975.
113. Mahloudji M, Teasdall RD, Adamkiewicz JJ, Hartmann WH, Lambird PA, McKusick VA: The genetic amyloidoses. Medicine 48:1, 1969.
114. Meretoja J, Natvig JB, Husby G: Amyloid-related serum protein (SAA) in patients with inherited amyloidosis and certain viral conditions. Scand J Immunol 5:169, 1976.
115. Meyerloff J: Familial Mediterranean fever: Report of a large family, review of the literature, and discussion of the frequency of amyloidosis. Medicine 59:66, 1980.
116. Wright JR, Calkins E, Breen WJ, Stolte G, Schultz RT: Relationship of amyloid to aging: Review of the literature and systematic study of 83 patients derived from a general hospital population . Medicine 48:39, 1969.
117. Calkins E, Binette JP, Wright JR, Matsuzaki M, Ozdemir I: Some clinical observations on the nature of amyloid. Trans Am Clin Climatol Assoc 81:34, 1970.
118. Powers JM, Spicer SS: Histochemical similarity of senile plaque amyloid to apudamyloid. Virchows Arch A Pathol 376:107, 1977.
119. Ishii T, Haga S: Immuno-electron microscopic localization of immunoglobulins in amyloid fibrils of senile plaques. Acta Neuropath 36:243, 1976.
120. Ishii T, Haga S, Shimizu F: Identification of components of immunoglobulins in senile plaques by means of fluorescent antibody technique. Acta Neuropath 32:157, 1975.
121. Bruni J, Bilbao JM, Pritzker KPH: Vascular amyloid in the aging central nervous system. Can J Neuro Sci 4:239, 1977.
122. Mandybur TI: The incidence of cerebral amyloid angiopathy in Alzheimer's disease. Neurology 25:120, 1975.
123. Miyakawa T, Uehara Y: Observations of amyloid angiopathy and senile plaques by the scanning electron microscope. Acta Neuropathol 48:153, 1979.
124. Harman D, Eddy DE, Noffsinger J: Free radical theory of aging: Inhibition of amyloidosis in mice by antioxidants; possible mechanism. J Am Ger Soc 24:203, 1976.
125. Torack RM: Adult dementia: History, biopsy, pathology. Neurosurgery 4:434, 1979.

126. Okazaki H, Reagan TJ, Campbell RJ: Clinicopathologic studies of primary cerebral amyloid angiopathy. Mayo Clin Proc 54:22, 1979.
127. Hodkinson M, Pomerance A: The clinical significance of senile cardiac amyloidosis: A prospective clinico-pathological study. Q J Med 46:381, 1977.
128. Wright JR, Calkins E: Amyloid in the aged heart: Frequency and clinical significance. J Am Ger Soc 23:97, 1975.
129. Kunze W-P: Senile pulmonary amyloidosis. Pathol Res Pract 164:413, 1979.
130. Isobe T, Osserman EF: Patterns of amyloidosis and their association with plasma-cell dyscrasia, monoclonal immunoglobulins and Bence-Jones proteins. N Engl J Med 290:473, 1974.
131. Lender M, Rosenblueth M: Amyloidosis of the kidneys: Review of patients and literature. South Afr Med J 49:813, 1975.
132. Cohen AS: Amyloidosis. N Engl J Med 277:628, 1967.
133. Child JS, Levisman JA, Abbasi AS, MacAlpin RN: Echocardiographic manifestations of infiltrative cardiomyopathy. Chest 70:6, 1976.
134. Swanton RH, Brooksby IAB, Davies MJ, Coltart DJ, Jenkins BS, Webb-Peploe MM: Systolic and diastolic ventricular function in cardiac amyloidosis. Am J Card 39:658, 1977.
135. Ridolfi RL, Bulkley BH, Hutchins GM: The conduction system in cardiac amyloidosis. Clinical and pathologic features of 23 patients. Am J Med 62:677, 1977.
136. Cassidy JT: Cardiac amyloidosis. Two cases with digitalis sensitivity. Ann Int Med 55:989, 1961.
137. Smith RRL, Hutchins GM: Ischemic heart disease secondary to amyloidosis of intramyocardial arteries. Am J Card 44:413, 1979.
138. Smith RRL, Hutchins GM, Moore GW, Humphrey RL: Type and distribution of pulmonary parenchymal and vascular amyloid. Am J Med 66:96, 1979.
139. Rubio PA, Farrell EM, Lehane DE: Primary liver amyloidosis producing obstructive jaundice. S Med J 72:891, 1979.
140. Pear BL: Big heart, tongue, and kidneys—stiff intestines. JAMA 241:58, 1979.
141. Battle WM, Rubin MR, Cohen AS, Snape WJ: Gastrointestinal-motility dysfunction in amyloidosis. N Engl J Med 301:24, 1979.
142. Kelly Jr JJ, Kyle RA, O'Brien PC, Dyck PJ: The natural history of peripheral neuropathy in primary systemic amyloidosis. Ann Neurol 6:1, 1979.
143. Rubinow A, Cohen AS: Skin involvement in generalized amyloidosis. A study of clinically involved and uninvolved skin in 50 patients with primary and secondary amyloidosis. Ann Intern Med 88:781, 1978.
144. Milutinovich J, Wu W, Savory J: Periorbital purpura after renal biopsy in primary amyloidosis. JAMA 242:2555, 1979.
145. Wiernik PH: Amyloid joint disease. Medicine 51:465, 1972.
146. Katz GA, Peter JB, Pearson CM, Adams WS: The shoulder-pad sign—a diagnostic feature of amyloid arthropathy. N Engl J Med 288:354, 1977.
147. Furie B, Voo L, McAdam KP, Furie BC: Mechanism of acquired factor X deficiency and systemic amyloidosis. N Engl J Med 304:827, 1981.
148. McPherson RA, Onstad JW, Ugoretz RJ, Wolf PL: Coagulopathy in amyloidosis: Combined deficiency of factors IX and X. Am J Hem 3:225, 1977.
149. Greipp PR, Kyle RA, Bowie EJW: Factor X deficiency in primary amyloidosis. N Engl J Med 301:1050, 1979.
150. Shemer J, Messer GY, Pras M, Gafni J: Amyloid in urinary sediments as a diagnostic technique. Ann Intern Med 90:61, 1979.
151. Pras M, Zaretzky J, Frangione B, Franklin EC: AA protein in a case of "primary" or "idiopathic" amyloidosis. Am J Med 68:291, 1980.

152. Cornwell III GG, Husby G, Westermark P, Natvig JB, Michaelsen TE, Skogen B: Identification and characterization of different amyloid fibril proteins in tissue sections. Scand J Immunol 6:1071, 1977.

153. Wright JR, Calkins E, Humphrey RL: Potassium permanganate reaction in amyloidosis. Lab Invest 36:274, 1977.

154. van Rijswijk MH, van Heusden CWGJ: The potassium permanganate method. Am J Pathol 97:43, 1979.

155. Kyle RA, Spencer RJ, Dahlin DC: Value of rectal biopsy in the diagnosis of primary systemic amyloidosis. Am J Med Sci 36:501, 1966.

156. Schroeder JF, Billingham ME, Rider AK: Cardiac Amyloidosis—Diagnosis by Transvenous Endomyocardial Biopsy. Am J Med 59:269, 1975.

157. Cohen HJ, Lessin LS, Hallal J, Burkholder P: Resolution of primary amyloidosis during chemotherapy. Studies in a patient with nephrotic syndrome. Ann Intern Med 82:466, 1975.

158. Bradstock K, Clancy R, Uther J, Basten A, Richards J: The successful treatment of primary amyloidosis with intermittent chemotherapy. Aust N Z J Med 8:176, 1978.

159. Schwartz RS, Cohen JR, Schrier SL: Therapy of primary amyloidosis with melphalan and prednisone. Arch Intern Med 139:1144, 1979.

160. Mehta AD: Regression of amyloidosis in multiple myeloma. Br J Clin Proc 32:358, 1978.

161. Buxbaum JN, Hurley ME, Chuba J, Spiro T: Amyloidosis of the AL type. Am J Med 67:867, 1979.

162. Cohen HJ: Combination chemotherapy for primary amyloidosis reconsidered. Ann Intern Med 89:572, 1978.

163. Kyle RA, Greipp PR: Primary systemic amyloidosis: Comparison of melphalan and prednisone versus placebo. Blood 52:818, 1978.

164. Michael J, Jones NF: Spontaneous remissions of nephrotic syndrome in renal amyloidosis. B Med J 1:1592, 1978.

165. Dikman SH, Kahn T, Gribetz D, Churg J: Resolution of renal amyloidosis. Am J Med 63:430, 1977.

166. Falck Hans M, Törnroth T, Skrifvars B, Wegelius O: Resolution of renal amyloidosis secondary to rheumatoid arthritis. Acta Med Scand 205:651, 1979.

167. Rey C, Escribano JC, Vidal MT: Retroperitoneal paraganglioma and systemic amyloidosis. Cancer 43:702, 1979.

168. Cohen AS, Bricetti AB, Harrington JT, Mannick JA: Renal transplantation in two cases of amyloidosis. Lancet 2:513, 1971.

169. Jones MB, Adams JM, Passer JA: Amyloidosis in a renal allograft in familial Mediterranean fever. Ann Intern Med 87:579, 1977.

170. Ravid M, Robson M, Kedar (Keizman) I: Prolonged colchicine treatment in four patients with amyloidosis. Ann Intern Med 87:568, 1977.

171. Kuhlbäck B, Falck H, Törnroth T, Wallenius M, Lindström BL, Pasternack A: Renal transplantation in amyloidosis. Acta Med Scand 205:169, 1979.

172. Light PD, Hall-Craggs M: Amyloid deposition in a renal allograft in a case of amyloidosis secondary to rheumatoid arthritis. Am J Med 66:532, 1979.

173. Kennedy CL, Castro JE: Transplantation for renal amyloidosis. Transplantation 24:382, 1977.

174. Jacob ET, Bar-Nathan N, Shapira Z, Gafni J: Renal transplantation in the amyloidosis of familial Mediterranean fever. Arch Intern Med 139:1135, 1979.

175. Ari JB, Zlotnik M, Oren A, Berlyne GM: Dialysis in renal failure caused by amyloidosis of familial Mediterranean fever. Arch Intern Med 136:449, 1976.

176. Shirahama T, Cohen AS: Blockage of amyloid induction by colchicine in an animal model. J Exp Med 140:1102, 1974.
177. Wright DG, Wolff SM, Fauci AS, Alling DW: Efficacy of intermittent colchicine therapy in familial Mediterranean fever. Ann Intern Med 86:162, 1977.
178. Kedar (Keizman) I, Greenwald M, Ravid M: Treatment of experimental murine amyloidosis with dimethyl sulfoxide. Eur J Clin Invest 7:149, 1977.
179. Ravid M, Kedar (Keizman) I, Sohar E: Effect of a single dose of dimethyl sulphoxide on renal amyloidosis. Lancet 1:730, 1977.
180. van Rijswijk MH, Donker AJM, Ruinen L: Dimethylsulphoxide in amyloidosis. Lancet 1:207, 1979.
181. Hanai N, Ishihara T, Uchino F, Imada N, Fujihara S, Ikegami J: Effects of dimethyl sulfoxide and colchicine on the resorption of experimental mayloid. Virchows Arch A Pathol 384:45, 1979.
182. Franklin EC: Immunopathology of the amyloid disease. Hosp Prac 15:70, 1980.
183. Cohen AS: An update of clinical, pathologic, and biochemical aspects of amyloidosis. Int J Dermatol 20:515, 1981.
184. Glenner GG: The bases of the staining of amyloid fibers: Their physico-chemical nature and the mechanism of their dye-substrate interaction. Prog Histochem Cytochem 13:1, 1981.
185. Benson MD: Partial amino acid sequence homology between an heredofamilial amyloid protein and human plasma prealbumin. J Clin Invest 67:1035, 1981.
186. Skinner M, Cohen AS: The prealbumin nature of the amyloid protein in familial amyloid polyneuropathy (FAP)-Swedish variety. Biochem Biophys Res Com 99:1326, 1981.
187. Tawara S, Araki S, Toshimori K, Nakagawa H, Ohtaki S: Amyloid fibril protein in type I familial amyloidotic polyneuropathy in Japanese. J Lab Clin Med 98:811, 1981.
188. Dalakas MC, Engel WK: Amyloid in hereditary amyloid polyneuropathy is related to prealbumin. Arch Neurol 38:420, 1981.
189. Gorevic PD, Franklin EC: Amyloidosis. Ann Rev Med 32:261, 1981.
190. Breathnach SM, Melrose SM, Bhogal B, de Beer FC, Dyck RF, Tennent G, Black MM, Pepys MB: Amyloid P component is located on elastic fibre microfibrils in normal human tissue. Nature 293:652, 1981.
191. Natigv JB, Westermark P, Sletten K, Husby G, Michaelsen T: Further structural and antigenic studies of light-chain amyloid proteins. Scand J Immunol 14:89, 1981.
192. Marhaug G, Husby G: Characterization of human amyloid-related protein SAA as a polymorphic protein: Association with albumin and prealbumin in serum. Clin Exp Immunol 45:97, 1981.
193. Bausserman LL, Herbert PN, McAdam KPWJ: Heterogeneity of human serum amyloid A proteins. J Exp Med 152:641, 1980.
194. Morrow JF, Stearman RS, Peltzman CG, Potter DA: Induction of hepatic synthesis of serum amyloid A protein and actin. Proc Natl Acad Sci USA 78:4718, 1981.
195. Kyle RA: Amyloidosis, Parts 1, 2 and 3. Int J Dermatol 19:537, 1980, 20:20, 1981, 20:75, 1981.
196. Ratz JL, Bailin PL: Cutaneous amyloidosis. J Am Acad Dermatol 4:21, 1981.
197. Fujihara S, Glenner GG: Primary localized amyloidosis of the Genitourinary Tract. Lab Invest 44:55, 1981.
198. Finn DG, Farmer JC Jr: Management of amyloidosis of the larynx and trachea. Arch Otolaryngol 108:54, 1982.
199. Huston DP, McAdams KP, Balow JE, Bass R, DeLellis RA: Amyloidosis in systemic lupus erythematosus. Am J Med 70:320, 1981.

200. Vanley CT, Aguilar MJ, Kleinhenz RJ, Lagio MD: Cerebral amyloid angiopathy. Hum Pathol 12:609, 1981.
201. Wright JR, Calkins E: Clinical-pathologic differentiation of common amyloid syndromes. Medicine 60:429, 1981.
202. Glenner GG: Amyloidosis: The hereditary disorders, including Alzheimer's disease. J Lab Clin Med 98:807, 1981.
203. Siqueira-Filho AG, Cunha CLP, Tajik AJ, Seward JB, Schattenberg TT, Giuliani ER: M-mode and two-dimensional echocardiographic features in cardiac amyloidosis. Circulation 63:188, 1981.
204. Tyberg TI, Goodyer AVN, Hurst VW, Alexander J, Langou RA: Left ventricular filling in differentiating restrictive amyloid cardiomyopathy and constrictive pericarditis. Am J Card 47:791, 1981.
205. Ribinow A, Skinner M, Cohen AS: Digoxin sensitivity in amyloid cardiomyopathy. Circulation 63:1285, 1981.
206. Giacchino R, Stratta P, Aprato A, Belardi P, Mazzucco G, Cirone U, De Filippi PG, Segoloni G, Vercellone A, Picolli G: Renal amyloidosis and treatment with dimethyl-sulphoxide (DMSO). Min Nefr 27:559, 1980.

Pathology of Immunoglobulins: Diagnostic and
Clinical Aspects, pages 325–382
© 1982 Alan R. Liss, Inc., 150 Fifth Avenue, New York, NY 10011

12

Unusual Manifestations of Plasma-Cell Dyscrasia

Waldemar Pruzanski, MD

INTRODUCTION

Plasma-cell dyscrasia denotes excessive, usually uncontrolled, proliferation of plasmalymphocytic clone(s) of cells that are capable of synthesizing homogeneous immunoglobulins—M-components. Such proliferation, also called monoclonal gammopathy, is usually malignant, although in some instances a very prolonged stationary phase or even regression in the rate of synthesis of an M-component may occur, thus undermining the classical definition of a malignant process [19]. Until about a quarter of a century ago only two diseases, multiple myeloma and macroglobulinemia of Waldenström, belonged to the group of monoclonal gammopathies. Subsequently, benign monoclonal gammopathy and heavy chain diseases were added to this group. Today, a great variety of conditions with monoclonal gammopathy have been described. The discovery of clinically atypical or intermediate forms makes the diagnosis often difficult and uncertain. It has been recognized that B-cell neoplasia can present with a variety of clinical manifestations that do not conform to the orthodox nomenclature and that a new classification based on the combination of immunologic, enzymatic, biochemical, and genetic markers is required. An attempt to develop such modern classification has already been made [218], but a more definitive one is needed. Recognizing these limitations, this chapter by virtue of necessity attempts to describe rather than to explain various unusual manifestations of plasma cell dyscrasias.

PLASMA-CELL DYSCRASIA WITH MULTIPLE M-COMPONENTS

The great majority of patients with plasma cell dyscrasia (PCD) have only one M-component in the serum, and when Bence Jones proteinuria occurs, the type of Bence Jones protein (BJP) is identical to the light chain of the circulating M-component.

PCD with multiple M-components (MMC) may be defined as a condition where more than one M-component is synthesized by the immunoglobulin (Ig)-producing cells [1,4,8,24,26,27,33,46,49,50,53,57,58,63,67,68,71,83 85, 87, 88, 111, 116, 117, 121, 123, 130, 134a, 138, 155, 163, 177, 184, 193, 202, 215, 219, 224, 227, 232, 235, 251, 252a, 256, 259, 263, 264, 271, 280, 283]. The heavy (H) and/or light (L) chains of these M-components should exhibit at least minimal differences, even if they belong to the same class and/or type.

The incidence of MMC is low, ranging from 0.14% to 3.2% [134a]. Only 4 sera with two M-components were found among 500 sera with M-components (0.8%) [138]. In other series, MMC was noted in 0.5% of 789 sera with M-components [4] and in 1.7% of the sera from 870 myeloma patients [232]. However, the incidence of MMC is probably underestimated. Two M-components may have similar (Fig. 1) or identical (Fig. 2) electrophoretic mobility, thus, the presence of one spike on serum electropherogram does not rule out MMC. Furthermore, if the concentration is low, some M-components may not be visible on the electrophoretic strip. Thus, accurate diagnosis of MMC requires the use of numerous antisera specific to various H and L chains in each case of monoclonal gammopathy, regardless of the electrophoretic findings. Alternatively, the presence of several spikes does not necessarily denote MMC. For example, the presence of several molecular species of the same monoclonal immunoglobulin [256], postsynthetic deamination [85], an excess of L chains in the serum in addition to the whole-molecular M-component [283], or pseudospikes (nonimmunoglobulins) [280] cannot be classified as true MMC.

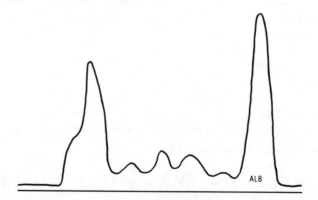

Fig. 1.   Serum electrophoresis. Spike of γ-mobility contained IgG/λ, 19 S IgM/λ, 7 S IgM/λ, and Bence Jones λ-type protein. ALB = albumin.

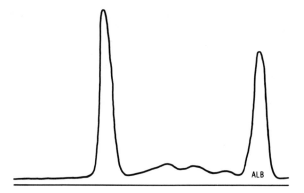

Fig. 2. Serum electrophoresis. Spike of γ-mobility contained IgG/κ, IgG/λ, and Bence Jones λ-type protein. ALB = albumin.

TABLE I. Plasma Cell Dyscrasia with Multiple M-Components

IgG/κ + IgG/κ [232][a]	IgM/κ + IgM/κ [87,88]
IgG/λ + IgG/λ [232]	IgM + IgE [227]
IgG/κ + IgG/λ [26,232,235,271]	IgG/κ(s)[b] + BJP/λ (u)[b] [155]
IgG/κ + IgA/κ [46,67,138,224,232]	IgG/λ(s) + BJP/κ(u) [63]
IgG/κ + IgA/λ [57]	IgA/κ(s) + BJP/λ + BJP/κ(u) [50]
IgG/λ + IgA/κ [138]	IgG + IgA + IgM [219]
IgG/λ + IgA/λ [232]	IgG₃/λ + IgA₁/κ + IgA₂/κ [202]
IgG/κ + IgM/κ	IgG/κ + IgA/κ + IgM/λ [116]
[163,193,219,232,251,263]	
IgG/κ + IgM/λ [24]	IgG/κ + IgG/λ + IgM/κ [33]
IgG/λ + IgM/λ [184,193,219]	BJP/λ(s) + BJP/λ and BJP/κ(u) [49,83]
IgG₁/κ + IgD/λ [177]	
IgA/κ + IgM/κ [68]	
IgA/λ + IgM/λ [193]	

[a]Reference.
[b]s = serum; u = urine.

Multiple gammopathy applies not only to the serum. The presence of one M-component in the serum and a different M-component in another fluid or in a tissue is classified as true MMC [58].

MMC may be represented by almost any combination of M-components of various classes of H chains and/or types of L chains (Tables I and II). Usually two M-components present as two separate spikes on serum electrophoretic strip [24,33,46,67,68,177,215] (Fig. 3) or in the urine [50,63,83]. In some instances, however, MMC may present as one spike in the serum

TABLE II. Plasma Cell Dyscrasia with M-Components and Heavy Chain Disease (HCD) Proteins

IgG/λ + γ-HCD [71][a]	IgM/κ + γ-HCD and BJP/κ (u) [121]
IgG₃/λ + γ₃-HCD [1]	IgM/κ + γ₃-HCD [264]
IgG₁/λ + γ₁-HCD [130]	IgM/λ + γ-HCD [259]
IgA/κ + μ-HCD [117]	

[a]Reference.

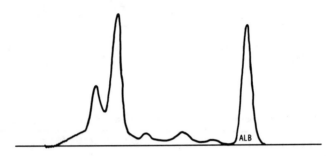

Fig. 3.   Serum electrophoresis. Two spikes, the slower one containing IgG/λ and the faster one IgM/λ. ALB = albumin.

[116] (Fig. 2) or in the urine [49]. Appearance of a new spike in the serum may follow the earlier one [33,163,177,224,235,271]. Similarly, BJP of one type may follow excretion of BJP of another type in the urine [33]. M-components in MMC may respond differently to chemotherapy (Fig. 4). In a case of IgG + IgG MMC, only one spike disappeared during chemotherapy [8]. In another case of MMC there were initially two spikes in the serum, representing IgD/λ and BJP/λ; both disappeared on chemotherapy. Later, when the patient was in remission, a new M-component, IgG₁/κ, developed and again chemotherapy was given. Subsequently, the concentration of IgG/κ M-component declined markedly, and at the same time the IgD/λ M-component reappeared [177].

MMC may be found in malignant and benign conditions as well as in apparently healthy individuals. Jensen described a healthy person who had three M-components—IgG, IgA, and IgM—in the serum [116]. Classical multiple myeloma (MM) was observed in patients with IgG + IgG [26,235], IgG + IgA [46,215,224], and IgG + IgM [163,251] MMC. Diagnosis of myeloma was made in patients with two different BJPs in the urine [49,50,63,83], discordant L chain types in the serum M-component and

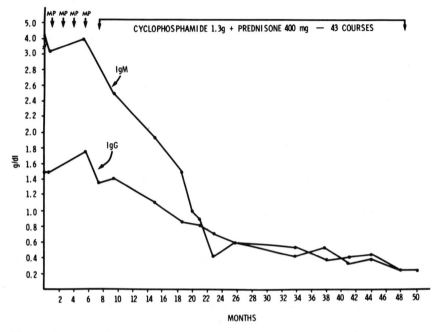

Fig. 4. Response of two M-components to chemotherapy. The conc ation of IgM was reduced to 50% of the pretreatment value in less than 14 months; of IgG in more than 22 months.

urinary BJP [155], IgG + IgD gammopathy [177], and in a patient with IgG/λ and γ-H chain disease (HCD) protein [71]. MM was diagnosed in a patient who had BJP type κ-protein in the serum and IgA/κ M-component in the cerebrospinal fluid [58].

In many other cases, however, the clinical picture did not conform to that of MM [134a]. More than 30 cases in which one of the M-components was IgM and the other belonged to either IgG, IgA, or IgE class have been reported [70a,193,227]. Only a few patients had MM. Three patients had a solitary plasmacytoma [184,193,219] and one had plasma-cell leukemia. In six patients the clinical picture was compatible with macroglobulinemia of Waldenström (MW). Two patients had lymphosarcoma and one had amyloidosis. None of the others had definite clinical manifestations of a malignant plasmalymphocytic disease [24,193,219]. Skin lesions, polyarthralgia, anemia, and chronic thyroiditis were observed. Plasma-cell leukemia was observed in a patient with IgM and γ-HCD protein [121]. Abdominal lymphoma was found in another patient with IgM and γ-HCD [259], whereas a third patient with the same combination of M-components did not have any obvious malignant disease and survived for more than 15 years [264].

A patient with IgG + IgA had polycythemia vera followed by anemia, azotemia, and bone marrow plasmacytosis [57]. IgG/κ + IgG/λ MMC was found in a patient with Von Recklinghausen's disease [271]. The same combination of M-components along with two BJPs, κ and λ, in the urine was reported in a child with type I dysgammaglobulinemia [33]. Children with severe combined immunodeficiency may occasionally have M-components in the serum before bone marrow transplantation; however, MMC is more common after the transplant. These M-components are usually transient [202].

Some patients with whole-molecular M-components and γ-HCD protein presented clinically with γ-HCD disease [1], while others had unusual clinical manifestations such as polyarthritis, vasculitis, hyperviscosity [130], or recurrent fever [111]. One patient with IgA M-component and μ-HCD presented with splenomegaly and ulcerating lesion over his earlobe [117].

It would appear that the *clinical picture in patients with MMC is not related directly to the type or class of serum M-components*. In several cases the condition resembled a collagen or an autoimmune disease. It is possible that M-components in these patients developed as a result of chronic antigenic stimulation and did not represent a malignant condition in the strict sense.

The pathogenesis of MMC is not clear. The simplest explanation would be that two separate B-cell clones proliferate simultaneously or sequentially as a result of one or more mitogenic insults. An alternative possibility is that one clone of cells produces two different polypeptide chains. These two alternatives have been studied by immunofluorescent techniques and by comparing multiple M-components for immunochemical and antigenic differences. In some patients with two M-components, the same myeloma cells produced both Igs. In the case of IgG + IgA MMC, plasmacytes from the bone marrow and from plasmacytomas contained both M-components [46]. In another patient with IgG$_1$/κ + IgG$_1$/λ MMC, the determinants of both κ- and λ-L chains were found in the same plasma cells [26]. In another patient with IgG + IgA + IgM MMC, single plasma cells contained two of three M-components [219]. Analysis of 141 sera with two M-components showed highly significant frequency of L chains of the same type on both M-components ($P < 0.005$). This suggested a linkage in the synthesis of the two proteins [27].

In other patients, however, two separate clones each synthesized one M-component [24,57,224,263]. In two patients with IgG + IgM MMC and in two others with IgG + IgA MMC, different clones of plasma cells produced individual M-components [24,57,224,263]. One patient with IgG/λ + IgA/λ MMC had three types of plasma cells in the bone marrow; two types produced one M-component each and another type produced both M-components [215].

In one patient, study of the L chains in IgG/κ + IgM/κ MMC showed identical peptide mapping, circular dichroism, and amino acid analysis. However, each M-component was synthesized by a separate clone. The authors concluded that a single type of L polypeptide chain was synthesized by two different clones [263]. In another case of IgM/λ + IgG/λ MMC, both M-components shared idiotypic determinants on the H and on the L chains. L chains, however, were not identical as examined by the peptide mapping [184]. Lack of identity of the L chains in three other cases of MMC was proven by differences in Inv and Oz markers [219]. In a case of two BJPs, κ and λ, in the urine, variable parts were found to be different [83].

Variable results were obtained as well when H chains were studied. In a patient with IgG + IgA MMC, both M-components shared idiotypic antigenic determinants but were produced by different plasma cell clones [224]. Similarity of idiotypic determinants was noted in IgG + IgA MMC [67,215]. In a case of $IgG_1/κ$ + $IgG_1/λ$ MMC, identical antigenic determinants were detected on the variable regions of the H chain of both M-components [26].

It seems, therefore, that MMC may be caused by either proliferation of several homogeneous clones of plasma cells or by production of several M-components by the same clone. In the case of sequential appearance of different M-components, a switch-over from production of one Ig to another may occur. Such a mechanism has been documented in animals.

PLASMA-CELL DYSCRASIA WITH HALF-MOLECULE M-COMPONENTS

In a few patients with PCD, IgG M-components composed of only one H and one L chain have been reported [22,23,98,119,226,237,238,239,246]. The clinical manifestations varied from patient to patient. A 76-year-old man had plasmacytic infiltrate in the lymph nodes, liver, and spleen, but not in the bone marrow. Serum and urine contained a γ-spike, which was shown to be an IgG/κ half-molecule with molecular weight of 75,000 daltons [98]. Another patient had plasma-cell leukemia and $IgG_1/κ$ half-molecules with $S_{20,w}$ value of 4.3 in the serum and urine. This M-component failed to precipitate with anti-Fc antiserum. The H chain had large deletion in $Cγ_3$ domain [237]. Another patient had MM and $IgG_1/κ$ half-molecules in the serum. The same M-component along with BJP type κ-protein was found in the urine. This M-component also failed to precipitate with anti-Fc antiserum and showed double precipitation line with anti-IgG antiserum [226].

Five patients with IgA half-molecules, two with κ- and three with λ-L chains, were reported [22,23,119,239,246]. There were three patients with MM, one with plasma-cell leukemia, and one with tuberculosis. In one patient with myeloma, IgA_1/κ half-molecules with $S_{20,w}$ value of 3.9 and molecular weight of 59,000 were detected, along with 7S IgA. In other cases molecular weights varied from 40,000 to 53,000 daltons. Anti-α antiserum showed double precipitation arc on serum immunoelectrophoresis (IEP) [246].

Several "broken" M-components have been found in patients with PCD. A 47-year-old patient with malignant lymphoma had IgM/κ M-component with $S_{20,w}$ value of 6.1 and molecular weight of 130,000 daltons. Immunochemical analysis characterized this M-component as $F(ab)_2\mu$ [54]. IgG_1/κ M-component with $S_{20,w}$ value of 5.4 and molecular weight of 125,000 daltons was observed in a patient with scleroderma-like disease. This M-component had deletions in both H and L chains [144]. Similar cases with deletions in the H and/or L chains and lower than normal molecular weight have subsequently been described.

NONSECRETORY MULTIPLE MYELOMA

Nonsecretory multiple myeloma (NSM) [5, 9, 15, 17, 18, 44, 51, 56, 65, 69a, 75, 81, 97, 107, 109, 118, 122, 126, 151, 152, 154, 162, 165, 167a, 172, 183,187,201,206,234,240,242,243,253,257,269,270] can be defined as otherwise typical myeloma where neither serum nor appropriately concentrated urine contains antigenically active M-components or their fragments that can be detected by the presently available techniques. The prevalence of NSM among the myelomas is about 1% [97]. In our series, four cases were diagnosed among more than 1200 myeloma patients. More than 90 cases of NSM have been reported, but not many were fully described. Age varied from 38 years to 79 years, mean 58.6 years, and median age of 59 years. About 60% of patients were males.

Subjective complaints were remarkably similar to secretory myeloma: backache, sciatic syndrome, and pain in the ribs were frequent complaints. Occasionally, hepato- and/or splenomegaly, pathological fractures, general weakness, and weight loss were the predominant clinical manifestations.

In 21 reported patients, more or less severe anemia was reported, whereas 17 patients had normal hemoglobin. Azotemia was reported in 8 of 19 patients and hypercalcemia in 8 of 25 examined patients. Osteolytic lesions were almost invariably multiple. Bone marrow, with only three exceptions, was heavily infiltrated with myeloma cells, which often completely replaced normal marrow elements. When counted in 28 patients, the myeloma cells were on average 53% of the bone marrow cells. In a few cases plasma-cell leukemia was observed [118,152,183,257]. Extraskeletal spread was reported in a few patients [59] and amyloidosis in one [9]. Immunoquantitation showed low

IgG, IgA, and IgM in 40 of 54 reported patients; in many others low γ-globulin was observed on electrophoretic strip.

Immunofluorescent study of myeloma cells in the bone marrow was reported in 65 patients. In 9, no intracellular proteins were detected (*nonproducers*) [69a,81,109,154,162,172,183,206], whereas in 56, positive identification of intracellular Igs was obtained (producers, *nonsecretors*) [5,9,17,107,118,152,154,165,167a,172,187,201,240,253,257,269,270, and others]. The intracellular Igs were IgG/κ, 26; IgG/λ, 3; IgA/κ, 2; IgA/λ, 9; IgA, 1; IgM, 1; κ-L chains, 11; λ-L chain, 1, IgD/κ, 1. In one instance, λ-L chains, μ- and λ-chains were found. Electron microscopic studies of myeloma cells in NSM almost invariably showed dilated, rough endoplasmic reticulum and prominent Golgi apparatus, even in the absence of intracellular Igs [118,152,240,270].

Survival in 17 patients, who subsequently died, was 3–96 months, mean 25.0 months. In 13 patients who were still alive at the time of reporting, survival was 3–120 months, mean 23.9 months. Thus, the statement that NSM carries the worst prognosis among myelomas [97] cannot be substantiated. It seems that there is *no significant clinical difference between NSM and secretory myeloma*. It can be concluded that since osteolytic lesions are invariably present in NSM, the excretion of osteoclast activating factor is not linked to the production or secretion of Igs.

The mechanism(s) preventing production and/or secretion of Igs from myeloma cells has not been elucidated. Faulty molecular machinery on DNA/RNA levels [240], secretion of nonantigenic Ig fragments [206] and several others have been proposed, but not yet proven. The evidence for the lack of secretion depends on the available techniques. In one instance when routine IEP was normal, sensitive radioimmunoassay detected homogeneous κ-chain polymer in the serum [234]. In some cases transient appearance of BJP in the serum [122], intermittent Bence Jones proteinuria [118,122] and late or transient appearance of IgA or IgG M-components was observed [118].

IgM MULTIPLE MYELOMA

In 1944, Waldenström described a new syndrome characterized by the presence of M-component, anemia, lymphadenopathy, hepatosplenomegaly, and a high incidence of hyperviscosity syndrome [261]. Subsequently this condition was called macroglobulinemia of Waldenström and the characteristic M-component was called IgM. Although the typical forms of MW and MM are clinically and prognostically quite different, several intermediate forms have been described such as plasmacytomas with IgM M-components, syndromes clinically typical for MW but with other than IgM M-components and osteolytic lesions in otherwise typical MW. In a series of 41 patients with MW, 8 had osteolytic lesions and 7 had prominent osteoporosis [258]. The plasmacytic nature of osteolytic lesions in MW has not always been ascertained, since in another series of 40 patients with MW, 3 had osteolytic lesions and in each the biopsy showed lymphosarcoma and not plasmacytoma [161].

One of the intermediate forms is clinically typical MM with IgM M-component, or so-called IgM myeloma. More than 40 cases have been reported, but not all of them have been well described [2,21,29,31,32,36, 37,66,93,96,97,102,140,188,210,216,223,252,258,262,265,268,279]. The incidence of IgM myeloma is about 0.5% [97]. We observed two such cases among about 1200 patients with MM and approximately 2200 M-components. In another series, 10 patients with IgM myeloma and 6 with extramedullary plasmacytoma and IgM M-component were observed among 204 IgM M-components, including 58 patients with MW [36].

In 25 patients with IgM myeloma, more or less complete clinical description was provided. Age varied from 43 to 76 years, mean 59 years. The proportion of men to women was 1:1. Nine patients complained of pain, mainly in the lower back; seven others suffered mostly from bleeding diathesis and anemia. Hepato- and/or splenomegaly and lymphadenopathy were quite common. In one case bilateral malignant exophthalmos due to orbital plasmacytic infiltrates was the main manifestation [252]. In one patient IgG M-component and plasmacytic infiltration of the bone marrow preceded development of IgM myeloma by 3 years [188]. In all patients osteolytic lesions were observed, with or without osteoporosis, and in all bone marrow was infiltrated, usually quite heavily, with plasma cells. The description of plasma cells in the bone marrow varied from "typical" plasmacytes [29,31,66,93,188,210,216,258,279], immature plasmacytes [21,37,252,258], myeloma cells [258, ours], plasmacytoid lymphocytes [21,223,265], to lymphoid reticulum cells [265]. An increase in the mast cells has also been noted [223]. In three cases immunofluorescent study identified IgM M-component in the plasma cells [258, ours]. Anemia was found in 17 patients, whereas only 2 had normal hemoglobin. Normal calcium level was reported in 6 patients and hypercalcemia in 8 others. Five patients had azotemia and 8 had normal renal function. IgG was low in 13 patients and normal in one. All 14 had low IgA. Bence Jones proteinuria was found in 23 patients. Serum hyperviscosity was noted in 8 patients. In 3 patients plasma cell leukemia was observed [223,265,268]. In two of them, IgM M-component was cryoprecipitable [223,265].

Patients with IgM myeloma were treated similarly to other myeloma patients. Occasionally chlorambucil was given either instead of or in addition to other chemotherapeutic agents.

The survival varied from 3 months to 8 years, mean 30.6 months. Four of 8 patients living at the time of reporting, and 5 of 8 patients who had died survived for longer than 2 years. Thus, the 24 months' survival rate was at least 70%.

Autopsies of patients with IgM myeloma usually showed histological picture indistinguishable from other myelomas [37,93,210,258]. Myeloma kidney [210] and frequent plasmacytic infiltration in various organs and tissues were observed [37,66,93,252,258,265,268]. Occasionally lympho-plasmacytic rather than typical plasmacytic infiltration was observed [93,265].

It seems, therefore, that the *incidence of organomegaly and lymphade-nopathy and the hyperviscosity syndrome is higher in IgM myeloma than in other classes of myeloma.* On the other hand, *the incidence of azotemia and hypercalcemia is higher than in MW.*

MULTIPLE MYELOMA WITH FEATURES OF WALDENSTRÖM'S DISEASE

Clinical differences between MM and MW have been well documented [129,194]. However, patients with M-components conventionally seen in myeloma may present clinically as MW [80]. Twelve such patients were reported [39,94,204,254,260; Pruzanski—personal observation]. There were 7 men and 5 women aged from 40 to 80 years, mean 62 years. They presented with general weakness, tiredness, pallor, visual disorders, and hemorrhagic dyscrasia. In 8 of 12 patients, hepato- and/or splenomegaly was detected and 4 had lymphadenopathy. Ten patients had anemia. Peripheral blood lym-phocytosis and elevated sedimentation rate were common and occasionally thrombocytopenia was observed. Five patients had positive Coombs' test [254,260]. There was no cryoglobulinemia. Serum hyperviscosity was re-corded in some patients [39,260; Pruzanski—personal observation]. In only one patient was hypercalcemia detected [Pruzanski—personal observation], and all but one patient [260] had normal renal functions. M-components were of IgA class in 5 patients and of IgG class in the remaining 7 patients. L chain type was reported in 5 patients, being κ in 4 and λ in 1 patient. Serum of one patient contained also BJP/κ protein [Pruzanski—personal observa-tion]. In 10 patients reduction in the concentration of polyclonal Ig was noted. Bence Jones proteinuria was recorded in 3 patients [39,260; Pru-zanski—personal observation]. Bone marrow aspirates invariably showed mixed infiltration, predominantly of lymphocytic type with an admixture of plasma cells and plasmacytoid lymphocytes. In one patient the marrow also contained 10% eosinophils [39]. Skeletal x-rays were normal in all 12 pa-tients. Seven patients were alive at the time of reporting, after a follow-up of from 6 months to 7 years [204,254; Pruzanski—personal observation]. Four patients had died after a follow-up of a few weeks up to 7 years [39,94,254]. No information was given on one case [260].

PLASMA-CELL DYSCRASIA WITH LEUKEMIC FEATURES

Plasma-cell leukemia (PCL) is a rare from of PCD. More than 100 cases of PCL have been reported [112,131,191,275,282]. The incidence of PCL among myeloma patients varies from less than 2% to 6% [112,131], the difference depending on the diagnostic criteria. Lower incidence was reported when the diagnosis of PCL was made only when peripheral blood plasma cells exceeded 20% of the while blood cell count [131]; higher incidence was noted when the acceptable number of plasma cells was over 10% [112].

Clinically, PCL resembles acute leukemia rather than MM, having less advanced bone disease, common infiltration of organs and tissues, prominent anemia, and frequent azotemia [16,112,131,191,275,282]. It may present from the beginning as an acute leukemia or may appear late in the course of MM [131,191,275]. In one series leukemia preceded more obvious manifestations of myeloma in twelve cases and followed myeloma in five [131].

Analysis of more than 100 patients with PCL showed that 65% were males. In a Japanese series of 13 patients, only males were found [112]. The age varied from 28 years to 82 years, mean age ranging in different series from 51 to 59.5 years. The clinical picture was dominated by general fatigue, tiredness, weight loss, and hemorrhagic manifestations. Skeletal pain occurred in about half of the patients, being less frequent than in MM. Hepatomegaly was recorded in 57%, splenomegaly in 46%, and lymphadenopathy in 28% of the patients. For comparison, liver enlargement was observed in about 20% and spleen enlargement in less than 5% of patients with MM [131]. Plasmacytic infiltrates in various organs and tissues are not rare in PCL.

Anemia, usually more marked than in myeloma patients, was noted in over 75% and thrombocytopenia was recorded in about 70% of patients with PCL. The total peripheral white blood count varied from normal to more than $250,000/mm^3$ with variable percentage of plasmacytes and plasmablasts in the peripheral blood. It was suggested that plasmacytes in PCL are smaller than in MM [112] and the nuclei are more immature [275]. Increase in the counts of lymphocytes, monoblasts, and occasionally eosinophils was also noted. Erythrocyte sedimentation rate was usually very high. Azotemia was found in more than 70% and hypercalcemia in 48% of patients, both being more frequent than in MM. In the majority of patients the bone marrow was heavily infiltrated with abnormal plasma cells. Plasmacytes of various maturity, plasmablasts, lymphocytoid plasmacytes and lymphocytes were observed in the bone marrow in PCL [191]. Radiologic surveys showed osteo-lytic lesions in 58% of patients, however when osteoporosis and pathologic fractures were included, the total incidence of skeletal abnormalities was close to 70%.

Electrophoretic abnormalities in serum proteins were observed in more than 90% of patients with PCL. Immunoelectrophoretic analysis was done in over 50 patients and showed IgG M-component in 43%, Bence Jones proteinemia in 33%, and other M-components in 22%. A few cases of IgD [16] and one of IgE M-components have been reported in PCL. Seventy percent of identified BJP in the serum were of the λ type. There is not enough information about L chain types of IgG or IgA M-components in PCL. Proteinuria was observed in over 75% of patients with PCL; 76% of patients with proteinuria had BJP in the urine, which was of λ-type in 60% and κ-type in 40%. When the data on serum and urinary proteins were combined, approximately 95% of patients with PCL were found to have some protein abnormality. This incidence is similar to that observed in MM.

Patients with PCL have been treated with various chemotherapeutic agents, irradiation, blood transfusions, etc. Therapeutic remissions were usually of short duration, from 1–3 months. Fifty percent or more of the patients sur-vived for less than one month from diagnosis [191,275]. However, in one series survival of 40% of patients for more than a year was reported [131]. In another group the mean survival from onset was 9.2 months and from diagnosis 7 months [112]. Prolonged survival of more than 4 years has been observed as well [282].

Autopsy usually showed widespread plasmacytic infiltrates in various or-gans and tissues. Occasionally, accumulations of plasma cells resembled plasmacytomas [191]. Amyloidosis was found in two patients only, and myeloma kidney was much less common than in MM.

PLASMA-CELL DYSCRASIA WITH OSTEOSCLEROTIC LESIONS

The majority of patients with MM present with osteolytic lesions and/or osteoporosis [132]. As a result of treatment and healing and occasionally after fractures, osteosclerotic reaction may be observed in the osteolytic lesions. Cases of MM presenting from the beginning with osteosclerotic lesions are very rare. About 80 such cases were reported [60,134a,203a]. The incidence of PCD with osteosclerotic lesions is not known, since their presence, especially when osteolytic lesions are found as well, may not necessarily be recorded. It seems, however, that the osteosclerotic process occurs in about 1% of patients with MM.

Clinical and laboratory data collected in 68 patients are presented in Table III [60]. Forty percent of patients had osteosclerotic lesions only, whereas

TABLE III. Data on 68 Patients with Plasma-Cell Dyscrasia and Osteosclerotic Lesions

Age	28-81 (mean 55.3)
Sex (M/F)	43/25
Skeletal pain	30/68 (44%)
Bone or soft tissue swelling	6/68 (9%)
Neurologic symptoms[a]	33/68 (49%)
Hepatomegaly	11/68 (16%)
Splenomegaly	7/68 (10%)
Lymphadenopathy	7/68 (10%)
ESR > 20 mm/h	18/30 (60%)
Anemia (Hb < 12.0 g/dL)	29/55 (53%)
Polycythemia (Hb ≥ 18.0 g/dL)	5/55 (9%)
Azotemia (BUN ≥ 30 mg/dL or Creatinine ≥ 1.5 mg/dL)	11/33 (33%)
Hypercalcemia (Ca ≥ 11 mg/dL)	3/37 (8%)
High alkaline phosphatase	7/37 (19%)
Hypoalbuminemia (< 3.5 g/dL)	10/38 (26%)
Serum M-component[b]	38/61 (62%)
Proteinuria	17/32 (53%)
Skeletal lesions ≤ 3	16/68 (24%)
> 3	52/68 (76%)

[a]30 had peripheral polyneuropathy.
[b]By electrophoresis.

60% had both lytic and sclerotic lesions. Comparison of these two groups showed that patients with sclerotic lesions only had less skeletal pain and bone swelling. Anemia was less pronounced and some patients had polycythemia. Azotemia and hypercalcemia were rare.

When the whole group of 68 patients was compared to MM in general, some striking differences were found. Early onset of the disease was significantly different from MM. Skeletal pain was less common, whereas hepato- and/or splenomegaly and lymphadenopathy were more common than in MM. Thirty of 68 patients developed peripheral polyneuropathy. The incidence of elevated sedimentation rate, anemia, azotemia, and hypercalcemia was lower than in MM. Mean survival time was less than 20 months from the first symptoms and 12 months from diagnosis.

The proposed mechanisms of bone destruction in MM are mechanical pressure of myelomatous infiltrates and secretion of the osteoclast-activating factor (OAF) by plasma cells. The mechanism of the osteosclerotic process has not been elucidated. In one patient, a high level of calcitonin was found in the plasma and the lymph nodes [211,212] and the authors proposed that hypercalcitoninemia may initiate the osteosclerotic process. However, in our patients a normal level of calcitonin was found in the serum [198]. The phenomenon of osteosclerosis may indicate either the failure of production of OAF by plasmacytes and/or an ability of the host to respond to the infiltration by malignant plasma cells by osteoblastic activity. This would reflect a host-tumor relationship different from that observed in MM in general. The differences in the clinical picture and laboratory manifestations between osteosclerotic myeloma and MM in general are in favor of this hypothesis.

PLASMA-CELL DYSCRASIA WITH PERIPHERAL POLYNEUROPATHY

Peripheral polyneuropathy (PPN) occurs rarely in PCD, the incidence being less than 1% [61]. Many single cases and a few small series have been reported, and the total number of cases is now well over 50 [61,134a,203a]. PPN usually is of a mixed motor-sensory type, involving all extremities and presenting histologically as demyelination and axonal degeneration.

Analysis of the clinical picture of 54 patients with PCD and PPN [61] has shown some significant differences as compared to MM in general [132]. There was higher prevalence of males (78%), and the patients were significantly younger than those with classic MM—48% being younger than 51 years at diagnosis.

The majority of patients presented initially with symptoms related to polyneuropathy; less than 15% complained of skeletal pain. Even at the time of diagnosis skeletal pain was a major complaint in only one third of the patients, as compared to about 70% of patients with MM in general; the difference being significant at $P < 0.001$. Physical findings were primarily related to the peripheral nerves. Mixed sensory-motor deficit was observed in over 80% of patients, whereas isolated motor or sensory deficits were seen in less than 20%. In about 70% of patients all four extremities were involved. Hepato- and/or splenomegaly were not common (< 10%), however lymphadenopathy was detected in 17% of cases, compared to 4% in myeloma in general.

Laboratory investigation showed anemia with hemoglobin of less than 12 g/dL in 45% of cases, compared to 62% of myeloma patients in general. There were 6 patients with polycythemia. Thrombocytopenia was not observed and white cell count was usually normal. Erythrocyte sedimentation rate was seldom high, being over 40 mm/h in only one third of the patients.

Azotemia was less frequent than in MM in general, 44% vs. 55%, and hypercalcemia was not observed in 21 examined patients. The total serum protein was elevated in less than one third of patients and electrophoresis showed an M-component in 45% of patients, contrasting with 76% in myeloma. Serum IEP as reported in 20 patients detected homogeneous IgG in 14, IgA in 3, BJP/λ in 1 and no abnormalities in 2 patients. L chains were identified on ten M-components and in all instances were of the λ-type. In only ten cases was urine electrophoresis reported, showing abnormal bands in three. Examination of cerebrospinal fluid (CSF) was reported in 40 patients and showed increased protein in 36 (90%). In 5 of 11 examined CSFs an M-component was found. In 23 of 24 examined CSFs the cell count was normal, and in 5 CSFs examined no plasma cells were found.

Bone marrow plasmacytosis was found in 98% of the patients showing both pleomorphism and increase in the number of plasma cells. Radiological study showed osteosclerotic lesions with or without osteolytic lesions in 55% of cases, whereas osteolytic lesions were observed in 24%. In the remaining patients, either osteoporosis or normal skeleton were observed.

Electromyographic and nerve conduction studies showed fibrillations, denervation potentials, and slow conduction. Histological studies showed axonal degeneration and demyelination in the peripheral nerves and neurogenic atrophy in the muscles.

Forty patients received chemotherapy and/or radiotherapy. Regression of neurological deficit was observed in 21 patients. Median survival from the first symptoms was 28 months and from diagnosis 20 months. The 5-year survival rate was 21% and 20%, respectively. These values are almost identical to those found in MM in general. Thirty-eight of 54 reported patients were dead at the time of reporting. Infection and respiratory failure were the most common causes of death. Autopsy was performed in 19 cases and was consistent with PCD in all of them. No amyloidosis was observed.

Although analysis of the whole series showed marked variability in the clinical picture, it seems that the patients with PCD and PPN are different from those with MM. Younger age, less common anemia, azotemia, and hypercalcemia, common osteosclerotic lesions, and high incidence of solitary plasmacytomas (26%) distinguish this group from typical MM.

TAKATSUKI'S SYNDROME

Recently, more than 60 patients with M-components, osteosclerotic skeletal lesions, mild bone marrow plasmacytosis, high incidence of solitary plasmacytomas, PPN, and a variety of autonomic nervous system, endocrine and cutaneous manifestations have been investigated in Japan [61,247,248,278]. Often these manifestations improved or disappeared after chemotherapy or resection of the plasmacytomas. Takatsuki suggested that this may be a new syndrome of PCD [247]. Patients with this syndrome present with darkening, thickening or swelling of the skin, hyperhidrosis, hypertrichosis, ascites, pleurisy, lymphadenopathy, gynecomastia, diabetes and clubbing. Only 6 of

54 non-Japanese patients with PCD and PPN had some manifestations of Takatsuki's syndrome [61]. No pathogenetic explanation of this syndrome can be provided at the present time. Interestingly enough, all M-components studied in Takatsuki's syndrome had λ-L chains. Such preponderance of λ-L chains has also been noted in IgD myeloma (90%), immunoglobulin-related amyloidosis (70%), and lichen myxedematosus (70%).

PLASMA-CELL DYSCRASIA WITH FANCONI SYNDROME

Fanconi syndrome (FS) is characterized by renal proximal tubular dysfunction and rickets or osteomalacia. Hypophosphatemia, hypopotassemia, low serum uric acid, glycosuria, aminoaciduria, phosphaturia, proteinuria, and hyperchloremic acidosis are characteristic for FS. Usually there is no azotemia, and glomerular filtration rate and distal tubular functions are normal.

Often patients with adult FS develop PCD, either a typical MM with osteolytic lesions or less characteristic proliferation of immature plasma cells and M-components but not bone destruction [6,25,34,45,48,55,59,62, 72, 76, 89, 90, 91, 101, 141, 153, 169, 203, 221, 228, 230, 231, 244, 276]. The relationship of FS to PCD has not been clarified. Since in almost all patients manifestations of FS preceded those of PCD, the possibility that FS causes prolonged antigenic stimulation that leads to the neoplastic proliferation cannot be ruled out.

Until now, more than 30 patients with FS and PCD have been reported. This review is based on information available in 29 patients, including three personal observations. There were 15 males and 14 females aged from 34 to 81 years, mean 55 years. In 18 patients the relationship in time between FS and PCD was mentioned, and in the majority of them manifestations of FS preceded PCD, sometimes for as long as 9 years [59,153; Pruzanski—personal observation]. Seldom were both conditions noted at the same time [45] and once Bence Jones proteinuria was recorded 16 years before the diagnosis [153].

Analysis of the whole group of 29 patients who had PCD associated with FS showed that only 9 patients met all criteria for FS and MM [25,62,101,153,231; Pruzanski—personal observation]. Ten other patients had typical Fanconi syndrome but some of the criteria for definite MM were missing. Normal or insufficient bone marrow aspirate and/or lack of typical skeletal abnormalities were the main diagnostic problems. All of them, however, had an M-component and/or Bence Jones proteinuria [55,72,90,91,153,169,203,244,276]. It is conceivable that some of them had myeloma, since normal marrow, especially when bone marrow aspiration is performed only once, or normal skeleton are not against the diagnosis. On the other hand, such patients may have had monoclonal gammopathy without progressive malignant disease. In two patients typical myeloma was diagnosed but some of the manifestations of FS were lacking. One of these two patients had azotemia and normal uric acid, potassium and phosphorus [228] and the other had azotemia and normal uric acid [45]. Both had glycosuria and proteinuria and other manifestations of FS. It is possible that when myelomatous changes in the kidneys complicate FS, azotemia and elevation of uric acid and electrolytes may counterbalance typically low level of these substances in the blood. In eight other patients not enough information was provided to classify them as typical or atypical cases [6,59,76,89,141,153,221,230].

The majority of patients complained of skeletal pain, mostly in the ribs, shoulders, back, pelvic areas, and legs. Often they reported muscular pain, ache, weakness, and extreme fatigue. Swaying, shuffling or waddling gait, weight loss, hemorrhagic phenomena and polyuria, and frequency and nycturia were quite common. Physical findings were usually limited to the musculoskeletal system, showing tenderness over the bones, muscular weakness and abnormal gait. Hepatosplenomegaly was observed in four patients. Seldom were the patients referred because of fractures.

Since detailed investigation was not reported in all patients, the incidence of various findings was calculated per number of patients who had the tests, and not per whole group (Table IV). Additional findings included elevated calcium in 2 of 24 patients (8%) and high alkaline phosphatase in 13 of 16 patients. Six of 17 patients had diabetic glucose tolerance test. Five of 23

TABLE IV. Plasma-Cell Dyscrasia with Fanconi Syndrome

Finding	Incidence
Hypophosphatemia	24/25 (96)[a]
Hypouricemia	19/21 (90)
Hypopotassemia	19/26 (73)
Hyperchloremia	10/22 (45)
Azotemia	16/24 (67)
Proteinuria	27/27 (100)
Glycosuria	29/29 (100)
Aminoaciduria	27/28 (96)
Serum M-component	15/16 (93)
Urinary M-components	25/25 (100)
Abnormal bone marrow	25/29 (86)
Osteoporosis	13/25 (50)
Osteolytic lesions	6/25 (25)
Osteomalacia and fractures	16/25 (67)

[a]Number found/number investigated (percentage).

patients had anemia, and elevated sedimentation rate was noted in 10 of 17 cases. White blood cell count was usually normal. In one patient plasma cells were observed in the peripheral blood [45] and another had lymphocytosis [72].

Proteinuria, up to 55 g/d, was recorded in all patients examined. Likewise, glycosuria, up to 50 g/d, was found in all patients. Amino-aciduria occasionally exceeded 3500 mg/24 h. Creatinine clearance test was reported in 14 patients and was low in all of them. Hyperchloremic acidosis was common. In some cases, failure to acidify the urine after ammonium chloride load was noted [203], others had normal acidification mechanism [153].

Serum electrophoresis showed an M-component in 8 patients, hypogammaglobulinemia in 4, and normal pattern in 12. No information was provided on the others. Serum IEP was reported in 15 patients: in 9 BJP κ-type proteinemia was found; in 3 IgG M-components (1 with κ- and 1 with λ-L chains, 1 not reported), in 1 IgA/κ M-component, and in 1 IgM M-component were observed. In 1 case the IEP pattern was normal.

Urine was tested for BJP by the heat test, by electrophoresis and/or by IEP in 28 patients and was abnormal in all. BJP heat test was positive in 23 of 25 patients (92%). Abnormal spikes were noted in all 24 examined urines. IEP showed BJP κ-type in 17 cases and BJP λ-type in 1. When immunological studies of the serum and urine were compiled, abnormal findings were recorded in 28 of 29 patients, whereas 1 showed low γ-globulin but was not studied further [59]. Immunoquantitation was reported in 14 patients; in all but 1 polyclonal Igs were suppressed. The results of bone marrow aspiration were reported in 28 patients. In 23, findings typical for myeloma were noted, with percentage of abnormal plasma cells varying from 9 to 98%, mean 32%. In 1 patient, bone marrow showed diffuse increase in lymphocytes, in another there were crystals in the macrophages. Two bone marrows were normal and 1 was unsuccessful.

Radiological study of the skeleton detected abnormalities in 21 of 24 patients. Osteoporosis was noted in 12, Milkman fractures in 9, osteomalacia in 9, fractures in 7 and osteolytic lesions in 6 patients [45,62,101,228; Pruzanski—personal observation].

Almost all patients were treated with various combinations of vitamin D, Shohl's mixture, potassium citrate or bicarbonate, calcium lactate, and sodium bicarbonate. At least 14 patients also received chemotherapy and/or cortisone or adrenocorticotropic hormone (ACTH).

The clinical course was reported in 25 patients. Eleven were alive at the time of reporting, surviving from 24 to 108 months, mean 57 months. Survival of 14 patients who had died was from 12 months to 288 months, mean 93 months. Death was usually caused by infection and occasionally by renal failure or gastrointestinal bleeding.

Autopsies or biopsies were obtained in 15 patients. The kidneys were involved in all of them. In 6 of 15 patients (40%) glomerular hyalinization, sclerosis, or hypercellularity were found. Proximal tubuli were involved in all patients, showing prominent atrophy, degeneration of the cells and often casts in the lumen. In 8 of 11 reported patients, interstitial areas showed fibrosis, giant cells and mononuclear cell infiltrates.

Diffuse plasmacytic infiltrates in the bone marrow and other organs were noted in some patients [45,55,62]. Liver cirrhosis was observed in three cases [55,62,72]. Amyloidosis was observed in three patients [72,153,228]: in one patient, amyloidosis involved peritoneum, esophagus, and heart [228], in another, tongue, colon, heart, and bone marrow were involved [153]; and the third patient had an unusual form of nodular amyloidosis involving primarily bone marrow, nodes, spleen, liver, and muscles [72]. In none of these three patients was amyloid found in the kidneys. In all three periamyloid plasmacytosis was observed.

In 14 patients, crystals were observed in various cells. Three patients had crystals in the plasma cells located in the bone marrow and various organs. Three other patients had crystals in the plasma cells and in the proximal tubular cells. Four patients had crystals in the proximal tubular cells only. Occasionally crystals were noted in the liver cells, interstitial spaces of the kidneys, macrophages, and extracellular spaces in the bone marrow and the lymph nodes.

In eight patients, crystals were described as needle- and rod-shaped, whereas in two they were cuboid and rectangular. The latter were noted in the macrophages and extracellular spaces in various organs [55] and in the cytoplasm of plasma cells [153]. In two patients crystals were merely described as birefringent and in two others as crystalline inclusions. Crystals were PAS-negative [55,72] and Congo red-negative [72]. They stained purple with phosphotungstic acid-hematoxilin [45,72] and were pink in hematoxilin-eosin stain [45]. Pale yellow color was observed in Mallory stain [62] and a dark purple color with Weigert's fibrin stain [228]. In one of our cases the crystals stained positively with toluidine blue. Their nature has not been identified.

Electron microscopy of the crystals showed osmiophilic laminated structures [141] composed of aggregates of electron-dense granular particles [72,153]. The measurements in one case were about 76,000 Å by 56,000 Å for the rod-shaped crystals and 80 Å for the granular particles [72].

We observed three patients with PCD and FS.

CASE 1

MH as a child had difficulty in walking and was always tired. As a teenager she was unable to play games or to dance, however her physical development was normal, she got married and delivered two children. At the age of 36, when she was treated for urinary tract infection, glycosuria was detected with normal blood sugar levels. Two years later she was hospitalized with right renal colic, polydypsia, polyuria, and nocturia. Intravenous pyelography showed bilateral renal calculi. At that time glycosuria 4 + and proteinuria 3 + were detected but not investigated. At the age of 40 the patient noticed pain in the shoulder girdles, chest wall, pelvis, and thighs. Her gait became swaying. Three years later she was hospitalized again. At that time she had normal glucose tolerance test, glycosuria of 31 g/24 h, proteinuria of 2 g/24 h and generalized aminoaciduria. BUN was 21 mg/dL, creatinine 1.1–1.8 mg/dL, CCT 53–61 mL/min, sodium 141 mEq/ L, potassium 4.2 mEq/L, chlorides 112 mEq/L, calcium 8.9 mg/dL, phosphorus 1.5 mg/ dL, uric acid 1.1 mg/dL, and arterial blood pH 7.26. γ-Globulin was low. Generalized demineralization of the bones with pseudofracture in the right scapula were found. An adult Fanconi syndrome was diagnosed and the patient was treated with polycitrate and phosphate solutions. In one month, she was able to walk without pain and two months later she reported full activity.

At the age of 46 she was admitted for right shoulder pain. An x-ray of the skeleton did not show any change. Serum protein electrophoresis showed hypogammaglobulinemia and there was an abnormal spike in urine electrophoresis. At that time renal biopsy was performed. It showed mild glomerular changes consisting of slight mesangial hyalinization and slight thickening of the basement membrane. Proximal tubular cells were swollen with flattening of the villous borders at the apex, increase in the number of lysosomes and Golgi apparatus, and appearance of many fine cytoplasmic vesicles. The cells contained crystalline inclusions, the majority being rod-shaped with angulated ends. They were laminated and tied loosely in their membrane-enclosed vesicles. They were localized in the lysosomes and/or endoplasmic reticulum (Figs. 5,6). For the next 7 years the patient felt well and was symptom-free. At the age of 53 she was hospitalized with a history of three months' pain in the back and both flanks, stiffness of fingers, and lumbosacral tenderness. An x-ray of the skeleton did not show any change. Bone marrow showed 5% of plasma cells, some with atypical features. There was still left renal calculus seen in the x-ray. Another renal biopsy was performed. For the next three years the patient was stable and suffered from only occasional back pain. She was treated with polycitrate solution and phosphate solution.

At the age of 56 she was readmitted with severe recurrent back pain, tenderness in the cervical, thoracic, and lumbar spine. Hemoglobin was 13.7 g/dL and white count and platelets were normal. Erythrocyte sedimentation rate was 23 mm/h. Intravenous pyelography showed multiple opaque stones in the left kidney. Bone marrow showed prominent plasmacytosis and an x-ray of the skeleton showed multiple osteolytic lesions in the skull, ribs, vertebrae, and pelvis. Proteinuria of 16.5 g/24 h was comprised predominantly of BJP κ-protein (Fig. 7). Serum lysozyme was 8.4 μg/mL (normal 5–15) and urinary lysozyme was 27 μg/mL (normal 0–2). In the next 12 months she received six courses of melphalan and prednisone, developed pancytopenia and was admitted again. Bone marrow showed 5% of atypical plasma cells and 5% of atypical mononuclear cells. Peripheral blood smear showed many lymphocytoid plasmacytoid cells. In the next 2 years the patient received seven courses of chemotherapy, which had to be given irregularly because of recurrent pancytopenia. Repeat bone marrow aspirate showed patchy infiltration by abnormal cells, with large pale cytoplasm and eccentric nuclei that could not be definitely identified. IEP detected BJP type κ-proteinemia (Fig. 7). IgG was 440 mg/dL (normal 1171 ± 255), IgA 50 mg/dL (normal 216 ± 86), and IgM 40 mg/dL (normal 135 ± 61). Urinalysis showed up to 22 g of protein/24 h, with albumin comprising less than 20% of the total protein. BJP κ-type protein amounted to 13.5 g/24 h and lysozyme was up to 108 mg/24 h (normal up to 5 mg/24 h).

At the age of 60 the patient was admitted again because of fever, sore throat, and productive cough. Hemoglobin was 9.0 g/dL, white count 1600/mm with 46% lymphocytes and 27% mononuclear cells. Platelets were 40,000/mm, creatinine was 1.3 mg/dL, calcium 9.1 mg/dL, and glucose between 399 and 460 mg/dL. Bone marrow showed 80% of large, primitive,

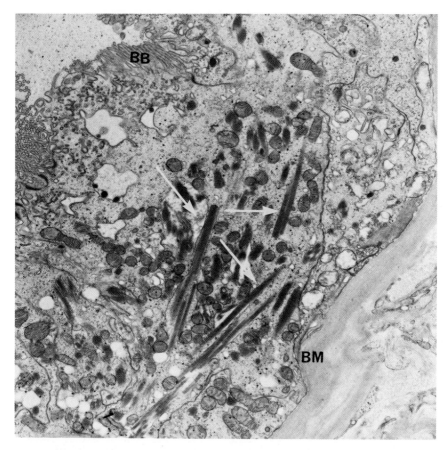

Fig. 5.   Electron micrograph of the proximal tubular cell in Fanconi syndrome (Case 1).
Numerous membrane-enclosed rod-shaped inclusions in the cytoplasm. BB = brush border,
BM = basement membrane, arrows = cytoplasmic inclusions. × 9000.

plasmacytoid, lymphocytoid cells. Peripheral blood smear showed 13% of atypical plasma
cells. The patient developed pneumonia, gram-negative sepsis, and coma, and died. Permission
for autopsy was not granted.

CASE 2

HDW, an 80-year-old woman, was hospitalized because of 27-lb weight loss in 1 year,
widespread bone pain, and fatigue. Two years earlier marked proteinuria and fractures of the
left femoral head and left patella were diagnosed. Six months prior to admission anemia with
hemoglobin of 7.0 g/dL and glycosuria were found. Examination showed general emaciation
and diffuse tenderness to percussion over the bones. There was no lymphadenopathy or organomegaly.

Hemoglobin was 7.3 g/dL, white blood cells and platelet counts were normal. Blood sugar

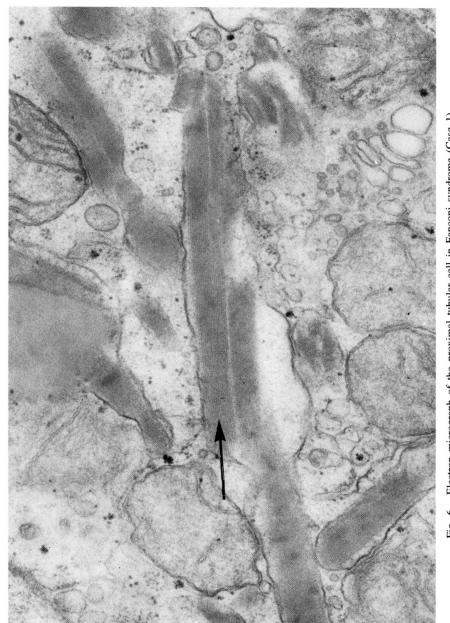

Fig. 6. Electron micrograph of the proximal tubular cell in Fanconi syndrome (Case 1). Arrow shows regular layering of the crystalline inclusions. × 44,000.

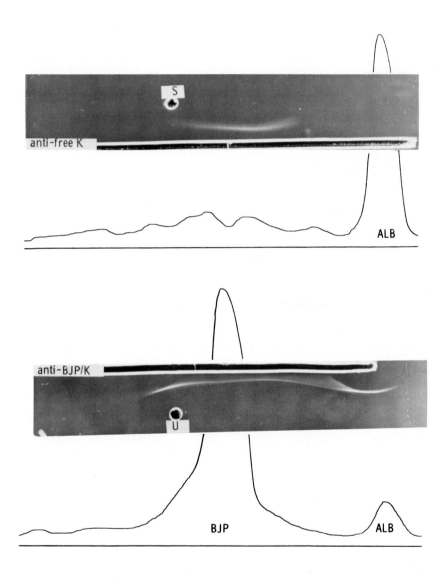

Fig. 7. Electrophoresis and immunoelectrophoresis from a patient with Fanconi syndrome (Case 1). ALB = albumin. S = serum; it showed free κ-light chains of α_2-mobility. U = urine; Bence Jones κ-type of α_2-mobility was detected.

was 80 mg/dL, sodium 142 mEq/L, potassium 2.8 mEq/L, chlorides 118 mEq/L, calcium 9.3 mg/dL, phosphorus 2.1 mg/dL, and uric acid 1.6 mg/dL Creatinine was 1.7–1.85 mg/dL. Blood pH was 7.27. Three hours glucose tolerance test was slightly abnormal. Plasma amino acids were normal. The total serum protein was 6.4 g/dL, albumin was 4.4 g/dL, γ-globulin was 0.48 g/dL, and electrophoretic strip was normal. IEP detected BJP κ-type in the serum. IgG was 370 mg/dL, IgA 47 mg/dL, and IgM 23 mg/dL. Serum lysozyme was 8.5 μg/ml (normal 5–15 μg/ml). Proteinuria, up to 8 g/24 h, was composed predominantly (70%) of BJP κ-protein of γ-mobility. There was glycosuria 3 + and prominent, generalized aminoaciduria. Urinary lysozyme was 27 μg/ml (normal 0–2 μg/ml). pH of the urine was 5.0–5.6. Ammonium chloride load test showed normal acidification. Creatinine clearance test was 25 mL/min. Bone marrow aspirate showed 30% abnormal-appearing plasma cells. Radiological survey of the skeleton showed severe osteoporosis and pathological fractures. The patient was treated with melphalan, phosphate, sodium bicarbonate, and potassium supplement. She was discharged and lost to follow-up.

CASE 3

LE, a 45-year-old man, was hospitalized because of pain in the ankles while walking and in the rib cage, which appeared 2 years prior to the admission. He experienced morning stiffness in his feet, hips, and spine, shortness of breath on exertion, and palpitations. He became thirsty, drinking more than 5 liters of fluid a day and had polyuria and nycturia. He suffered from severe headaches for which he took up to 20 tablets of ASA and 222s per day. There was a weight loss of 20 lb in 2 years.

Fifteen years earlier the patient had subtotal gastrectomy for ulcer and gastritis. At that time the urine was negative for glucose and protein. Three years earlier hypertension was found and treated with phenobarbital.

Examination revealed no significant distress. Blood pressure was 135/90mm Hg, pulse 100/min with atrial fibrillation. The liver was palpable 4 cm below the costal margin and the tip of the spleen was felt. There was tenderness to palpation in both ankles, right hip, and lower back. The rest of the examination was noncontributory. Laboratory tests showed hemoglobin of 14.9 g/dL. Creatinine was 1.1 mg/dL, potassium 3.4 mEq/L, chlorides 111 mEq/L, calcium 8.8 mg/dL, phosphorus 1.7 mg/dL, uric acid 1.4 mg/dL, glucose 90 mg/dL, alkaline phosphatase 21.3 King-Armstrong units. Glucose tolerance test curve was flat. The total serum protein was 8.9 g/dL. IgG/κ M-component of 1.92 g/dL was detected. Urine showed prominent glucosuria up to 49 g/24 h, proteinuria over 3 g/24 h, aminoaciduria 1630 mg/24 h. Creatinine clearance test was 62 mL/min. Bone marrow aspiration showed initially 10% normal-looking plasma cells. Later on the number of plasma cells increased to 19% and the majority were immature, often binucleated cells arranged in clumps. Skeletal survey showed osteoporosis.

A year later he was admitted to another hospital because of severe pain in the heels, thighs, back, shoulders, and arms. He took 20 ASA daily for one year and up to 10 222s for the last 2 months prior to admission. For a couple of weeks he was on steroids. There was an additional weight loss of 47 lb in the last year. Physical examination showed marked tenderness over the ribs, sacroiliac joints, and metatarsal heads. His gait was waddling. The liver was palpable 4 cm under the costal margin and the spleen tip was palpable. Diagnosis of adult Fanconi syndrome and plasmacytic neoplasia was made. At that time anemia with hemoglobin of 10.4 g/dL was noted. Platelets were 90,000/mm³. Creatinine increased to 3.6 mg/dL. M-component increased to 2.6 g/dL and IgA and IgM were reduced. Radiological survey showed Looser zones in the right femoral neck, calcaneal, and metatarsal bones, pathological fracture of the right sixth rib, and patchy areas of rarefaction in the calvarium, tibiae, fibulae, ulnae, and femoral bones. Two courses of cyclophosphamide and prednisone were given, but had to be discontinued because of leukopenia and sepsis.

A month later prominent increase in the urinary output was recorded, up to 12.5 L/24 h. Such diuresis continued for 5 days and then decreased to 3–6 L/24 h. Pitressine tannate, potassium phosphate, and K-lyte were administered, without any evident influence on the urinary output or specific gravity of the urine. Plasmapheresis was undertaken, with removal of 26 units of plasma in 1 month, but there was no change in the level of serum M-component or proteinuria. Subsequently the patient was started on intermittent courses of melphalan and prednisone. Three courses were given without influence on the concentration of serum M-component. The patient developed a rectal fistula, candidiasis, axillary, and perirectal abscesses. Septicemia associated with an interstitial pneumonia ensued and the patient died in coma at the age of 48 years. At autopsy the kidneys showed minimal glomerular changes consisting of mesangial hyalinization and thickening of the basement membrane. Ballooning of the proximal tubular cells was noted with large number of lysosomes and increase of the Golgi apparatus. Proximal tubular cells contained many cytoplasmic crystalloid inclusions, irregular in shape and poorly defined fibrillar internal structure. Occasionally they were needle-shaped and rarely had angulated ends (Figs. 8,9).

The liver showed slight fatty change. The hepatocytes contained abundant glycogen. The mitochondria were increased in number, enlarged and irregular in outline. Many hepatocytes contained stacks of rod-like crystalline inclusions. Additional findings were abundant plasma cells in the splenic pulp and plasmacytosis in the bone marrow.

PLASMA-CELL DYSCRASIA ASSOCIATED WITH LIPID ABNORMALITIES

Lipid abnormalities in patients with plasma-cell dyscrasia were noticed long ago. Low serum cholesterol in myeloma [222,225] and hypolipidemia resulting from the binding of IgG or IgA M-components to low-density lipoproteins [205] have been reported.

During the last three decades an association of PCD with hyperlipidemia, rather than hypolipidemia, and/or xanthomatosis has been described in more than 30 patients [12–14,42,69,77,95,99,113,115,120,128,142,143,145,146, 148,156,160,167,168,170,171,173,178,207,220,229,233,249,272]. Xanthomas were observed mainly on the skin and were of either plane or tuberous variety. Occasionally, visceral xanthomas were observed such as in the ribs [229]. In addition to xanthomas, xanthelasmas were observed in three patients [69,272]. In a few instances familial lipid abnormalities were recorded [42,120,173].

This review is based on investigation of 31 patients (Table V). There were 18 males and 11 females, aged from 31 to 75 years, mean 56 years; in 2, no sex or age were reported. Twenty-three patients met the clinical and/or autopsy criteria for MM, 5 had M-components but could not be classified with certainty as myeloma patients, 2 had cryoglobulinemia, and 1 had lymphoma with cryoprecipitable M-component. In some patients xanthomas preceded development of PCD [12,160,170,220,272], whereas in others both conditions developed simultaneously [171]. In one patient cryoglobulinemia was detected 5 years before development of tuberous xanthomas [69], in another hypergammaglobulinemic purpura developed first [220]. In several patients the main clinical manifestations were cold sensitivity, purpura, urticaria and Raynaud's phenomena [69,95,115,148,220]. In others, hyper-

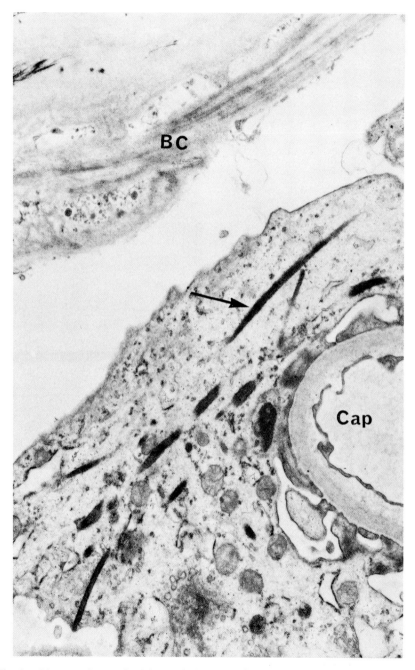

Fig. 8.   Electron micrograph of the renal glomerulus from a patient with Fanconi syndrome (Case 3). Swollen epithelial cells contained rod-like inclusions in the cytoplasm (arrow). BC = Bowman's capsule; Cap = capillary. × 17,950.

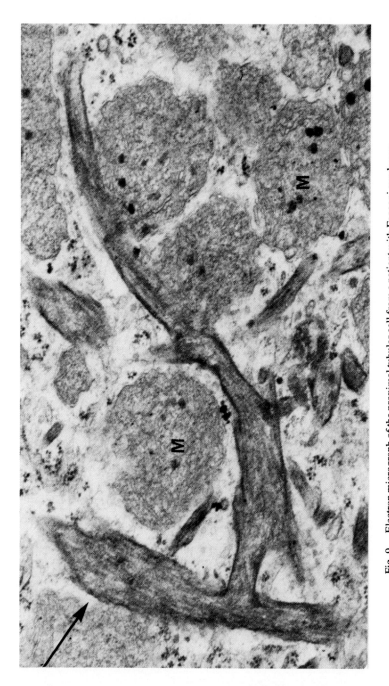

Fig. 9. Electron micrograph of the proximal tubular cell from a patient with Fanconi syndrome (Case 3). Branching inclusions showed filamentous structure (arrow). M = mitochondria. × 44,000.

TABLE V. Plasma-Cell Dyscrasia Associated with Lipid Abnormalities

	Multiple myeloma (23)	M-component (5)	Cryoglobulinemia (2)	Lymphoma (1)	Total (31)[a]
Plane xanthomas	11	2	—	—	13
Tuberous xanthomas	3	1	1	—	5
Normal skin	9	2	1	1	13
Hypercholesterolemia	17	5	—	—	22
Normal cholesterol	3	—	1	1	5
Elevated total lipids	9	3	—	—	12
Hypertriglyceridemia	8	1	—	—	9
Normal triglycerides	4	—	—	—	4
Bone marrow plasmacytosis[b]	19	3	1	—	23
Normal bone marrow	1	1	—	—	2
Skeletal abnormalities[c]	11	—	—	—	11
Normal skeleton	7	3	1	—	11
M-components—spike	7	2	1	1	11
IgG[d]	9	2	—	—	11
IgA[e]	7	1	—	—	8
IgM	—	—	1	—	1
Cryoglobulinemia	6	—	2	1	9

[a]Number of patients. If the total number for each variable does not add up to 31, it means that in some patients the finding was not reported.
[b]In all cases abnormal-looking plasma cells were observed.
[c]Osteolytic lesions and/or severe osteoporosis. In one patient osteolytic and osteosclerotic lesions were observed [99].
[d]Five with κ-light chains and four with λ-light chains.
[e]In only one light chains (κ) were typed.

viscosity syndrome was observed [95,115,207,249]. Several additional conditions such as diabetes and glomerulosclerosis [178], hepato- and/or splenomegaly [99,143,160,207], plasmacytoma with amyloid in the lesion [229], or chronic membranous proliferative glomerulonephritis [233] have been reported in some patients.

The usual finding was high cholesterol and/or triglycerides. In a few instances striking elevation of β-lipoproteins and especially of low-density lipoproteins (LDL) and very low density lipoproteins (VLDL) was observed [72,145,170,171,249]. Flotation experiments showed marked increase in < 1006 and 1006–1009 density fractions of lipoproteins [42]. Lipemic, turbid, or milky plasma was observed in some patients [12,42,99,142,207,272], in others, normal-looking plasma was found [115,160]. Amylase and lipase were usually normal [42]. Abnormal liver function tests were found in a few patients [178,272; Pruzanski—personal observation].

The association of lipids with the M-components was studied by several methods and formation of complexes was implicated in the majority of patients, especially when hyperlipemia was present [249]. Analytical ultracentrifugation of the serum has shown heavy substances with $S_{20,w}$ values reaching 38 [249]. In some instances the electrophoretic mobility of the lipids was found to correspond to that of an M-component [128,249]; in others it did not [42,272]. In a few cases of cryoglobulinemia, isolated cryoglobulin contained β-lipoproteins and cholesterol [148,249,272]. In one instance precipitation of IgM-lipoprotein (Lp) cryocomplex was markedly enhanced by addition of VLDL [148]. Complexes of Ig-Lp react with appropriate anti-Ig antisera such as in the case of IgA polymer-Lp complex [145]. In a few cases of IgA myeloma with hyperlipidemia, IgA M-components had antilipoprotein activity [13,14,113]. Such IgA extracted from the complex reacted with both α- and β-lipoproteins [14]. In other cases, IgA/κ and IgG/κ M-components did not have antibody activity against lipoprotein [128,207]. In one patient with nodular xanthomatosis, lipemia, delayed triglyceride, and cryolipoprotein removal and heparin binding to the M-component were observed [272]. In another patient with cryoglobulinemia, diffuse plane xanthomatosis, and normal lipids, cryoglobulin contained IgG together with β- and pre-β-lipoproteins, carotenoids, and cholesterol. Triglyceride turnover in this patient was normal [272].

Histological studies showed variable results. In a patient with diffuse plane xanthomatosis, immunofluorescent studies of the skin showed neither IgG nor lipoproteins [272]. In another patient, immunofluorescence of the skin from the involved areas showed both IgG and VLDL in the lipid-laden cells in the deep dermis. The normal skin was negative. Bone marrow showed cells containing IgG and lipoproteins [249]. In some cases perivascular accumulation of foaming histiocytes in the skin was noted [160]. Infiltration and obliteration of the arteries were found in a patient with myeloma, IgG/κ-lipoprotein cryocomplex and necrotizing vasculitis of the kidney and lungs [249].

The influence of a low-fat, low-cholesterol diet was disappointing. In some cases it reduced the level of cholesterol but did not influence the course of the disease. Cholestyramine, penicillamine, and thyroid hormones were not helpful either. However, chemotherapeutic agents were capable of reducing cholesterol and lipids and diminishing the size of xanthomas [115,249].

Familial predisposition for xanthomatosis was observed in a few patients. In one instance a patient had two sisters and one brother; one sister had hyperlipidemia and xanthomas and the brother had hyperlipidemia. None had PCD [42]. Another patient had three brothers with hyperlipidemia and high cholesterol but no PCD [120]. Familial hypercholesterolemia with xanthomatosis was reported in another patient [173].

The exact relationship of PCD to lipid abnormalities and development of xanthomas has not been elucidated. In some patients lipid abnormalities preceded in time clinical manifestations of PCD, in others the opposite was observed. It was suggested that M-components may release their lipid fraction in the skin capillaries, where it is subsequently phagocytized by dermal histiocytes, initiating formation of xanthomas. Alternatively, xanthomas may be secondary to cutaneous lymphoreticular proliferation. Whether or not plasma cells are capable of synthesizing and excreting lipids has not been clarified, although incorporation of ^{14}C-L-glutamic acid into both plasma cells and the lipids has been reported [170]. Since in the majority of instances lipoprotein M-component complexes were detected, the possibility that some M-components may have antibody activity against lipoproteins cannot be ruled out and is supported by experimental evidence [13,14,113,168,189]. In one instance an IgA M-component from a patient with MM, hyperlipidemia and xanthomatosis agglutinated sheep red blood cells and the agglutination was inhibited by choline. It is feasible that its activity was directed to the lipid hapten rather than to the protein moiety of the lipoprotein [168].

One patient with MM and hyperlipidemia was observed by us: AT, a 54-year-old man, was hospitalized because of ataxia, drowsiness, confusion, and radicular pain corresponding to the T_{7-8} level. The liver and spleen were palpable 13 cm and 10 cm below the costal margin, respectively. There were no xanthomas or xanthelasma. Hemoglobin was 9.0 g/dL, white blood cell count 9,000/mm^3, with 12% monocytes and 1% plasma cells in the differential count. Platelets were 140,000/mm^3. Calcium was 10.4 mg/dL, creatinine 2.7 mg/dL, uric acid 12.3 mg/dL, bilirubin 1.1 mg/dL, SGOT 71 IU, γ-GT 447 units, amylase 491 units (normal up to 75 units), alkaline phosphatase 560 units (normal < 185 units), cholesterol 424 mg/dL, and triglycerides 802 mg/dL. The fasting serum was milky. Prothrombin time was 13 seconds (control 15 seconds). The total serum protein was 11.2 g/dL, with albumin 3.9 g/dL and γ-mobility M-component of 4.6 g/dL. IEP identified this M-component as IgG/λ. IgG was 2502 mg/dL, IgA 28 mg/dL and IgM 14 mg/dL. Cryoglobulin test was negative and serum viscosity was 2.4 (normal < 1.9). Bone marrow was totally replaced by abnormal-looking plasma cells. Radiological survey of the skeleton was negative. Myelography showed a block at the midthoracic level. Cerebrospinal fluid contained numerous immature plasma cells and an IgG/λ M-component. The patient was treated with irradiation to the spinal cord, prednisone, and phenylalanine mustard. His recovery was quick, with disappearance of neurological signs and of confusion. His liver function tests, alkaline phophatase, cholesterol, and triglycerides promptly decreased to normal values. Incidentally, one year before onset of the disease the level of cholesterol and triglycerides was normal. There was no history of alcoholism or of any liver disease.

PLASMA-CELL DYSCRASIA WITH GAUCHER'S DISEASE

Several patients with Gaucher's disease and PCD have been reported [17,173,186,215a,255,274]. The incidence of such association is unknown. In a group of sixteen patients with Gaucher's disease, four had IgG/κ M-components [199]. These patients were aged 61 to 68 years. All had high γ-globulin, from 2.7 to 3.6 g/dL. Three out of four patients had normal percentage of plasma cells in the bone marrow, and in one patient plasmacytosis of 18% was found [199]. In one 68-year-old man, bone marrow showed a double infiltration by plasma cells and Gaucher's cells; by immunofluorescence the plasma cells were shown to contain an IgG M-component [173]. One case of Gaucher's disease and nonsecretory myeloma with intracellular IgD M-component was reported [17]. Another patient suffered from classical IgA/κ myeloma and Gaucher's disease [215a].

CLINICAL SPECTRUM OF COLD AGGLUTININS

Cold agglutinins (CA) are defined as antibodies which, by interacting with membrane antigens, agglutinate red blood cells in temperatures below that of the human body. It has only recently been recognized that CA are capable of attaching to and often killing and lysing many other types of mammalian cells and interfering with biological functions of living cells [195].

CA that appear during some infectious diseases are usually heterogeneous and have both κ- and λ-L chains, as tested by immunochemical assays. Patients with mycoplasma infections may occasionally have homogeneous IgM/κ CA. Usually, serum electrophoresis shows diffuse hypergammaglobulinemia, whereas IEP of CA eluted from red blood cells shows heterogeneous IgM. In contrast, CA from patients with malignant lymphoplasmacytic diseases and chronic cold agglutinin disease (CCAD) are homogeneous. Serum electrophoresis in such patients usually shows a narrow band, whereas IEP detects an M-component, usually IgM, with either κ- (common) or λ- (rare) L chain. Most CA are IgM, but IgA and IgG CA have also been described in patients with CCAD. In infectious mononucleosis, CA were found to be either IgG or mixed IgG/IgM. In some areas of Melanesia, 'endemic' CA affecting up to 75% of the population were detected. Although the majority of these CA are heterogeneous IgM with anti-I activity, some homogeneous IgM have also been observed.

H chains of various IgM CA were found to share antigenic determinants not found on IgM without CA activity. These specific antigenic determinants were found on both anti-I and anti-i IgM CA and also on IgA CA. Amino acid sequence studies of the L chains of several CA showed marked similarities in the part forming antigen-combining site. The distribution of κ-chain subtypes on CA was also different from that on ordinary IgM showing predominance of the Vk_{111} subtype.

Cold agglutinins interact with a group of antigens located in the membrane of red blood cells. These antigens are glycoproteins or glycolipids, related in structure to A, B, H, and Lewis antigens. With a few exceptions, adult red blood cells have an I antigen, whereas cord cells have i antigen on the surface. Consequently, CA reacting predominantly with adult red blood cells are called anti-I and those reacting more with cord red cells are called anti-i. Seldom do CA react equally with adult and cord blood cells, and then their specificity is directed towards other antigens. Such non-I, non-i antigens have been identified and are called $Pr_{1,2,3}$ and Gd [208]. Recently a new antigen, tentatively called Sa, was discovered [209].

Anti-I CA are physiologically found in the serum of healthy individuals; however, their titer is low, usually less than 1:64, and they are active only at low temperatures. Their biological significance has not been clarified. In pathological situations the titer of CA is usually high and the thermal amplitude may be wide. The highest temperature at which CA is binding to the corresponding antigen precludes its clinical significance. Some CA may react at or above 20°C or even above 30°C.

Most monoclonal CA are found in patients with lymphoplasmacytic disorders. They may be slowly progressive as in CCAD or rapid as in reticulum cell sarcoma (Table VI).

CCAD is probably a variant of MW[1], in which the IgM M-component has CA activity. Histological features of CCAD are similar to those of MW. In CCAD, CA usually have I-specificity, whereas in other lymphoprolifer-

[1]Ed. note: See also [285].

TABLE VI. Diseases in Which Cold Agglutinins May Occur

Monoclonal cold agglutinins	Polyclonal cold agglutinins
Chronic cold hemagglutinin disease	Mycoplasma pneumonia
Macroglobulinemia of Waldenström	Infectious mononucleosis
Hodgkin's and non-Hodgkin's lymphoma	Cytomegalovirus infection
Chronic lymphocytic leukemia	Listeriosis
Chronic myelogenous leukemia	Mumps orchitis
Kaposi's sarcoma	Subacute bacterial endocarditis
Plasmacytoma and multiple myeloma	Syphilis
Severe combined immunodeficiency[a]	Tropical diseases (trypanosomiasis, malaria, tropical eosinophilia)
Mycoplasma pneumonia (rare)	Collagen vascular and immune complex diseases
	Angioimmunoblastic lymphadenopathy

[a]In association with a leukemia-like B lymphocyte proliferation.

ative disorders with CA they are either anti-I or anti-i. Clinical manifestations related to CA are dependent on the exposure to cold. As blood flows through the capillaries of the skin and subcutaneous tissues, its temperature may fall a few degrees if the ambient temperature is low. If the CA is active at these temperatures, it agglutinates the cells and fixes complement. Obstruction of the circulation follows and results in acrocyanosis. The toes, earlobes, and tip of the nose, as well as the fingers may be affected. Gangrene occurs only infrequently because the agglutination is rapidly reversible on warming of the affected parts. CA may also cause hemolytic anemia which is often mild, since C3b inactivator is present in the blood. The degree of hemolysis is related to the rate of fixation of C3. In the cold, the capacity of C3b inactivator is exceeded and red cells with C3b on their surface are either rosetted and phagocytosed or (after fixation of the remaining complement components) lysed, resulting in hemoglobinemia and hemoglobinuria.

Management of the patient with CCAD is often difficult and depends on the maintenance of an ambient temperature above the maximum temperature at which his CA reacts. If the antibody has high thermal amplitude, warming of the patient is often insufficient to prevent hemolysis. Steroids and/or splenectomy are less useful than in patients with warm antibody autoimmune hemolytic anemia. Chemotherapeutic agents such as chlorambucil or cyclophosphamide are beneficial in chronic management, but they are of no value in an acute condition. Penicillamine and plasmapheresis were used in some patients. Blood transfusions should be given when severe anemia develops but transfused cells, unprotected by C3b, are more susceptible to lysis than the patient's own cells. Washed, packed red cells only should be transfused. Crossmatching should be done strictly at 37°C to avoid reactions due to autoantibody and thus allowing the detection of red cell alloantibodies. When blood is being transfused, it is advisable to warm the patient as well as the transfused blood.

Exhaustive plasmapheresis may be used in life-threatening hemolysis to quickly remove significant quantities of antibody, however massive agglutination of blood once it is removed from the patient may make the procedure technically difficult. Plasmapheresis can be carried out successfully by using a blood warmer to keep the blood at 37°C as it is being withdrawn from the patient. It is then advisable to centrifuge the blood at 37°C, remove the plasma containing most of the antibody and rewarm the cells to 37°C with the blood warmer before returning them to the patient.

It has recently been discovered that CA of various specificities react with antigens on the membrane of many types of normal and neoplastic cells. *In vitro,* in the presence of complement, the interaction of CA with these cells leads to cell death and sometimes to lysis. CA were found to be cytotoxic to normal human peripheral and tonsillary T and B lymphocytes, thymocytes, polymorphonuclears, macrophages, and monocytes [197]. CA also agglutinate platelets in the cold [196]. The presence of antigens interacting with CA was found in the kidney, fibroblasts, and several other tissues. Cytotoxic activity of CA against lymphoblasts, chronic lymphocytic leukemia cells, myeloblasts and some neoplastic cells has also been documented.

It seems, therefore, that the antigens interacting with CA are common to many, if not to all, types of mammalian cells. This makes the question about the physiological role of CA even more significant.

PLASMA-CELL DYSCRASIA WITH POLYCYTHEMIA VERA

The association of PCD with polycythemia vera (PV) has been reported by several investigators [57,61,78,84,92,125,139,154a,236]. The incidence of this association among PCD in general has not been estimated. Six patients were found among 41 patients with PCD, peripheral neuropathy and osteosclerotic lesions (15%) [61], but none were reported among 869 cases of MM [132]. In 12 of 20 described patients the diagnosis of MM could be made with certainty. Four of 12 had osteolytic lesions [84,92,139], 5 had osteosclerotic lesions [61], and 2 had mixed osteosclerotic and osteolytic lesions in the skeleton [61,236]. Eight patients presented with peripheral polyneuropathy [61,139,154a]. Another patient presented with hepatosplenomegaly, bone marrow infiltrate, and cord compression due to plasmacytoma [78].

In eight patients, the diagnosis of MM could not be definitely made because of either normal skeleton or a lack of sufficient information. However, all of them had plasmacytic infiltrate of the bone marrow and an M-component or Bence Jones proteinuria. The clinical course and prognosis of MM with PV seem to be similar to myeloma in general, but the series is too small to draw statistically significant conclusions.

PLASMA-CELL DYSCRASIA WITH PERNICIOUS ANEMIA

Although the association of pernicious anemia (PA) with PCD has been noted [30,79,105,127,137,179,185], the incidence of such association has not been estimated. In a group of 69 patients with MM, 5 (7%) had PA (137) but no larger series were analysed. Over 30 patients with PCD and PA have been reported [185]. The age varied from 43 to 86 years, mean 72 years. Sixty percent of the patients were women. The majority of patients suffered from MM; however, some others had M-components without evidence for myeloma [30,127,137]. In some patients atrophic gastritis [185] and in others carcinoma of the stomach [30] was noted. One patient had a history of carcinoma of the colon, cancer of the tongue, and parathyroid adenoma. She developed PA and had IgG/κ M-component without evidence for myeloma [127]. M-components were of IgG class [79,127,185], IgA [30,105,185], or IgM [30,137].

It seems that the clinical picture of MM with PA does not differ from that of myeloma in general. A few patients had autoimmune conditions such as myxedema or rheumatoid arthritis [30]. Presence of antiparietal cells and antithyroid microsomal antibodies was documented in some patients [30,127]. Therapy with vitamin B_{12} usually had a favorable effect on the anemia [137].

Association of PA with PCD seems to occur usually in elderly patients. Since PA is an antibody-mediated condition, its relationship to PCD may be explained by two alternative, but not mutually exclusive, mechanisms. Chronic antigenic stimulation, which leads to continuous antibody production, may trigger imbalanced proliferation of plasma-cell clones. In such a case PA should precede the development of PCD, as has happened in several cases. On the other hand, development of PCD may lead to the excessive use of vitamin B_{12} by malignant cells. Alternatively, some M-components may have antibody activity against the intrinsic factor.

PLASMA-CELL DYSCRASIA WITH PYROGLOBULINEMIA

The term "pyroglobulinemia" was coined by Martin and Mathieson in 1953 [157] and denotes precipitation or gelation of the serum on heating, usually at 56°C. In distinction to cryoglobulinemia, which is usually reversible on heating, pyroglobulinemia is irreversible on cooling. Neither further heating nor cooling of the serum was found to change the gel, with the exception of one case where further heating above 56°C dissolved the pyroglobulin [273]. Such behaviour resembled BJP and indeed a search for this protein was made in many cases of pyroglobulinemia. In some cases, BJP was found in the urine [70,106,110,158,181] or in the serum [110], but none was detected in other patients [38,110,158,181,182].

Although pyroglobulinemia usually occurs in plasmalymphocytic proliferative diseases with M-components (Table VII), it was also observed in other diseases and even in healthy individuals. Pyroglobulins were detected among IgG, IgM, and IgA M-components of both κ- and λ-types [28, 38, 43, 64, 70, 74, 86, 106, 110, 149, 157, 158, 159, 164, 180, 181, 182, 241, 245,266,273,284] (Table VIII). The proportion of M-components with κ-type L chains to those with λ-type L chains was found to be 2.3:1. Analytical ultracentrifugation of M components with pyroglobulin property showed the following values: 4 IgG were 7 S each; 1 IgA had 12.3 and 16.1 S units; another had 15.5, 17, and 20 S units. Six IgM had 19 S, whereas 6 others were heavier, with $S_{20,w}$ units between 21 and 26. Seven sera with pyroglobulinemia also contained cryoglobulin [110,158,164,266]. In four instances the same Ig shared cryoprecipitable and pyroprecipitable properties. In three other cases cryoglobulins were complexes of IgM/IgG type. Only the IgM parts of these complexes had the property of pyroprecipitation. No rheumatoid factor activity was found [149,164].

In a few instances biochemical studies of the sera containing pyroglobulin and/or of the purified protein were performed. The property of pyroprecipitation was found to reside on the H chains of Igs [38,181,284]. Four IgM pyroglobulins lost their precipitability when they were reduced to monomeric form by treatment with 2-mercaptoethanol. Reassociation to pentameric form restored pyroprecipitation [182,241]. In several other cases of IgM pyrog-

TABLE VII. Clinical Conditions in 56 Patients with Pyroglobulinemia

Multiple myeloma	27
Macroglobulinemia of Waldenström	11
Plasma-cell leukemia	1
Lymphosarcoma	4
Chronic lymphocytic leukemia	1
Cancer	1
Systemic lupus erythematosus	1
No definite diagnosis	7
Healthy individuals	3

TABLE VIII. Breakdown of 23 Cases of Pyroglobulinemia According to Class and Type of M-component

IgM/κ	10 ⎫	
IgM/λ	5 ⎭	15 (65%)
IgG/κ	4 ⎫	
IgG/λ	1 ⎭	5 (22%)
IgA/κ	2 ⎫	
IgA/λ	1 ⎭	3 (13%)

lobulinemia, 2-mercaptoethanol had no effect [110,159]. In three cases 3% NaCl inhibited pyroprecipitation of IgM, yet enhanced it in another case [110].

IgA pyroglobulins were not influenced by 2-mercaptoethanol [110,245], whereas treatment with 5.0 mol/L guanidine HCl, glycine buffer pH 3.0, phosphate buffer pH 9.0 [245], or with 3% NaCl [110] inhibited or abolished pyroprecipitation. In another case of 16 S IgA/λ pyroglobulin, which was also a cryoglobulin, reduction to 6.7 monomers abolished both cryo- and pyroprecipitation [266].

In a few cases of IgG pyroglobulinemia, 2-mercaptoethanol did not abolish this property [110,181]. Partial or complete inhibition of pyroprecipitation was achieved by 0.3 mol/L glycine buffer, pH 6.2 (181), 3% NaCl (110), 6M urea, and by sodium dodecyl sulphate (284). Since SDS is an amphiphile, the authors speculated that pyroprecipitation is hydrophobic in nature. It seems, however, that pyroprecipitability is a complex phenomenon that may not necessarily be identical in all cases. Whereas polymeric form seems to be essential in IgM and in some IgA pyroglobulins, no such prerequisite is necessary in IgG pyroglobulins. The influence of pH and molarity on pyroprecipitation implies that tertiary structure, folding of the molecule and electrical charges, may play a role in the induction of pyroglobulinemia.

The incidence of pyroglobulinemia varies, depending on the type of assessed patients. In a series of 260 M-components, 8 were pyroglobulins (3%) [110]; 2 were found among 202 cases of myeloma (1%) and 6 among 44 cases of macroglobulinemia (14%) [110]. The clinical picture, laboratory data and survival in myeloma and macroglobulinemia with pyroglobulinemia are similar to those without pyroglobulinemia. A few cases of hyperviscosity syndrome were reported [159,245,266; Pruzanski—personal observation]. At the present time, *pyroglobulinemia seems to be a laboratory phenomenon only,* but more studies are necessary to understand its nature and significance.

PLASMA-CELL DYSCRASIA WITH LYSOZYME-PRODUCING CELL DYSCRASIA

In 1966, Osserman and Lawlor reported on the presence of large amounts of lysozyme (LZM) (muramidase) in the sera and urines of patients with mono and myelomonocytic leukemia (174) (Fig. 10). This discovery inspired further studies that identified monocytic-macrophage series as the source of production and secretion of LZM, described lysozyme nephropathy, characterized physico-chemical properties of human LZM, and identified the role of LZM in defense mechanisms against infection. The role of LZM in resistance against neoplasia has also been suggested.

Osserman was the first to notice occurrence of lysozyme-producing cell dyscrasia (LPCD) and PCD in the same patient [175]. He proposed that LZM and Igs are interrelated, serving as mediators of macrophage and plasma-cell functions in a general defense system [176].

LPCD and PCD may be related in several ways: 1) Myeloma or macro-globulinemia may terminate in myelomonocytic leukemia; 2) both diseases may appear simultaneously; 3) monocytic or myelomonocytic leukemias may present with M-components. An example of the first group is a patient with

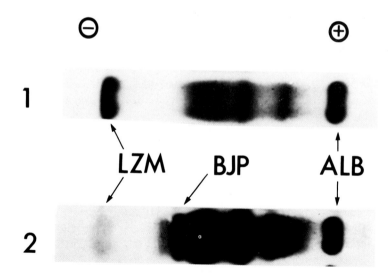

Fig. 10. Electrophoretic pattern of two urines: 1) Myelomonocytic leukemia, 2) Fanconi syndrome. ALB = albumin; LZM = lysozyme; BJP = Bence Jones protein.

L chain disease who developed amyloidosis and terminal monocytic leukemia with marked lysozymuria [175]. Analysis of 58 cases of MM terminating in acute leukemia showed that in 23 patients (40%), the leukemia was of myelomonocytic or myelomonoblastic type [213]. Invariably MM preceded leukemia by intervals ranging from $1^1/_2$ months to 9 years, and all patients received chemotherapy, usually melphalan [213]. Some had chromosomal abnormalities in the plasma cells [103]. By 1978 more than 100 patients with MM who developed leukemia were reported. Monocytic and myelomonocytic varieties were disproportionately frequent [214].

The relationship of leukemia to MM is not clear. Acute leukemia may well be a part of the natural history of MM and may be recorded more frequently because of longer survival of the patients on chemo- and/or radiotherapy. On the other hand, the possibility that the therapy *per se* may have neoplastic effect cannot be dismissed at the present time [20,133,134]. Thus it is important to document cases of PCD which either develop simultaneously or convert into LPCD without being treated. Cleary et al. reported such a patient who developed MM and myelomonocytic leukemia prior to chemotherapy [41]. This 64-year-old man had an IgA/κ M-component, low IgG and IgM, and white blood cell count of 34,500 mm^3 with 18% monocytes and 27% monoblasts. His bone marrow showed double infiltrate with 25% monoblasts and 10–20% immature plasma cells. Both serum and urinary LZM were elevated. There were no osteolytic lesions in the skeleton and no Bence Jones proteinuria. The patient died but no autopsy was performed.

Myelomonocytic leukemia developed in another untreated patient with MW [217]. This 68-year-old woman initially presented with 61% lymphocytes in the peripheral blood, IgM/κ in the serum and BJP/κ in the urine. Four years later she developed leukocytosis of 45,100/mm^3, with the majority of cells belonging to the monocytic series. Serum and urinary LZM were high. Bone marrow showed a mixture of monoblasts and plasmacytes. Interestingly enough, the patient subsequently developed widespread osteolytic lesions and died with renal failure and disseminated intravascular coagulation syndrome. In retrospect, it was probably a case of IgM myeloma.

Ligorsky et al. described a patient with diffuse, poorly differentiated lymphocytic lymphoma and IgM/κ M-component who developed acute myelomonocytic leukemia [147]. This 69-year-old man presented with lymphadenopathy, organomegaly, and anemia. White blood cell differential showed 62% lymphocytes and 18% monocytes. Immunofluorescence detected IgM in the plasma cells and in the monocytic leukemic cells, in the latter probably as a product of ingestion. Only one course of cyclophosphamide was given. Subsequently, the patient's peripheral blood showed 88% of immature granulocytes and monocytes and the bone marrow became infiltrated with immature granulocytic and monocytic cells. Prominent lysozymuria was observed and the patient died in renal failure. At autopsy no evidence for lymphoma was found. Plasma cells and plasmacytoid lymphocytes in the marrow and various tissues contained IgM/κ in the cytoplasm.

The first two patients with LPCD and IgG M-component without myeloma were reported by Osserman [175]. IgG M-components in LPCD were later reported by other investigators [10,73,190,281]. Poulik reported a patient with monocytic leukemia and IgG_1/κ M-component in the serum. Bone marrow showed 1–3% plasma cells, some atypical. Urine of the patient contained not only IgG but also Fc, F^1c, and Fab fragments [190]. Incidentally, such breakdown of IgG molecules in the urine was reported in patients with myelomonocytic leukemia who did not have M-components [192]. Bernard described a patient with chronic myelomonocytic leukemia, IgG/κ M-component, and reduced IgA and IgM in the serum (10). Bone marrow did not show plasmacytic infiltrate and skeletal survey was normal. In the patient with myelomonocytic leukemia described by Finkle, LZM formed a complex with IgG/λ M-component. There was no evidence for myeloma [73]. Pruzanski (unpublished report) observed 5 patients with M-components among more than 150 patients with LPCD. There were 2 patients with IgG/λ, 1

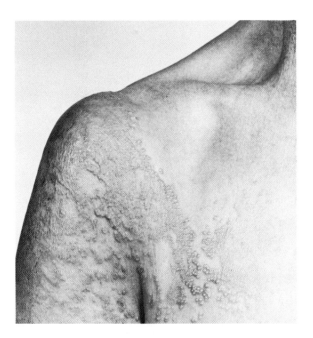

Fig. 11. Lichen myxedematosus with IgG/κ M-component. Confluent papular erythema with discrete, firm papules over the skin. (Reproduced with permission [52].)

with IgG/κ, 1 with IgM/κ, and 1 with transient BJP/κ proteinuria (Fig. 10). None had any evidence for MM and the level of polyclonal Igs was normal or elevated. Allen described a patient with myelomonocytic leukemia, IgM/κ M-component in the serum, BJP/κ in the urine, and hypercalcemia, but no evidence for MM or MW [3]. It seems that an association between PCD and LPCD is more than fortuitous, but the pathogenetic mechanisms of this association remain to be elucidated.

PLASMA-CELL DYSCRASIA WITH LICHEN MYXEDEMATOSUS

Lichen myxedematosus (papular mucinosis) is a rare skin condition which usually has a prolonged benign course (Figs. 11, 12). Several clinical types have been described: 1) a generalized lichenoid eruption with papules all over the body, especially face, neck, upper trunk, hands and forearms; 2) a discrete papular eruption on the trunk and extremities; 3) localized or generalized lichenoid plaques; and 4) a combination of urticarial plaques and nodular eruption.

Patients with lichen myxedematosus (LM) almost invariably have an M-component in the serum. Until now about 40 such patients have been reported

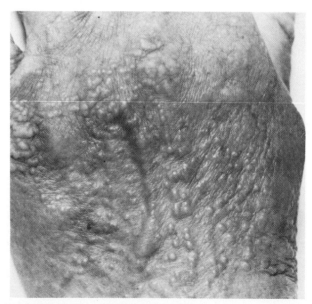

Fig. 12. Lichen myxedematosus with IgG/κ M-component. Peau-d'orange-like papular erythema and discrete papules on dorsum of left hand. (Reproduced with permission [52].)

[11,52,124,129a]. Males composed 65% of this group and the age varied from 23 to 68 years, mean 48 years. Hematological data were normal in almost all patients, anemia and elevated erythrocyte sedimentation rate being very rare. A few patients had mild eosinophilia.

The total serum protein and albumin levels were usually normal. Serum protein electrophoresis usually detected M-components with a very slow (cathodal) mobility. The concentration of M-components was almost always low, ranging from 0.4–1.1 g/dL, mean 0.85 g/dL. Higher level was occasionally observed and denoted the presence of MM [11]. Altogether three patients were diagnosed as MM and one as MW, the rest did not have sufficient evidence for malignancy. In 37 cases, the M-components were typed and were IgG in 35, IgA in 1, and IgM in 1 patient. Almost all M-components had λ-L chains [52]. In one instance an IgG/λ M-component had a molecular weight of 110,000 daltons and deletion of a part of Fd was suspected [124]. The concentration of polyclonal Igs remained usually normal. Proteinuria was only seldom observed. Occasionally mild plasmacytosis was observed in the bone marrow, however more prominent infiltration was noted in 3 patients. In two instances plasma cells from normal-looking bone marrow synthesized in vitro an M-component. No osteolytic lesions were detected and only a few patients had osteoporosis. In 3 of 18 instances, when the skin was tested by immunofluorescence, the presence of IgG was documented. In one instance, IgG was synthesized in the skin tissue culture despite a negative immunofluorescence test. One patient had amyloidosis along with papular mucinosis.

Autopsies were performed in a few instances. In a 35-year-old man who died following progressive mental deterioration, deposits of Mayer's mucicarmine-positive material were found around eccrine sweat glands, in cutaneous nerve bundles, in the wall of cutaneous blood vessels, in the heart vessels, in the perivascular connective tissue of the kidney and Bowman's capsules, in adrenal glands, and in the pancreas. The mucinous material in the perivascular spaces and in the connective tissue was often accompanied by fibroblastic proliferation.

In another patient, a 36-year-old man, numbness of all extremities and incoordination progressed to paralysis and coma and terminated in death. At autopsy, mucicarmine-positive material was detected in the renal papillae, bronchial epithelium and ductal epithelium of the pancreas. The brain showed multiple infarctions. Thus, deposits of mucicarmine-positive material similar to those found in the skin are also present in internal organs in some or maybe all patients with LM. It is feasible to conclude that LM is a systemic rather than solely a cutaneous disease.

The relationship of LM to PCD has not been clarified. The presence of M-components in many patients with this disease implies abnormal proliferation of the plasma-lymphocytic cells of B lineage. As in other PCD, steroids and immunosuppressive agents seem to be the drugs of choice. Indeed, in some patients treated with these drugs subjective and objective improvement was achieved [129a]. In others, however, no obvious improvement was observed and some deteriorated rapidly and died. The disease seems to have a prolonged 'benign' course, different from that of MM. There is no study available of the functional characteristics of T and B lymphocytes in this disease; thus, the significance of Ig abnormalities in LM remains to be elucidated.

PLASMA-CELL DYSCRASIA WITH PYODERMA GANGRENOSUM

Pyoderma gangrenosum (PG) is an ulcerative skin disease. The lesions are single or multiple, characterized by fast development, initially as plaques or pustules then spreading with ulceration and necrosis in the central areas. Necrotic ulcers are usually surrounded by an inflamed area. The pathogenesis of PG is unknown, but its association with several conditions such as leukemia, arthritis, or inflammatory bowel diseases has been well documented [100].

Until 1978, 21 cases of PG with M-components had been reported [35,100]. There were 15 IgA, 5 IgG, and 1 IgM [35,47,100,166,250]. Immunoquantitation showed either normal or slightly reduced polyclonal Ig [47,250]. Bone marrow aspirates showed moderate increase in normal-looking plasma cells [250] or a definite increase in abnormal-looking plasmacytes [100,166]. In some cases PCD presented as a typical MM [166]; in other cases no definite evidence for myeloma was found. Imhof reported a patient with PG and IgG_3/κ M-component who developed 4 years later typical myeloma with plasma-cell leukemia. Another patient with PG developed azotemia and died. Postmortem showed generalized amyloidosis with predominant involvement of the liver, spleen, and kidneys [108]. There is no specific therapy for PG and there is not enough information as to the evolution of M-component in these patients. The relationship of PG to PCD has not been elucidated.

PLASMA-CELL DYSCRASIA WITH SYSTEMIC CAPILLARY LEAK SYNDROME

Systemic capillary leak syndrome (SCLS) [7,40,82,104,114, 135,136,150,200,267,277] presents with recurrent episodes of generalized angioedema and shock caused by increase in systemic capillary permeability [7]. During the attacks there is a shift of up to 70% of plasma volume, with water, electrolytes, and proteins from the intravascular to extravascular space. Each attack lasts for about 1–3 days. The patients characteristically suffer from myalgias, perspiration, lacrimation, hoarseness, and excessive thirst.

In nine such patients, γ-mobility M-components have been observed [7,40,82,114,135,136,150,200,267,277]. The age of these patients varied from 34 to 45 years, mean 40.3 years. There were five males and three females, and in one patient the sex was not reported. In two, serum protein electrophoresis showed γ-mobility spikes but no immunological identification was performed (40,267). In seven others the M-components were identified as IgG, with κ-L chains in four and λ-L chains in two, while in one L chains were not identified. In one of these patients serum electrophoresis showed no spike; however, IgG_2/λ homogeneous protein was detected by IEP. For this reason, in patients with SCLS who had normal serum electrophoresis [104], the existence of homogeneous Igs could not be ruled out. In some patients IgA and IgM were low [135], whereas in others normal polyclonal Igs were found [7,114]. Bone marrow aspiration and postmortem material did not show plasmacytic infiltrates or other signs of myeloma, although in one patient an increase in plasmacytes to 6% was noted in the bone marrow [114]. The relationship of PCD to SCLS has not been elucidated. In one case, injection of the patient's plasma into the patient and into animals failed to provoke an attack. No pericapillary deposits of IgG were found in the skin [7].

Although the pathogenesis of SCLS has not been clarified, the presence of homogeneous immunoglobulins in the serum denotes profound aberration of the immunologic surveillance system. Further study is needed to explain the link between capillary permeability and plasma-cell dyscrasia.

REFERENCES

1. Adlersberg JB, Grann V, Zucker-Franklin D, Frangione B, Franklin EC: An unusual case of a plasma cell neoplasm with an IgG3λ myeloma and γ3 heavy chain disease protein. Blood 51:85, 1978.
2. Adner PL, Wallenius G, Werner I: Macroglobulinemia and myelomatosis. Acta Med Scand 168:431, 1960.
3. Allen EL, Metz EN, Balcerzak SP: Acute myelomonocytic leukemia with macroglobulinemia, Bence Jones proteinuria and hypercalcemia. Cancer 32:121, 1973.
4. Ameis A, Ko HS, Pruzanski W: M Components—A review of 1242 cases. Can Med Assoc J 114:889, 1976.
5. Arend WP, Adamson JW: Nonsecretory myeloma. Immunofluorescent demonstration of paraprotein within bone marrow plasma cells. Cancer 33:721, 1974.
6. Arlet J, Vidal R, Sebbag D: Un cas de maladie de Kahler avec syndrome de Looser-Milkman (Syndrome de Fanconi De L'adulte). Rev Rhum 32:380, 1965.
7. Atkinson JP, Waldmann TA, Stein SF, Gelfand JA, MacDonald WJ, Heck LW, Cohen EL, Kaplan AP, Frank MM: Systemic capillary leak syndrome and monoclonal IgG gammopathy. Medicine 56:225, 1977.
8. Axelsson U: The plasma cells of the bone marrow in myelomatosis treated with Alkeran (Melphalan). Scand J Haematol 3:123, 1966.

9. Azar HA, Zaino EC, Pham TD, Yannopoulos K: 'Nonsecretory' plasma cell myeloma: Observations on seven cases with electron microscopic studies. Am J Clin Pathol 58:618, 1972.

10. Barnard DL, Burns GF, Gordon J, Cawley JC, Barker CR, Hayhoe FGJ, Smith JL: Chronic myelomonocytic leukemia with paraproteinemia but no detectable plasmacytosis. A detailed cytological and immunological study. Cancer 44:927, 1979.

11. Bataille R, Rosenberg F, Sany J, Serre H, Meynadier J, Guilhou JJ, Baldet P, Barneon G: Association d'une mucinose papuleuse et d'un myelome multiple IgG lambda. Sem Hop Paris 54:865, 1978.

12. Beaumont JL, Jacotot B, Beaumont V, Marnet J, Vilain C: Myelome, hyperlipidemie et xanthomatose. Nouv Rev Fr Hematol 5:507, 1965.

13. Beaumont JL, Jacotot B, Vilain C, Beaumont V: Myelome, hyperlipidemie et xanthomatose. III. Un syndrome du a la presence d'un auto-anticorps anti-β lipoproteine. Nouv Rev Fr Hematol 5:787, 1965.

14. Beaumont JL, Poullin MF, Jacotot B, Beaumont V: Myelome et hyperlipidemie. IV. Nature de l'activite specifique antilipoproteine. Nouv Rev Fr Hematol 7:481, 1967.

15. Bedou G, Le Goff P, Besson G, Balnguernon P, Garré H: Myelome non excretant revele par une compression medullaire. Sem Hop Paris 50:2477, 1974.

16. Ben-bassat I, Frand UI, Isersky C, Ramot B: Plasma cell leukemia with IgG paraprotein. Arch Intern Med 121:361, 1968.

17. Benjamin D, Joshua H, Djaldetti M, Hazaz B, Pinkhas J: Nonsecretory IgD-kappa multiple myeloma in a patient with Gaucher's Disease. Scand J Haematol 22:197, 1979.

18. Bentegat MJ, De Cacqueray-Joigny C, Henry P, Moreau F, Dermendrail V, Jallon MP: La notion de myelome non-excretants ou hypoexcretants. Bordeaux Medicale 9:101, 1976.

19. Bergsagel DE, Pruzanski W: Immunoglobulins in diagnosis and monitoring of neoplasia. In Herberman RB, McIntire KR (eds): "Immunodiagnosis of Cancer, Part 1." New York: Marcel Dekker, Inc., 1979, p 450.

20. Bergsagel DE, Bailey AJ, Langley JR, MacDonald RN, White DF, Miller AB: The chemotherapy of plasma-cell myeloma and the incidence of acute leukemia. N Engl J Med 301:743, 1979.

21. Berman HH: Waldenström's macroglobulinemia with lytic osseous lesions and plasma-cell morphology. Am J Clin Pathol 63:397, 1975.

22. Bernier GM, Berman JH: IgA/2. Plasma cell leukemia with urinary excretion of IgA half-molecules. Clin Res 24:444A, 1976.

23. Biewenga J, Van Loghem E: IgA half-molecules in human myeloma. In: "Protides of Biological Fluids." (Proc. of the 25th Colloquium.) Oxford: Pergamon Press, 1978, p 899.

24. Bjerrum OJ, Stud M, Weeke B: Two M components (γGK and γML) in different cells of the same patient. Scand J Haematol 5:215, 1968.

25. Bontoux D, Alcalay M, Liere C, Baloin Ph, Frocrain C: Syndrome de Fanconi de l'adulte au cours d'une maladie des chains kappa. Rev Rhum 43:384, 1976.

26. Bouvet JP, Buffe D, Oriol R, Liacopoulos P: Two myeloma globulins IgG1-κ and IgG1-λ, from a single patient (Im). Immunology 27:1095, 1974.

27. Bouvet JP, Feingold J, Oriol R, Liacopoulos P: Statistical study on double paraproteinemias. Evidence for a common cellular origin of both myeloma globulins. Biomedicine 22:517, 1975.

28. Brachfeld J, Myerson RM: Pyroglobulinemia. Diagnostic clue in multiple myeloma. JAMA 161:865, 1956.

29. Bureau Y, Senelar R, Barriere H, Bureau B, Litoux P, Bray B: Macroglobulinémie au cours d'une maladie de Kahler. Presse Med 76:961, 1968.

30. Burnier E, Zwahlen A, Cruchaud A: Nonmalignant monoclonal immunoglobulinemia, pernicious anemia and gastric carcinoma. A model of immunologic dysfunction. Report of two cases and review of the literature. Am J Med 60:1019, 1976.
31. Burns GF, Cawley JC, Barker CR, Worman CP, Raper CGL, Hayhoe FGJ: Differing surface marker characteristics in plasma cell dyscrasias with particular reference to IgM myeloma. Clin Exp Immunol 31:414, 1978.
32. Burns GF, Worman CP, Roberts BE, Raper CGL, Barker CR, Cawley JC: Terminal B cell development as seen in different human myelomas and related disorders. Clin Exp Immunol 35:180, 1979.
33. Bushell AC, Whicher JT, Yuille T: The progressive appearance of multiple urinary Bence-Jones proteins and serum paraproteins in a child with immune deficiency. Clin Exp Immunol 38:64, 1979.
34. Butler EA, Flynn FV: The proteinuria of renal tubular disorders. Lancet II:978, 1958.
35. Callen JP, Taylor WP: Pyoderma gangrenosum—a literature review. Cutis 21:61, 1978.
36. Carter P, Koval JJ, Hobbs JR: The relation of clinical and laboratory findings to the survival of patients with macroglobulinaemia. Clin Exp Immunol 28:241, 1977.
37. Case records of the Massachusetts General Hospital, Case 31–1972. N Engl J Med 287:243, 1972.
38. Cattaneo R, Bazzi C, Simonati V, Balestrieri G: Studio Immunochimico di tre casi di piroglobulinemia. Prog Immunobiol Standard 4:199, 1970.
39. Child JA, Franklin IM, Warren JV, Cawley JC, Roberts BE, Burns GF, Roach TC: Pleomorphic B cell neoplasm with monoclonal IgA secretion. Cancer 40:2948, 1977.
40. Clarkson B, Thompson D, Horvith M, Luckey EH: Cyclical edema and shock due to increased capillary permeability. Am J Med 29:193, 1960.
41. Cleary B, Binder RA, Kales AN, Veltri BJ: Simultaneous presentation of acute mye-lomonocytic leukemia and multiple myeloma. Cancer 41:1381, 1978.
42. Cohen L, Blaisdell RK, Djordjevich J, Ormiste V, Dobrilovic L: Familial xanthomatosis and hyperlipidemia and myelomatosis. Am J Med 40:299, 1966.
43. Collier FC, Reich A, King JW: Multiple myeloma. A report of four cases demonstrating Bence-Jones proteinemia found during routine complement-fixation tests. N Engl J Med 247:969, 1951.
44. Coltman CA Jr: Multiple myeloma without a paraprotein. Report of a case with ob-servations on chromosomal composition. Arch Intern Med 120:687, 1967.
45. Constanza DJ, Smoller M: Multiple myeloma with the Fanconi syndrome. Study of a case with electron microscopy of the kidney. Am J Med 34:125, 1963.
46. Costea N, Yakulis VJ, Libnoch JA, Pilz CG, Heller P: Two myeloma globulins (IgG and IgA) in one subject and one cell line. Am J Med 42:630, 1967.
47. Cream JJ: Pyoderma gangrenosum with a monoclonal IgM red cell agglomerating factor. Br J Dermatol 84:223, 1971.
48. Da Costa SFG, Relvas MESA, Halpern MJ, Da Silva JAF: Contribuições para o estudo da patologia quimica de um caso de mieloma associado ao sindroma de Fanconi. Gaz Med Portuguesa 13:583, 1960.
49. Dalal FR, Winsten S: Double light-chain disease: A case report. Clin Chem 25:190, 1979.
50. Dammacco F, Trizio D, Bonomo L: A case of IgAκ-myelomatosis with two urinary Bence-Jones proteins (BJκ and BJλ) and multiple chromosomal abnormalities. Acta Haematol 41:309, 1969.
51. Dammacco F, Miglietta A, Ferrannini A, Antonaci S: Il problema de mieloma 'non-secernente.' Haematologica (Pavia) 58:816, 1973.

52. Danby FW, Danby CWE, Pruzanski W: Papular mucinosis with IgG(κ) M component. Can Med Assoc J 114:920, 1976.
53. Danon F, Clauvel JP, Seligmann M: Les "Paraproteines" de type IgG et IgA en dehors de la maladie de Kahler. Rev Franc Etudes Clin Biol 12:681, 1967.
54. De Coteau WE, Calvanico NJ, Tomasi TB Jr: Malignant lymphoma with a monoclonal F(ab)μ fragment. Clin Immunol Immunopathol 1:190, 1973.
55. Dedmon RE, West JH, Schwartz TB: The adult Fanconi syndrome. Report of two cases, one with multiple myeloma. Med Clin North Am 47:191, 1963.
56. Delbarre F, Siguier F, Godeau P, Saporta L, Seligmann M, Hurez D: La maladie de Kahler à plasmocytes 'non-excretants.' Ann Med Interne (Paris) 121:537, 1970.
57. Dittmar K, Kochwa S, Zucker-Franklin D, Wasserman LR: Coexistence of polycythemia vera and biclonal gammapathy (γGκ and γAλ) with two Bence Jones proteins (BJκ and BJλ). Blood 31:81, 1968.
58. Dotten D, Pruzanski W: Multiple myeloma with discordant M-components in the serum and cerebrospinal fluid. Arch Intern Med 14:1374, 1981.
59. Dragsted PJ, Hjorth N: The association of the Fanconi syndrome with malignant disease. Dan Med Bull 3:177, 1956.
60. Driedger H, Pruzanski W: Plasma cell neoplasia with osteosclerotic lesions. A study of five cases and a review of the literature. Arch Intern Med 139:892, 1979.
61. Driedger H, Pruzanski W: Plasma cell neoplasia with peripheral polyneuropathy. A study of five cases and a review of the literature. Medicine 59:301, 1980.
62. Engle RL, Wallis LA: Multiple myeloma and the adult Fanconi syndrome. I. Report of a case with crystal-like deposits in the tumor cells and in the epithelial cells of the kidney. Am J Med 22:5, 1957.
63. Engle RL, Nachman RL: Two Bence Jones proteins of different immunologic types in the same patient with multiple myeloma. Blood 27:74, 1966.
64. Englis M, Englisova M: Pyroprecipitation dans un cas de myelome. Nouv Rev Fr Hematol 8:264, 1968.
65. Fabia F, Burnichon J, Cornillot P: Essai d'interpretation physiopathologique du myeloma 'non-excretant.' Pathol Biol (Paris) 22:617, 1974.
66. Fagiolo E: Plasmocytoma with IgM paraproteinemia. A case report. Acta Haematol 55:123, 1976.
67. Fair DS, Krueger RG, Gleich GJ, Kyle RA: Studies on IgA and IgG monoclonal proteins derived from a single patient. I. Evidence for shared individually specific antigenic determinants. J Immunol 112:201, 1974.
68. Fateh-Moghadam A, Beil E, Borchers H, Asamer H, Raab Ch: Plasmazytom, Macroglobulinämie Waldenström und Morbus Paget bei einem Patienten mit IgAκ + IgMκ-Doppelparaproteinämie und Bence-Jones-Protein (Typ κ). Blut 21:146, 1970.
69. Feiwel M: Xanthomatosis in cryoglobulinaemia and other paraproteinaemias with report of a case. Br J Dermatol 80:719, 1968.
69a. Ferraris AM, Haupt E, Ratti M: Multiple myeloma without detectable Ig synthesis. Acta Haematol 62:257–261, 1979.
70. Fine JM, Dormont J, Creyssel JPhMR, Groulade J, Debray-Sachs M: Etudes sur la nature d'une pyroglobuline sèrique observée au cours du myelome. Rev Fr Etudes Clin Biol 6:864, 1961.
70a. Fine JM, Gorin NC, Gendre JP, Petitpierre JC, Labro-Bryskier MTh, Lambin P: Simultaneous occurrence of clinical manifestations of myeloma and Waldenström's macroglobulinemia with monoclonal IgG lambda and IgM kappa in a single patient. Acta Med Scand 209:229, 1981.

71. Fine JM, Zakin MM, Faure A: Myelome avec paraproteine serique γG et elimination urinaire d'un fragment de γG despourvous de chaines legeres. Rev Fr Etud Clin Biol 13:175, 1968.
72. Finkel PN, Kronenberg K, Pesce AJ, Pollak VE, Pirani CL: Adult Fanconi syndrome, amyloidosis and marked κ-light chain proteinuria. Nephron 10:1, 1973.
73. Finkle HI, Brownlow K, Elevitch FR: Monoclonal IgG-lysozyme (muramidase) complex in acute myelomonocytic leukemia: An unusual finding. Am J Clin Pathol 60:936, 1973.
74. Fisher B, Schaer LR, Messinger S: The occurrence of pyroglobulins in unsuspected myeloma. Am J Clin Pathol 40:291, 1963.
75. Forssman O, Nilsson G: A case of myeloma with flaming plasma cells but no significant M-compound in serum or urine. Acta Med Scand 181:33, 1967.
76. Fournier A, Bernaudin JF, Kremski J, Hirbec G, Berry JP, Lagrue G, Hazard J: Quadriparesie hypokaliemique revelatrice d'un syndrome de Fanconi et d'un myelome. Nouv Presse Med 4:2983, 1975.
77. Frame B, Pachter MR, Nixon RK: Myelomatosis with xanthomatosis. Ann Intern Med 54:134, 1961.
78. Franzen S, Johansson B, Kaigas M: Primary polycythaemia associated with multiple myeloma. Acta Med Scand 179 (suppl 445):336, 1966.
79. Fraser KJ: multiple myeloma and pernicious anemia. Med J Aust 1:298, 1969.
80. Fudenberg HH, Virella G: Multiple myeloma and Waldenström macroglobulinemia: Unusual presentations. Semin Hematol 17:63, 1980.
81. Gach J, Simar L, Salmon J: Multiple myeloma without M-type proteinemia. Report of a case with immunologic and ultrastructure studies. Am J Med 50:835, 1971.
82. George C, Regnier B, Le Gall JR, Gastinne H, Carlet J, Rapin M: Hypovolaemic shock with oedema due to increased capillary permeability. Intensive Care Med 4:159, 1978.
83. Gibaud A, Gibaud H: Another case of double light chain disease. Clin Chem 25:644, 1979.
84. Giertsen JC: Polycythaemia vera with multiple myeloma. Report of a case. Acta Pathol Microbiol Scand 38:439, 1956.
85. Goldrosen MH, Pruzanski W, Freedman MM: Structural and immunological study of two IgG myeloma proteins from a single patient. Immunochemistry 9:387, 1972.
86. Hammarsten G, Lindgren G, Olhagen B, Ordell R: Hyperglobulinemia with a unique thermolabile γ-component. Report of a case. Acta Med Scand 123:50, 1945.
87. Hannestad K, Eriksen J, Christensen T, Harboe M: A serum with two IgM M-components of different combining specificity. Immunochemistry 7:861, 1970.
88. Hannestad K, Sletten K: Multiple M components in a single individual. III. Heterogeneity of M-components in two macroglobulinemia sera with antipolysaccharide activity. J Biol Chem 246:6982, 1971.
89. Harrison JF, Blainey JD, Hardwicke J, Rowe DS, Soothill JF: Proteinuria in multiple myeloma. Clin Sci 31:95, 1966.
90. Harrison JF, Blainey JD: Adult Fanconi syndrome with monoclonal abnormality of immunoglobulin light chain. J Clin Pathol 20:42, 1967.
91. Headley RN, King JS Jr, Cooper MR, Felts JH: Multiple myeloma presenting as adult Fanconi syndrome. Clin Chem 18:293, 1972.
92. Heinle EW Jr, Sarasti HO, Garcia D, Kenny JJ, Westerman MP: Polycythemia vera associated with lymphomatous diseases and myeloma. Arch Intern Med 118:351, 1966.
93. Heron JF, Guaydier G, Loyau G, Laniece M, Mandart JC, Borel B, L'Hirondel JL, Dumas M, Foucault JP: Myelome a IgM. A propos d'une observation. Sem Hop Paris 52:2549, 1976.
94. Hijmans W: Waldenström's disease with an IgA paraprotein. Acta Med Scand 198:519, 1975.

95. Hill RM, Mulligan RM, Dunlop SG: Plasma cell myeloma associated with high concentration of plasma lipoprotein. Am J Pathol 24:688, 1948.

96. Hobbs JR: Disturbances of the immunoglobulins. Sci Basis Med Ann Rev p 106, 1966.

97. Hobbs JR: Immunochemical classes of myelomatosis. Including data from a therapeutic trial conducted by a Medical Research Council working party. Br J Haematol 16:599, 1969.

98. Hobbs JR, Jacobs A: A half-molecule Gκ plasmacytoma. Clin Exp Immunol 5:199, 1969.

99. Hollan SR, Solti V: Grape cell plasmacytoma associated with lipaemia and dynamic changes in the serum protein pattern. Acta Med Acad Sci Hung 20:249, 1964.

100. Holt PJA, Davies MG, Saunders KC, Nuki G: Pyoderma gangrenosum. Clinical and laboratory findings in 15 patients with special reference to polyarthritis. Medicine 59:114, 1980.

101. Horn ME, Knapp MS, Page FT, Walker WHC: Adult Fanconi syndrome and multiple myelomatosis. J Clin Pathol 22:414, 1969.

102. Hörner H: Makroglobulinamie Waldenström mit osteolitische Herden. Klin Wochenschr 33:1110, 1955.

103. Hossfeld DK, Holland JF, Cooper RG, Ellison RR: Chromosome studies in acute leukemias developing in patients with multiple myeloma. Cancer Res 35:2808, 1975.

104. Horwith M, Hagström JWC, Riggins RCK, Luckey EH: Hypovolemic shock and edema due to increased capillary permeability. JAMA 200:101, 1967.

105. Hrnčiř Z, Mazak J, Matěja F, Vanăsek J, Tichý M: Coincidence of pernicious anemia and IgA-κ myeloma. A clinical model of the relation between autoimmune disease and tumour from immunocompetent tissue. Neoplasma 17:197, 1970.

106. Huisman THJ, van der Wal B, Groen A, and van der Sar A: Investigations on a heat-coagulable globulin in the blood of a patient with multiple myeloma. Clin Chim Acta 1:525, 1956.

107. Hurez D, Preud'homme JL, Seligmann M: Intracellular "monoclonal" immunoglobulin in non-secretory human myeloma. J Immunol 101:263, 1970.

108. Imhof JW, Vleugels Schutter GJN, Hart HCh, Zegers BJM: Monoclonal gammopathy (IgG) and chronic ulcerative dermatitis (phagedenic pyoderma). Acta Med Scand 186:289, 1969.

109. Indiveri F, Barabino A, Santolini ME, Santolini B: 'Nonsecretory' multiple myeloma. Report of a case. Acta Haematol 51:302, 1974.

110. Invernizzi F, Cattaneo R, Rosso di san Secondo V, Balestrieri G, Zanussi C: Pyroglobulinemia. A report of eight patients with associated paraproteinemia. Acta Haematol 50:65, 1973.

111. Isobe T, Osserman EF: Plasma cell dyscrasia associated with the production of incomplete (? deleted) IgGλ molecules, gamma heavy chains and free lambda chains containing carbohydrate: Description of the first case. Blood 43:505, 1974.

112. Isobe T, Ikeda Y, Imura H, Ohta H: Plasma cell leukemia. A clinical study of 13 cases, with a demonstration of small-sized plasma cells. Acta Haematol Japonica 40:529, 1977.

113. Jacotot B, Nguyen-Trong T, Beaumont JL: Myélome, hyperlipidémie et xanthomatose. II. Recherches complementaires sur l'association entre la paraproteine et les lipoproteines légéres. Nouv Rev Fr Hematol 5:777, 1965.

114. Jacox RF, Waterhouse C, Tobin R: Periodic disease associated with muscle destruction. Am J Med 55:105, 1973.

115. James W III, Harlan WR: Plasma cell disease and xanthomatosis. Trans Am Clin Climatol Assoc 79:115, 1967.

116. Jensen K, Birger Jensen K, Olesen H: Three M-components in serum from an apparently

healthy person. Scand J Haematol 4:485, 1967.

117. Josephson AS, Nicastri A, Price E, Biro L: Hμ chain fragment and monoclonal IgA in a lymphoproliferative disorder. Am J Med 54:127, 1973.

118. Joyner MC, Cassuto J-P, Dujardin P, Schneider M, Ziegler G, Euller L, Masseyeff R: Non-excretory multiple myeloma. Br J Haematol 43:559, 1979.

119. Kang YS, Shim BS: An abnormal human IgA half-molecule. Biochim Biophys Acta 484:326, 1977.

120. Kayden HJ, Franklin EC: Interaction of myeloma gamma globulin with human beta-lipoprotein (P). Circulation 26:659, 1962.

121. Keller H, Spengler GA, Skvaŕil F, Flury W, Noseda G, Riva G: Zur frage der heavy chain disease. Ein Fall von IgG-heavy-chain-Fragment und IgM-Typ-κ-Paraproteinämie mit Plasmazellenleukämie. Schweiz Med Wochenschr 100:1012, 1970.

122. Kim I, Harley JB, Weksler B: Multiple myeloma without initial paraproteins. Am J Med Sci 264:267, 1972.

123. Kistner S, Nørberg R: The simultaneous occurrence of two different myeloma proteins. Scand J Clin Lab Invest 17:321, 1965.

124. Kitamura W, Matsuoka Y, Miyagawa S, Sakamoto K: Immunochemical analysis of the monoclonal paraprotein in Scleromyxedema. J Invest Dermatol 70:305, 1978.

125. Klemm D, Grusnick D, Weinreich J, Hauswaldt Ch, Hunstein W: Paraproteinämie und plasmaretikuläre Zellproliferation bei Polycythemia vera. Acta Haematol 38:240, 1967.

126. Klepping CL, Destaing F, Duzer A, Villand J, Carli PM, Seigneuric C: Nouvelle observation de myelome non-excretant. Lyon Medicale 228:131, 1972.

127. Ko HS, Minkarious EF: Immunologic abnormalities in a patient with multiple neoplasms. Can Med Assoc J 114:917, 1976.

128. Koga S, Kozura M, Hirayama C, Ibayashi H: An unusual lipid-protein complex observed in an IgG myeloma patient. Clin Chim Acta 54:169, 1974.

129. Krajny M, Pruzanski W: Waldenström's macroglobulinemia: Review of 45 cases. Can Med Assoc J 114:899, 1976.

129a. Krebs A, Muller A: Lichen myxoedematosus und multiples myelom vom Typ IgG/kappa. Hautarzt 31:649–653, 1980.

130. Kretschmer RR, Pizzuto J, Gonzales J, Lopez M: Heavy chain disease, rheumatoid arthritis and cryoglobulinemia. Clin Immunol Immunopathol 2:195, 1974.

131. Kyle RA, Maldonado JE, Bayrd ED: Plasma cell leukemia. Report on 17 cases. Arch Intern Med 133:813, 1974.

132. Kyle RA: Multiple myeloma: Review of 869 cases. Mayo Clin Proc 50:29, 1975.

133. Kyle RA, Pierre RV, Bayrd ED: Multiple myeloma and acute myelomonocytic leukemia. Report of four cases possibly related to melphalan. N Engl J Med 283:1121, 1970.

134. Kyle RA, Pierre RV, Bayrd ED: Multiple myeloma and acute leukemia associated with alkylating agents. Arch Intern Med 135:185, 1975.

134a. Kyle RA, Robinson RA, Katzmann JA: The clinical aspects of biclonal gammopathies. Review of 57 cases. Am J Med 71:999, 1981.

135. Larcan A, Calamai M, Heully MC, Helmer J: Choc cyclique par exageration de la permeabilite capillaire. Responsabilité probable d'une immunoglobuline G. Presse Med 77:1931, 1969.

136. Larcan A, Laprevote HC, Lambert H: Cyclical shock with hyperglobulinemia. Bibl Anat 13:343, 1975.

137. Larsson SO: Myeloma and pernicious anemia. Acta Med Scand 172:195, 1962.

138. Laurell CB, Snigurowicz J: The frequency of kappa and lambda chains in pathologic serum γG, γA, γD and γμ immunoglobulins. Scand J Haematol 4:46, 1967.

139. Lawrence JH, Rosenthal RL: Multiple myeloma associated with polycythemia: Report of four cases. Am J Med Sci 218:149, 1949.

140. Leb L, Grimes ET, Balogh K, Merritt JA Jr: Monoclonal macroglobulinemia with osteolytic lesions. A case report and review of the literature. Cancer 39:227, 1977.

141. Lee DBN, Drinkard JP, Rosen VJ, Gonick HC: The adult Fanconi syndrome. Observations on etiology, morphology, renal function and mineral metabolism in three patients. Medicine 51:107, 1972.

142. Lennard-Jones JE: Myelomatosis with lipaemia and xanthomata. Br Med J 1:781, 1960.

143. Levin WC, Aboumrad MH, Ritzmann SE: γ-Type I myeloma and xanthomatosis. Arch Intern Med 114:688, 1964.

144. Lewis AF, Bergsagel DE, Bruce-Robertson A, Schachter RK, Connell GE: An atypical immunoglobulin. Blood 32:189, 1968.

145. Lewis LA, Page IH: An unusual serum lipoprotein-globulin complex in a patient with hyperlipemia. Am J Med 38:286, 1965.

146. Lewis LA, Van Ommen RA, Page IH: Association of cold-precipitability with β-lipoprotein and cryoglobulin. Am J Med 40:785, 1966.

147. Ligorsky RD, Axelrod AR, Mandell GH, Palutke M, Prasad AS: Acute myelomonocytic leukemia in a patient with macroglobulinemia and malignant lymphoma. Cancer 39:1156, 1977.

148. Linscott WD, Kane JP: The complement system in cryoglobulinemia. Interaction with immunoglobulins and lipoproteins. Clin Exp Immunol 21:510, 1975.

149. Lipman IJ: Pyroglobulinemia. An unusual presenting sign in multiple myeloma. JAMA 188:1002, 1964.

150. Löfdahl CG, Sölvell L, Laurell AB, Johansson BR: Systemic capillary leak syndrome with monoclonal IgG and complement alterations. A case report on an episodic syndrome. Acta Med Scand 206:405, 1979.

151. Löffler H, Knopp A, Krecke HJ: Cases of multiple myeloma (plasmacytoma) "without paraprotein". Ger Med Mth 12:226, 1967.

152. Mabry RJ, Shelburne J, Cohen HJ: In vitro kinetics of immunoglobulin synthesis and secretion by nonsecretory human myeloma cells. Blood 50:1031, 1977.

153. Maldonado JE, Velosa JA, Kyle RA, Wagoner RD, Holley KE, Salassa RM: Fanconi syndrome in adults. A manifestation of a latent form of myeloma. Am J Med 58:354, 1975.

154. Mancilla R, Davis GL: Nonsecretory multiple myeloma. Immunohistologic and ultrastructural observations on two patients. Am J Med 63:1015, 1977.

154a. Maeda K, Abraham JP, Nalini J: Polycythemia vera associated with IgA myeloma; clinical study of three cases. Blood 58:167a, 1981.

155. Mannik M, Kunkel HG: Classification of myeloma proteins, Bence Jones proteins and macroglobulins into two groups on the basis of common antigenic characters. J Exp Med 116:859, 1962.

156. Marien KJC, Smeenk G: Plane xanthomata associated with multiple myeloma and hyperlipoproteinemia. Br J Dermatol 93:407, 1975.

157. Martin WJ, Mathieson DR: Pyroglobulinemia (heat coagulable globulin in the blood). Proc Staff Meet Mayo Clin 28:545, 1953.

158. Martin WJ, Mathieson DR, Eigler JO: Pyroglobulinemia: Further observations and review of 20 cases. Proc Staff Meet Mayo Clin 34:95, 1959.

159. McCann SR, Zinneman HH, Oken MM, Leary MC, Swaim WR, Moore M: IgM pyroglobulinemia with erythrocytosis presenting as hyperviscosity syndrome. I. Clinical features and viscometric studies. Am J Med 61:316, 1976.

160. McKenzie AW: Plane xanthoma, hypercholesterolaemia and myelomatosis. Proc R Soc Med 57:889, 1964.
161. MacKenzie MR, Fudenberg HH: Macroglobulinemia: An analysis for forty patients. Blood 39:874, 1972.
162. McLaughlin H, Farrelly PA, Melinn M: Non-paraprotein producing myeloma. Ir J Med Sci 145:181, 1976.
163. McNutt DR, Fudenberg HH: IgG myeloma and Waldenström macroglobulinemia. Arch Intern Med 131:731, 1973.
164. Meltzer M, Franklin EC: Cryoglobulinemia. A clinical and laboratory study. Am J Med 40:837, 1966.
165. Menkes CJ, Herreman G, Preud'homme JL, Godeau P, Delbarre F: Myélome à plasmocytes non excrétants. Nouv Presse Med 1:309, 1972.
166. Möller H, Waldenström JG, Zettervall O: Pyoderma gangrenosum (dermatitis ulcerosa) and monoclonal (IgA) globulin healed after melphalan treatment. Acta Med Scand 203:293, 1978.
167. Moschella SL: Plane xanthomatosis associated with myelomatosis. Arch Dermatol 101:683, 1970.
167a. Mossler JA, Wortman J, Reeves W, McCarty KS Jr: Intracytoplasmic IgM in a nonsecretory myeloma. Arch Pathol Lab Med 105:165–166, 1981.
168. Mullinax F, Himrod B, Berry ER: Myeloma protein with specific binding of choline. Clin Res 18:429, 1970.
169. Muntendam DH: Multipele myelomatosis en het syndroom van De Toni-Fanconi. Ned Tijdschr Geneeskd 102:1690, 1958.
170. Neufeld AH, Halpenny GW, Morton HS: Beta-2 lipoprotein myelomatosis. Can J Biochem 42:1499, 1964.
171. Neufeld AH, Morton HS, Halpenny GW: Myelomatosis with xanthomatosis multiforme. Can Med Assoc J 91:374, 1964.
172. Nilsson K, Killander D, Killander J, Mellstedt H: Short-term tissue culture of two nonsecretory human myelomas. A morphological and functional study. Scand J Immunol 5:819, 1976.
173. Osserman EF, Takatsuki K: Plasma cell myeloma: Gamma globulin synthesis and structure. Medicine 42:357, 1963.
174. Osserman EF, Lawlor DP: Serum and urinary lysozyme (muramidase) in monocytic and monomyelocytic leukemia. J Exp Med 124:921, 1966.
175. Osserman EF: The association between plasmacytic and monocytic dyscrasias in man: Clinical and biochemical studies. In Killander J (ed): "Gamma Globulins. Structure and Control of Biosynthesis." Nobel Symposium 3. Stockholm: Almqvist and Wiksell, 1967, pp 573–583.
176. Osserman EF: Postulated relationships between lysozyme and immunoglobulins as mediators of macrophage and plasma cell functions. Adv Pathobiol 4:98, 1976.
177. Oxelius VA: Alternating appearance of IgD and IgG myeloma protein during treatment. Scand J Haematol 8:439, 1971.
178. Özer FL, Telatar H, Telatar F, Müftüoglu E: Monoclonal gammopathy with hyperlipidemia. Am J Med 49:841, 1970.
179. Panders DJT, Leeksma CHW: Pernicieuze anemie met paraproteinemie. Ned Tijdscher Geneeskd 107:811, 1963.
180. Patterson R, Nelson VL, Pruzansky JJ: Pyroglobulinemia: Some characteristics of a heat labile protein. Immunology 9:477, 1965.
181. Patterson R, Weiszer I, Rambach W, Roberts M, Suszko IM: Comparative cellular and immunochemical studies of two cases of pyroglobulinemia. Am J Med 44:147, 1968.

182. Patterson R, Roberts M, Rambach W, Falleroni A: An IgM pyroglobulin associated with lymphosarcoma. Am J Med 48:503, 1970.
183. Pedraza MA: Plasma-cell leukemia with unusual immunoglobulin abnormalities. Am J Clin Pathol 64:410, 1975.
184. Penn GM, Kunkel HG, Grey HM: Sharing of individual antigenic determinants between a γG and a γM protein in the same myeloma serum. Proc Soc Exp Biol Med 135:660, 1970.
185. Perillie PE: Myeloma and pernicious anemia. Am J Med Sci 275:93, 1978.
186. Pinkhas J, Djaldetti M, Yaron M: Coincidence of multiple myeloma with Gaucher's disease. Isr J Med Sci 1:537, 1965.
187. Pinkus GS, Said JW: Specific identification of intracellular immunoglobulin in paraffin sections of multiple myeloma and macroglobulinemia using an immunoperoxidase technique. Am J Pathol 87:47, 1977.
188. Potier J, Thomas M, Laniece M, Ramon P, Jame P: Dysglobulinémie monoclonale à précédée d'une gammapathie monoclonale à IgG. Nouv Presse Med 5:274, 1976.
189. Potter M: Myeloma proteins (M-components) with antibody-like activity. N Engl J Med 284:831, 1971.
190. Poulik MD, Berman L, Prasad AS: "Myeloma protein" in a patient with monocytic leukemia. Blood 33:746, 1969.
191. Pruzanski W, Platts ME, Ogryzlo MA: Leukemic form of immunocytic dyscrasia (plasma cell leukemia). A study of ten cases and a review of the literature. Am J Med 47:60, 1969.
192. Pruzanski W, Platts ME: Serum and urinary protein, lysozyme (muramidase) and renal dysfunction in mono- and myelomonocytic leukemia. J Clin Invest 49:1694, 1970.
193. Pruzanski W, Underdown B, Silver EH, Katz A: Macroglobulinemia-myeloma double gammopathy. A study of four cases and a review of the literature. Am J Med 57:259, 1974.
194. Pruzanski W: Clinical manifestations of multiple myeloma: Relation to class and type of M component. Can Med Assoc J 114:896, 1976.
195. Pruzanski W, Shumak KH: Biologic activity of cold-reacting autoantibodies. N Engl J Med 297:538, 583, 1977.
196. Pruzanski W, Shumak KH: Cold agglutinins for platelets. N Engl J Med 298:402, 1978.
197. Pruzanski W, Roelcke D, Armstrong M, Manly MS: Pr and Gd antigens on human B and T lymphocytes and phagocytes. Clin Immunol Immunopathol 15:631, 1980.
198. Pruzanski W, Williams C: Role of calcitonin in osteosclerosis of myeloma. Arch Intern Med 140:1554, 1980.
199. Pratt PW, Estren S, Kochwa S: Immunoglobulin abnormalities in Gaucher's disease. Report of 16 cases. Blood 31:633, 1968.
200. Preston GM, Rees JR, Spathis GS: A man with cyclical edema. Guy's Hosp Rep 111:69, 1962.
201. Preud'homme JL, Hurez D, Danon F, Brouet JC, Seligmann M: Intracytoplasmic and surface-bound immunoglobulins in 'nonsecretory' and Bence-Jones myeloma. Clin Exp Immunol 25:428, 1976.
202. Rádl J, vd Berg P: Transitory appearance of homogeneous immunoglobulins—"paraproteins"—in children with severe combined immunodeficiency before and after transplantation treatment. Protides Biol Fluids 20:263, 1973.
203. Rawlings W Jr, Griffin J, Duffy T, Humphrey R: Fanconi syndrome with lambda light chains in urine. N Engl J Med 292:1351, 1975.
203a. Reitan JB, Pape E, Fosså, SD, Julsrud O-J, Stettnes ON, Solheim OP: Osteosclerotic myeloma with polyneuropathy. Acta Med Scand 208:137–144, 1980.

204. Resegotti L, Palestro G, Coda R, Dolci C, Poggio E, Leonardo E: Waldenström-like immunocytic lymphoma with IgG serum M component. Acta Haematol 58:38, 1977.
205. Riesen W, Noseda G, Bütler R: Anti-β-lipoprotein activity of human monoclonal immunoglobulins. Vox Sang 22:420, 1972.
206. River GL, Tewksbury DA, Fudenberg HH: "Nonsecretory" multiple myeloma. Blood 40:204, 1972.
207. Roberts-Thomson PJ, Venables GS, Onitiri AC, Lewis B: Polymeric IgA myeloma, hyperlipidemia and xanthomatosis: A further case and review. Postgrad Med J 51:44, 1975.
208. Roelcke D: Actual aspects of cold agglutination. Ric Clin Lab 7:11, 1977.
209. Roelcke D, Pruzanski W, Ebert W, Römer W, Fischer E, Lenhard V, Rauterberg E: A new human monoclonal cold agglutinin Sa recognizing terminal N-acetylneuraminyl groups on the cell surface. Blood 55:677, 1980.
210. Roujeau JC, Bisson M, Segond P, Massias P: Myelome a IgM. Sem Hop Paris 52:2277, 1976.
211. Rousseau JJ, Franck G, Grisar T, Reznik M, Heynen G, Salmon J: Osteosclerotic myeloma with polyneuropathy and ectopic secretion of calcitonin. Eur J Cancer 14:133, 1978.
212. Rousseau JJ, Heynen G, Franck G: Role of calcitonin in osteosclerosis of myeloma. Arch Int Med, 1980 (in press).
213. Rosner F, Grünwald H: Multiple myeloma terminating in acute leukemia. Report of 12 cases and review of the literature. Am J Med 57:927, 1974.
214. Rosner F: Multiple myeloma and acute leukemia: Review of 104 cases. Blood 52 (suppl 1):273(A), 1978.
215. Rudders RA, Yakulis V, Heller P: Double myeloma. Production of both IgG type lambda and IgA type lambda myeloma proteins by a single plasma cell line. Am J Med 55:215, 1973.
215a. Ruestow PC, Levinson DJ, Catchatourian R, Srekanth S, Cohen H, Rosenfeld S: Coexistence of IgA myeloma and Gaucher's disease. Arch Int Med 140:1115, 1980.
216. Said G, Henon P, Guérin A, Kahn MF, Dorfmann H, de Séze S: Un cas de maladie de Kahler a IgM globuline. Rev Rhum 39:140, 1972.
217. Salberg D, Kurtides S, McKeever WP: Monomyelocytic leukemia in an untreated case of Waldenström macroglobulinemia. Arch Intern Med 137:514, 1977.
218. Salmon SE, Seligmann M: B-cell neoplasia in man. Lancet 2:1230, 1974.
219. Sanders JH, Fahey JL, Finegold I, Ein D, Reisfeld R, Berard C: Multiple anomalous immunoglobulins. Clinical, structural and cellular studies in three patients. Am J Med 47:43, 1969.
220. Savin RC: Hyperglobulinemic purpura terminating in myeloma, hyperlipemia and xanthomatosis. Arch Dermatol 92:679, 1965.
221. Scheele C: Light chain myeloma with features of the adult Fanconi syndrome: Six years remission following one course of Melphalan. Acta Med Scand 199:533, 1976.
222. Schless GL: Serum cholesterol-globulin complex in multiple myeloma. Am J Med Sci 235:562, 1958.
223. Schwarz JA, Hufnagl HD, Jost H, Scheurlen PG: Subleukämischer Verlauf einer Makroglobulinämie Waldenström mit Osteolysen: IgM-kappa-Kryoglobulin mit antinuklearer Aktivität und μ-Kettenfragment. Klin Wochenschr 51:900, 1973.
224. Scolari L, Vaerman JP, Castigli E, Voliani D, Salsano F, Masala C, Di Guglielmo R: Late appearance of an IgA (k) monoclonal protein in a patient with IgG (k) multiple

myeloma: Sharing of idiotypic specificities between the two serum proteins. Scand J Immunol 8:201, 1978.

225. Seitanidis BA, Shulman G, Hobbs JR: Low serum cholesterol with IgA myelomatosis. Clin Chim Acta 29:93, 1970.

226. Seligmann M, Mihaesco E, Chevalier A, Miglierina R: Immunochemical study of a human myeloma IgG₁ half molecule. Ann Immunol 129:855, 1978.

227. Shirakura T, Takekoshi K, Umi M, Kanazawa K, Okabe H, Inoue T, Imamura Y: Waldenström's macroglobulinemia with IgE M-component. Scand J Haematol 21:292, macroglobulinemia with IgE M-component. Scand J Haematol 21:292, 1978.

228. Short IA, Smith JP: Myelomatosis associated with glycosuria and aminoaciduria. Scott Med J 4:89, 1959.

229. Short MH: Multiple myeloma with xanthoma formation. Arch Pathol 77:400, 1964.

230. Siame JL, Sebert JL, Delcambre B, D'erhougues JR: Le syndrome de Fanconi de l'adulte son association au myelome multiple (à propos d'un cas). Lille Med 23:428, 1978.

231. Sirota JH, Hamerman D: Renal function studies in an adult subject with the Fanconi syndrome. Am J Med 16:138, 1954.

232. Skvaril F, Juricic D, Spengler GA, Morell A: The IgG subclass distribution in double M-component sera. Protides Biol Fluids 20:273, 1972.

233. Sobel AT, Antonucci M, Intrator L, Bernard D, Beaumont JL, Lagrue G: Association d'une gammapathie monoclonale, d'une glomerulopathie chronique et d'une hyperlipidémie auto-immune. Nouv Presse Med 5:2375, 1976.

234. Sølling K, Sølling J, Jacobsen NO, Thomsen OF: Nonsecretory myeloma associated with nodular glomerulosclerosis. Acta Med Scand 207:137, 1980.

235. Spengler GA, Steinberg AG, Skvaril F: Development of a second monoclonal immunoglobulin G in a patient with late manifestation of myeloma. Acta Med Scand 192:309, 1972.

236. Spickard A: Multiple myeloma with myelofibrosis and with polycythemia vera: Further evidence of a relationship between the myeloproliferative disorders. Bull Johns Hopkins Hosp 107:234, 1960.

237. Spiegelberg HL: Human myeloma IgG half-molecules. Catabolism and biological properties. J Clin Invest 56:588, 1975.

238. Spiegelberg HL, Heath VC, Lang JE: IgG Half-molecules: Clinical and immunologic features in a patient with plasma cell leukemia. Blood 45:305, 1975.

239. Spiegelberg HL, Fishkin BG: Human myeloma IgA half-molecules. J Clin Invest 58:1259, 1976.

240. Stavem P, Frøland SS, Haugen HF, Lislerud A: Nonsecretory myelomatosis without intracellular immunoglobulin. Immunofluorescent and ultramicroscopic studies. Scand J Haematol 17:89, 1976.

241. Stefanini M, McDonnell EE, Andracki EG, Swansbro WJ, Durr P: Macropyroglobulinemia: Immunochemical studies in three cases. Am J Clin Pathol 54:94, 1970.

242. Stein H, Kaiserling E: Myeloma producing nonsecretory IgM and secretory IgG. Scand J Haematol 12:274, 1974.

243. Stites DP, Whitehouse MJ: Evolution of multiple myeloma with non-secreted paraproteins. Clin Res 23:283A, 1975.

244. Suau E, Fedou R, Laens J: Osteomalacie par syndrome de Fanconi de l'adulte secondaire à une maladie de Kahler agammaglobulinemique. Rev Med Toulouse 8:401, 1972.

245. Sugai S: IgA pyroglobulin, hyperviscosity syndrome and coagulation abnormality in a patient with multiple myeloma. Blood 39:224, 1972.

246. Sukarabayashi I, Kin K, Kawai T: Human IgA₁ half-molecules: Clinical and immunologic features in a patient with multiple myeloma. Blood 53:269, 1979.

247. Takatsuki K, Yodoi J, Wakisaka K et al: Plasma cell dyscrasia with polyneuritis and an endocrine anomaly: Endocrinological study of a new syndrome. Folia Endocrinol Jpn 50:567, 1974.

248. Takatsuki K, Uchiyama T, Sagawa K, Yodoi J: Plasma cell dyscrasia with polyneuropathy and endocrine disorder: Review of 32 patients. Excerpta Medica, Intern Cong Series no 415, Topics in Hematology. Proc 16th Int Cong Hematol, Kyoto, Sept. 5–11, 1976, p 454.

249. Taylor JS, Lewis LA, Battle JD, Butkus A, Robertson AL, Deodhar S, Roenigk HH: Plane xanthoma and multiple myeloma with lipoprotein-paraprotein complexing. Arch Dermatol 114:425, 1978.

250. Thompson DM, Main RA, Beck JS, Albert-Recht F: Studies on a patient with leucocytoplastic vasculitis, 'pyoderma gangrenosum' and paraproteinemia. Br J Dermatol 88:117, 1973.

251. Tischendorf FW, Heckner F: Atypisches Plasmozytom mit γG₃κ-γMκ - Doppelparaproteinämie Bence-Jones-Protein (Typ κ) und Lysozymurie. Hämatol Bluttransfus 8:162, 1969.

252. Trecan G, Dufier JL, Blatrix Ch, Aftimos G, Saraux H, Thomas M: Exophthalmie maligne bilaterale révélatrice d'un myelome multiple a IgM. Sem Hop Paris 53:1867, 1977.

252a. Tung E, Kuan TK, Litman GW, Wang AC: Three monoclonal immunoglobulins, an IgG₂(κ), an IgM(κ) and an IgM/A hybrid, in one patient. I. isolation and characterization. Immunology 44:257, 1981.

253. Turesson I, Grubb A: Non-secretory or low-secretory myeloma with intracellular kappa chains. Acta Med Scand 204:445, 1978.

254. Tursz T, Brouet J-C, Flandrin G, Danon F, Clauvel J-P, Seligmann M: Clinical and pathologic features of Waldenström's macroglobulinemia in seven patients with serum monoclonal IgG or IgA. Am J Med 63:499, 1977.

255. Tyson MC, Grossman WI, Tuchman LR: Gaucher's disease (with elevated serum acid phosphatase level) masquerading as cirrhosis of the liver. Am J Med 37:156, 1964.

256. Vaerman JP, Johnson LB, Mandy W, Fudenberg HH: Multiple myeloma with two paraprotein peaks: An instructive case. J Lab Clin Med 65:18, 1965.

257. Van Camp B, De Bock B, Peetermans M: Non-secretory myeloma: Immunological studies during treatment with melphalan, methotrexate and prednisolone. Br J Haematol 35:670, 1977.

258. Vermess M, Pearson KD, Einstein AB, Fahey JL: Osseous manifestations of Waldenström's macroglobulinemia. Radiology 102:497, 1972.

259. Virella G, Monteiro JMN, Lopes-Virella MF, Soares AD, Fudenberg HH: Asynchronous development of two monoclonal proteins (IgMλ and γ₁ chains) in a patient with abdominal lymphoma. Cancer 39:2247, 1977.

260. Vladutiu AO, Sielski L: Macroglobulinemia or multiple myeloma? Lancet 1:1122, 1973.

261. Waldenström J: Incipient myelomatosis or "essential" hyperglobulinemia with fibrinogenopenia—new syndrome? Acta Med Scand 117:216, 1944.

262. Waldenström J: Hypergammaglobulinemia as a clinical hematological problem: A study in the gammopathies. Prog Hematol 3:266–293, 1962.

263. Wang AC, Wang IYF, McCormick JN, Fudenberg HH: The identity of light chains of monoclonal IgG and monoclonal IgM in one patient. Immunochemistry 6:451, 1969.

264. Wang AC, Arnaud P, Fudenberg HH, Creyssel R: Monoclonal IgM cryoglobulinemia

associated with gamma-3 heavy chain disease: Immunochemical and biochemical studies. Eur J Immunol 8:375, 1978.

265. Wanner J, Siebenmann R: Über eine subakut verlaufende osteolytische Form der Makroglobulinämie Waldenström mit Plasmazellen-leukämie. Schweiz Med Wochenschr 87:1243, 1957.

266. Watanabe A, Kitamura M, Schimizu M: Immunoglobulin A (IgA) with properties of both cryoglobulin and pyroglobulin. Clin Chim Acta 52:231, 1974.

267. Weinbren I: Spontaneous periodic oedema. A new syndrome. Lancet 2:544, 1963.

268. Welton J, Walker SR, Sharp GC, Herzenberg LA, Wistar R Jr, Creger WP: Macroglobulinemia with bone destruction. Am J Med 44:280, 1968.

269. Whicher JT, Davies JD, Grayburn JA: Intact and fragmented intracellular immunoglobulin in a case of non-secretory myeloma. J Clin Pathol 28:54, 1975.

270. Wille LE, Førre Ø, Mathiesen PMS, Hovig T, Sorteberg K: "Non-secretory" plasma cell dyscrasia with normal serum immunoglobulins. Acta Med Scand 204:437, 1978.

271. Wille LE, Østborg J: Development of biclonal gammopathy in a patient with von Recklinghausen's neurofibromatosis. Acta Med Scand 205:243, 1979.

272. Wilson DE, Flowers CM, Hershgold EJ, Eaton RP: Multiple myeloma, cryoglobulinemia and xanthomatosis. Distinct clinical and biochemical syndromes in two patients. Am J Med 59:721, 1975.

273. Wodniecki J, Machalski M: A case of pyroglobulinaemia in the course of multiple myeloma. Wiadomosci Lekarskie 20:503, 1967.

274. Wolf P: Monoclonal gammopathy in Gaucher's disease. Lab Med 4:28, 1973.

275. Woodruff RK, Malpas JS, Paxton AM, Lister TA: Plasma cell leukemia (PCL): A report on 15 patients. Blood 52:839, 1978.

276. Worthington JW Jr, Mulder DW: Progressive muscular weakness and pain as symptoms of adult Fanconi syndrome. Neurology 9:475, 1959.

277. Yamamoto H, Yoshioka N, Watanabe T, Suzuki A, Hara T, Kawamura A, Itoh C: IgG-κ monoclonal gammopathy and systemic capillary leak syndrome. Proc 4th Int Cong Immunol, Paris, July 1980.

278. Yodoi J, Takatsuki K, Wakisaka K: Association of atypical myeloma, polyneuropathy, pigmentation and gynecomastia. A possible new syndrome. Acta Haematol Jpn 36:363, 1973.

279. Zarrabi MH, Stark RS, Kane P, Dannaher CL, Chandor SB: IgM myeloma—part of the spectrum of B-cell neoplasia. Blood 52 (suppl 1):282, 1978(A).

279a. Zarrabi MH, Stark RS, Kane P, Dannaher CL, Chandor S: IgM myeloma, a distinct entity in the spectrum of B-cell neoplasia. Am J Clin Pathol 75:1, 1981.

280. Zawadzki ZA, Edwards GA: Pseudoparaproteinemia due to hypertransferrinemia. Am J Clin Pathol 54:802, 1970.

281. Zawadzki ZA, Edwards GA: Nonmyelomatous monoclonal immunoglobulinemia. Prog Clin Immunol 1:105, 1972.

282. Zawadzki ZA, Kapadia S, Barnes AE: Leukemic myelomatosis (plasma cell leukemia). Am J Clin Pathol 70:605, 1978.

283. Zinneman HH, Seal US: Double spike in myeloma serum due to retention of light chains. Arch Intern Med 124:77, 1969.

284. Zinneman HH, Seal US: The role of hydrophobic bonding in the thermoprecipitation of a pyroglobulin. J Lab Clin Med 78:979, 1971.

285. Ritzmann SE: Immunoglobulin Abnormalities. In Ritzmann SE, Daniels JC (eds): "Serum Protein Abnormalities: Diagnostic and Clinical Aspects," 2nd printing. New York: Alan R. Liss, Inc., 1982, pp 440–443.

Index